Psychology and sociology applied to medicine

THIRD EDITION

AN ILLUSTRATED COLOUR TEXT

Commissioning Editor: Michael Parkinson / Timothy Horne
Development Editor: Ailsa Laing
Project Manager: Nancy Arnott
Designer: Erik Bigland
Illustrations Manager: Merlyn Harvey
Illustrators: Robert Britton, Roger Penwill, Graham Chambers and Graham Banks

Psychology and sociology applied to medicine

THIRD EDITION

AN ILLUSTRATED COLOUR TEXT

Edited by

Beth Alder BSc PhD CPsychol FBPsS
Emeritus Professor
Napier University
Edinburgh, UK

Charles Abraham BA DPhil CPsychol FBPsS
Professor of Psychology
Department of Psychology
University of Sussex, Brighton, UK

Edwin van Teijlingen MA MEd PhD
Professor of Maternal & Perinatal Health Research
School of Health & Social Care
Bournemouth University, UK

Mike Porter BA MPhil
Senior Lecturer
General Practice Section
Division of Community Health Sciences
College of Medicine and Veterinary Medicine
University of Edinburgh, UK

Foreword by

Keith Millar PhD CPsychol FBPsS
Professor of Medical Psychology
Faculty of Medicine, Glasgow University , UK

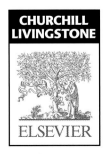

CHURCHILL
LIVINGSTONE

ELSEVIER

Edinburgh   London   New York   Oxford   Philadelphia   St. Louis   Sydney   Toronto   2009

CHURCHILL LIVINGSTONE
ELSEVIER

First edition 1999
Second edition 2004
Third edition 2009

ISBN-13   978-0-443-06787-7

British Library Cataloguing in Publication Data
A catalogue record for this book is available from the British Library

Library of Congress Cataloging in Publication Data
A catalog record for this book is available from the Library of Congress

Notice
Neither the Publisher nor the Editors assume any responsibility
for any loss or injury and/or damage to persons or property arising out of or related to any use of the material contained in this
book. It is the responsibility of the treating practitioner, relying on
independent expertise and knowledge of the patient, to determine
the best treatment and method of application for the patient.
The Publisher

your source for books,
journals and multimedia
in the health sciences

www.elsevierhealth.com

Working together to grow libraries in developing countries

www.elsevier.com | www.bookaid.org | www.sabre.org

ELSEVIER   BOOK AID International   Sabre Foundation

The
publisher's
policy is to use
**paper manufactured
from sustainable forests**

Printed in China

Contributors

Charles Abraham BA DPhil CPsychol FBPsS
Professor of Psychology, Department
of Psychology, University of Sussex,
Brighton, UK

Beth Alder BSc PhD CPsychol FBPsS
Emeritus Professor, Napier University,
Edinburgh, UK

Amanda Amos BA MSc PhD
Professor of Health Promotion,
Public Health Sciences, Division of
Community Health Sciences, University
of Edinburgh, UK

Jacqueline M. Atkinson BA PhD CPsychol
HonMFPHM
Professor of Mental Health Policy,
Public Health and Health Policy,
Division of Community Based Sciences,
University of Glasgow, UK

Susan Ayers PhD CPsychol
Senior Lecturer in Health Psychology,
Psychology Department, University of
Sussex, Brighton, UK

Pamela J. Baldwin BA MPhil PhD
CPsychol (deceased)
Clinical Psychologist, Working Minds
Research, Astley Ainslie Hospital,
Edinburgh, UK

Robin Banerjee BA DPhil CPsychol
Senior Lecturer in Psychology,
Department of Psychology, University
of Sussex, Brighton, UK

Lloyd Carson MA PhD CPsychol CSci
AFBPsS
Lecturer in Psychology, Division of
Psychology, School of Social and
Health Sciences, University of Abertay,
Dundee, UK

Jennifer Cleland BSc(Hons) MSc PhD
DClinPsychol
Senior Clinical Lecturer in Medical
Education and Primary Care, School
of Medicine, University of Aberdeen,
Foresterhill, Aberdeen

Sarah Cunningham-Burley BSocSc PhD
Professor of Medical and Family
Sociology and Co-Director, Centre for
Research on Families and Relationships,
Public Health Sciences, University of
Edinburgh, UK

George Deans BSc MSc PhD CPsychol
Consultant Clinical Psychologist and
Honorary Clinical Senior Lecturer,
Department of General Practice and
Primary Care, University of Aberdeen
Medical School, UK

Diane Dixon BSc(Hons) BA(Hons) PhD
CPsychol
Lecturer in Health Psychology,
Department of Psychology, University
of Stirling, Stirling, UK

Morag L. Donaldson MA PhD
Senior Lecturer in Psychology,
School of Philosophy, Psychology
and Language Sciences, University of
Edinburgh, UK

Andrew Eagle DClin Psychol CPsychol
Consultant Clinical Psychologist,
CNWL NHS Foundation Trust,
London, UK

Winifred Eboh PhD RNT PgCLT BSc(Hons)
RM RGN
Lecturer, School of Nursing and
Midwifery, The Robert Gordon
University, Aberdeen, UK

Helen Eborall BSc MSc
Research Psychologist, General Practice
and Primary Care Research Unit,
Department of Public Health and
Primary Care, Institute of Public Health,
Cambridge, UK

Tom Farsides BA MSc MA PhD
Lecturer, Department of Psychology,
University of Sussex, UK

Elizabeth Ford MA DPhil
Research Fellow, Department of
Psychology, University of Sussex,
Brighton, UK

Fiona French MA
Research and Development Officer,
NHS Education for Scotland,
Foresterhill, Aberdeen, UK

Alan Garnham MA DPhil
Professor of Experimental Psychology,
School of Life Sciences, Department
of Psychology, University of Sussex,
Brighton, UK

Richard Hammersley MA PhD
Professor of Social Psychology, Health
and Social Services Institute, University
of Essex, UK

Sarah E. Hampson PhD
Department of Psychology, University
of Surrey, UK and Oregon Research
Institute, Eugene, Oregon, USA

Linda Headland MA(Hons)
Director, ELCAP, Edinburgh, UK

Mike Hepworth BA AcSS (deceased)
Reader in Sociology, University of
Aberdeen, UK

Jane Hopton MA PhD HonMFPHM
Honorary Research Fellow,
General Practice,
University of Edinburgh,
Edinburgh, UK

Kathy Jenkins BSc MSc
Honorary Lecturer, Division of
Community Health Sciences, University
of Edinburgh, UK

Gail Johnston BSocSc PhD, DipDistrict
Nursing, CertEd for Health Professionals
Project Manager, Belfast, UK

Marie Johnston PhD, BSc DipClinPsych
CPsychol FBPsS FRSE FMedSci AcSS
Professor in Psychology, College of Life
Sciences and Medicine and Institute of
Applied Health Sciences, University of
Aberdeen, UK

Fiona Jones MSc PhD BA DipPsychol
Senior Lecturer in Health and
Occupational Psychology, Institute of
Psychological Sciences, University of
Leeds, Leeds, UK

Michael P. Kelly BA(Hons) MPhil PhD
HonMFPHM
Professor, Director of Research and
Information, The Health Development
Agency, London, UK

Jenny Kitzinger BA MA PhD
Professor, School of Journalism, Media
and Cultural Studies, Cardiff University,
UK

Susan Llewelyn PhD FBPsS
Director Oxford Doctoral Course in
Clinical Psychology,
University of Oxford, UK

Hannah M. McGee PhD RegPsychol FpsSI
CPsychol AFBPsS
Professor, Director, Health Services
Research Centre, Department of
Psychology, Royal College of Surgeons
in Ireland, Dublin, Ireland

Susan Michie MPhil DPhil CPsychol FBPsS
Professor of Health Psychology,
Department of Psychology, University
College London, UK

Kenneth Mullen MA MLitt PhD
Lecturer in Medical Sociology, Section
of Psychological Medicine, Division of
Community-based Sciences, University
of Glasgow, UK

Ronan O'Carroll BSc MPhil PhD CPsychol
AFBPsS
Professor of Psychology, Department of
Psychology, University of Stirling, UK

Foreword

Forewords are those parts of books that are rarely read – take it from me as a reader of many books but few Forewords. The fact that you, kind reader, are reading this Foreword and no doubt looking forward eagerly to the similarly neglected Preface, makes you a highly unusual, undoubtedly gifted and discerning person who is kind to children, old people and animals. In fact just the sort of person who will appreciate and benefit from this book.

What can one say about a book that, within only ten years, is now in its third edition? The fact that a third edition is necessary is a fact that itself speaks volumes; and, yes, the feeble pun is deliberate. The need for this third edition reflects how Psychology and Sociology continue to make inroads to inform practice and research in medicine. If anything is a testament to the integration of Psychology and Sociology within the medical curriculum, this book is it. The successful format remains of brief and easily assimilated two-page "spreads" where key topics are discussed, clinically-relevant examples are given, and the reader is challenged to consider their implications. The authors have been careful to revise their contributions in light of recent research findings and current theoretical thinking. Whilst the target audience is medical undergraduate students, the text will be equally at home on the shelves of those who teach the subject and, indeed, those health professionals in other disciplines who appreciate the relevance of Psychology and Sociology to their practice and teaching and wish to gain a contemporary view.

The world has changed radically in the ten years since the first edition appeared in 1998, and in ways that, directly and indirectly, impact on the health and well-being of us all. The third edition reflects those changes, most notably in the case of two new spreads: "Health: a global perspective" and "Health: a rural perspective". The global issues are the world events that change, subvert or derail the best laid plans of national governments – described memorably by Britain's last old-style avuncular and patrician prime minister Harold McMillan as "Events, dear boy, events". Those events, whether mass murder in New York, Madrid, London and elsewhere, natural disasters or the collapse of stock markets, bring distress, misery and hardship to many tens of thousands. The consequences for public and individual health and psychological well-being hardly need description, but it is health professionals who must be aware of those consequences and the evidence-based interventions that can help: this book provides them with such information. More positively, the information and communications revolution which continues apace despite the economic hiccup of the burst "dot. com bubble" brings significant benefits via "e-Health" and "Tele-health" mentioned in the new spread addressing rural perspectives of health. The internet provides previously unimagined immediate access to information about our health, symptoms and self-care and equips us better when we seek the advice of health professionals. Whether, however, this has had the unfortunate downside of adding to the worries of the already "worried well" and increased their consulting rates remains to be seen.

The past ten years have also seen major advances in functional and structural magnetic resonance imaging (MRI) of the brain which have provided remarkable insights as to 'how we work' in terms of our cognitive and emotional processes. This third edition devotes a section of the spread on "Memory Problems" to brain imaging: the technique was not mentioned in the earlier editions. We will certainly be reading much more about imaging in subsequent editions of this book.

This third edition has moved on and kept up to date but retains the basic strength of the earlier editions in making clear the contribution of Psychology and Sociology to understanding the processes behind the individual's behaviour in health and illness, and the overarching influence of our socio-economic background, culture and ethnicity. Medical students who read this book and engage with its ethos of active learning will profit from a deeper understanding of the people who will become their patients and an insight to their own motivations and aspirations in becoming medical practitioners.

Of course there is self-interest here. You, the medical students who are reading this textbook, will be those who, in ten or twenty years time, will be ministering to the present authors and Foreword writer as we succumb to the decline that awaits us all – the cells wildly out of control, the weary and failing heart or the deepening fog and confusion of the good Dr Alzheimer. But as you are the sort of people who read Forewords, we have the reassurance that we will be in good hands.

Keith Millar PhD, CPsychol, FBPsS
Professor of Medical Psychology
Section of Psychological Medicine
University of Glasgow Medical School

Preface to Third Edition

The first edition of *Psychology and Sociology Applied to Medicine* was published in 1999, and the second in 2004. The second edition was reprinted several times and was very well received by reviewers, and medical and health-care students. The third edition has given us the opportunity to add recent advances and expand into new areas. We have again updated the text, graphs and figures and added some chapters and omitted others. We have recruited new expert authors who have been involved in educating students in the health professions.

The views expressed in the prefaces of the previous editions still hold. As new medical curricula are developed in the UK and worldwide, it is recognised that an understanding of psychological and sociological processes is crucial to optimal individual care and effective national healthcare policies. These issues are central to core teaching in the medical and healthcare professions. An increasingly educated patient population and use of the web emphasises the need for greater interpersonal skills amongst health professionals, and the importance of communication to understanding and initiating behaviour change.

Medical curricula in the UK and elsewhere include psychology and sociology in integrated modules dealing with care and treatment in relation to particular physiological systems or diseases. *Psychology and Sociology Applied to Medicine* makes health psychology and medical sociology accessible to medical and healthcare students. This text also integrates psychological and sociological research findings with the delivery of care and treatment in healthcare settings. We have included recent references and often selected illustrative studies from medical and health journals rather than psychology or social science journals.

This book has been designed and written primarily to take account of the needs of students who are embarking on the various integrated systems-based and problem-based medical courses. Our material is presented in accessible, two-page 'spreads'. Each spread addresses a discrete topic with its own case study, questions for further thought and key points. However, the spreads are cross-referenced so that the book also forms an integrated whole. Of course, none of these topics can be adequately covered in two pages, but the spreads provide a good introduction and an overview of each topic. Spreads include key references which may be followed up, but individual course organisers and tutors will undoubtedly want to recommend further reading which links the material to their particular courses or modules.

The teaching and learning of psychology and sociology in relation to health, illness and medicine is often hampered by two important factors. First, psychology and sociology (unlike biomedical sciences) deal with aspects of our everyday experience. It is all too easy to believe that we already know what there is to be known about such familiar issues as, for example, 'Why don't people take their doctor's advice?' However, there is a body of research evidence which allows us to make informed judgements. Secondly, the very fact that people attempt to understand and make sense of their personal and social worlds makes it difficult to conduct behavioural and social research without, in some way, influencing what they tell us and their behaviour. Researchers have endeavoured to overcome this by using standardised assessments of health outcomes, and qualitative research has allowed those using health services to have their own voice.

Thus, for example, asking patients whether they took their medication or not may, if not carefully asked, elicit responses which patients think researchers want to hear rather than their real reasons. Asking doctors why patients don't take their medicines may prompt doctors to think about their own part in the process and so change their behaviour. Such opportunities for bias and influence make it particularly important for students to think critically and to check the assumptions, methods and findings of different research studies.

The references have been included not just to encourage students to read more deeply into a topic, but also to think critically about the reasoning and the evidence presented. Both psychology and sociology are enlivened by debate and discussion. Details of research studies are often given in boxes and students are encouraged to be critical. Evidence-based medicine is a concept that is as applicable to behavioural science as it is to clinical practice.

The book begins with a description of the bio-psycho-social model, which underpins the approach taken throughout the book. The remaining spreads are arranged into nine sections beginning with a description of normal human development and common health problems associated with the life-span. The second section addresses the question 'How does the person develop?' and focuses on the development of some key psychological processes, for example the development of language, personality and sexuality. The third section seeks to address the question 'In what ways are our behaviour and health constrained by the social contexts within which we live?' and also includes spreads on the concepts and measurement of health, illness and disease. Section 4 presents a more specific discussion of how social and personal factors interact to influence our risk of ill-health. Issues of illness prevention and health promotion are discussed in terms of both the behaviour of individuals and the behaviour of government and large organisations.

Section 5 shifts the perspective from health promotion to illness behaviour and focuses on what people do when they feel ill or anxious about their health and on their experience of consultations and of hospitals. Section 6 selects a number of specific disorders and examines how people experience and respond to them. In Section 7 ways in which people cope with illness and disability are described, including a new spread on counselling.

Section 8 examines some of the problems and issues associated with different ways of organising health services. Two new spreads have been added on International Perspective and Rural Health, and Section 9 has been extensively revised to review the experience of being a medical student and a trainee doctor, concluding with a discussion of basic professional and ethical issues.

It is doubtful whether any introductory textbook could cover such a wide range of topics comprehensively and we are aware of some important topics which have not been covered, and others which have received more of a psychological than a sociological approach, and vice-versa. We hope, however, that the breadth of coverage and the style of presentation will be attractive to students, stimulate their interest in the psychosocial aspects of health, illness and medical practice, and encourage them to pursue their interests in greater depth.

We were very sad that Pamela Baldwin and Mike Hepworth died before this third edition was planned. Their names remain attached to those chapters that have required only revision and updating.

Some editorial control has been exercised by the editors, but final responsibility for each spread has been left to individual authors. Our thanks to our authors for responding so willingly to our comments and suggestions, and for writing to such a tight word limit.

B.A. C.A. E.v.T. M.P.

Contents

Illness behaviour and the doctor–patient encounter

Illness and disability

Coping with illness and disability

How do health services work?

How do you fit into all this?

The biopsychosocial model

As future doctors, you will be looking forward to working face to face with patients – making sense of complex signs and symptoms, requesting and interpreting diagnostic tests, deciding on diagnoses, discussing their implications with patients and agreeing treatment and longer-term management for those who have chronic diseases that cannot be cured. You may also find yourselves involved in trying to prevent, or at least delay, the onset of disease through screening programmes, opportunistic screening and secondary prevention (see pp. 64–65 and 68–69).

The World Health Organization defined health as 'a state of complete physical, mental and social well-being and not merely the absence of disease or infirmity' (World Health Organization, 1948).

This definition emphasizes psychological and social aspects of health (see pp. 38–39). Any comprehensive framework for understanding health and health care services must embrace both psychological and sociological aspects of well-being and their interactions with biological processes (see pp. 38–39). Health depends on our perceptions, beliefs and behaviour and how these interact with physical systems such as the endocrine, immunological and cardiovascular systems. At the same time our perceptions and behaviours are shaped by our social context. Understanding how social, psychological and biological processes interact to create differences in health is what is meant by adopting a *biopsychosocial* perspective (Schwartz, 1980), as illustrated in the case study.

Bartholomew et al. (2006: 9) advocated a 'social ecological' model of health and health behaviours which includes

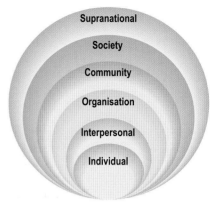

Fig. 1 Influences on health (from Bartholomew et al., 2006, with permission).

individual and social determinants of perception and behaviour (Fig. 1). For example, in the UK, where the wealthiest 10% of the population own more than half of all wealth, the difference in life expectancy between the poorest and richest areas is about 10 years (Shaw et al., 2005). Thus just knowing where someone is born (e.g. the northern UK or even which part of a city) allows us to make useful predictions about how long they will live, illustrating how our societal context shapes our well-being and health.

Our health and the health of a population more generally may also be significantly affected by public policy and legislation. For example, evaluating the law banning smoking in public places, Sargent et al. (2004) found that myocardial

---

Case study

Mr Brown is being interviewed by a small group of third-year medical students and telling them about his experience of heart disease (see pp. 106–107). He is 65 years old and married with two children and two grandchildren. He was born in a relatively poor part of the city and was one of four children living with their parents in a two-bedroomed third-floor tenement flat (see pp. 54–55). They ate what they regarded as good food: 'the best: eggs, butter, meat' as their mother worked as a cook and domestic for a local wealthy family. All six of them smoked (see pp. 84–85). He left school at 16 and went to work as bus driver and his ability led him to be promoted to operations manager – 'quite a demanding and stressful job' (see pp. 56–57).

Mr Brown first began to experience episodes of mild chest pain in his early 40s and when he went to see his doctor he was strongly advised to stop smoking. However, he did not stop because, as he saw it, he wasn't *that* ill (see pp. 72–75, 78–79, 88–91). He had his first heart attack when he was 45, describing it as 'crushing pain; as if a ton of bricks had landed on my chest'. In hospital, he had a second heart attack (see pp. 102–103), and he needed coronary bypass surgery which was successful (see pp. 104–105). He was discharged but has developed angina which has got worse over the years. Further surgery was not possible.

He finds it difficult to collect his newspaper from the local shop and takes tablets to help him cope with the pain and breathlessness. When he takes them first thing in the morning to help him get up they give him a headache and he has to take it easy until the side-effect wears off. He tells the students that he has taken two to get to the interview – one to get him to the doctor's practice, and another to get up the stairs to the room itself. He's got pain now as he's a bit nervous and stressed (see pp. 148–149).

Mr Brown explains he has changed a lot since his heart attack and become a lot more patient and relaxed, less irritable, adding by way of illustration, 'I used to shoo the pigeons off the windowsill, now I feed them' (see pp. 20–21). He is also concerned for his wife because she's a fairly anxious person at the best of times and she worries about him. He feels he can't give up living but is all too aware that this exacerbates her anxiety (see pp. 112–113). The best example he gives of how he manages his life is when, in answer to a question about how he's been recently, he describes a day the previous week when he showed his grandchildren a local historical tourist attraction. They were going to catch a bus but his son-in-law decided that it was such a nice day so they would walk. So Mr Brown, who has a great love of history and doesn't want to disappoint his grandchildren or make a fuss, walks with them, mostly uphill, but taking frequent strategic breaks to describe other local historical and interesting sites while he gets his breath back and the angina subsides. He manages the outing this way but then has to spend the next three days, exhausted, in his bed (see pp. 50–51, 136–137). This interview today is his first day out since that outing. When the students presented this case study, a member of staff was overheard to comment: 'stupid patient'.

Apart from the psychosocial issues relating directly to Mr Brown and his disease, the case illustrates the importance of understanding how lifestyle and material disadvantage (see pp. 44–45), often experienced early in life, are important life-course risk factors for disease in later life (Davey Smith et al., 1997).

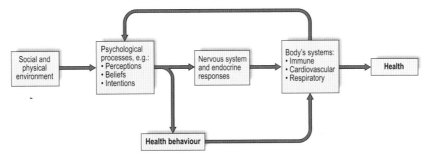

Fig. 2 Illustrative biopsychosocial pathways.

infarction admissions to a hospital fell significantly over 6 months during a smoking ban in public places, whereas surrounding areas (without a ban) experienced non-significant increases. Thus political action and legislation can sometimes be more effective in changing people's health behaviour than individual-level intervention.

At a more local level, community culture and resources may shape health-related behaviour and health. For example, the North Karelia project (in Finland) included education on smoking, diet and hypertension using widely distributed leaflets, radio and television slots (see pp. 52–53) and education in local organizations. Voluntary-sector organizations, schools and health and social services were involved and staff training was provided. The intervention included educating school pupils about the health risks of smoking and the social influences which lead young people to begin smoking as well as training them how to resist such social influences. This comprehensive intervention was found to be effective: 15 years later, smoking prevalence was 11% lower amongst intervention participants compared to controls (Vartiainen et al., 1998).

There are many examples of how insights from psychological research can help health care professionals with specific patient groups. For example, while adolescents have near-adult intellectual abilities and soon acquire adult physical abilities, neurological development continues into young adulthood and it has been suggested that adolescents' cognitions and hence behaviours tend to be more impulsive and less risk-averse than adults, because of this delay in brain development (Steinberg, 2007). Thus, compared to adults, adolescents tend to have poorer impulse regulation and heightened motivational drive in relation to rewards. Consequently, adolescents with chronic conditions are as likely, or more likely, to engage in risky health behaviour as healthy adolescents. This can have serious implications, e.g. adolescents suffering from asthma or cystic fibrosis who smoke are at increased risk of pulmonary deterioration. Smoking also accelerates the development of cardiovascular disease in individuals with diabetes and lupus. Yet health professionals report less confidence and competence in dealing with adolescents than with other age groups (Sawyer et al., 2007). This strongly indicates a need to improve training for health care professionals in relation to care of, and health promotion for, adolescents, particularly those with chronic conditions.

Educational interventions with health care professionals have been found to enhance health impact. For example, a randomized controlled trial of an education programme for general practitioners focusing on social and physical activity promotion as well as prescribing and vaccination practices for elderly patients showed that patients in the intervention group increased walking by an average of 88 minutes every 2 weeks, spent more time on pleasurable activities, and had better self-rated health than those in the control group (Kerse et al., 1999). Similarly, understanding how people plan actions and remember them can increase adherence amongst older patients. People who form 'if–then' plans are more likely to act on an intention in a specified context (Gollwitzer, 1999) (see pp. 76–77). Findings such as these demonstrate that educational interventions for general practitioners and other health care professionals can have substantial effects on public health targets.

Understanding people's interpersonal context can also help health care professionals to offer more effective care. For example, stressful relationships have an impact on people's immune functioning and health (Fig. 2). Indeed, stress has been found to have multiple effects on health (see pp. 126–127), including slowing wound healing (Kiecolt-Glaser et al., 1995), which is vital to the recovery processes. Consequently, helping patients cope with stressful relationships, e.g. through referral to counselling or therapy (see pp. 132–135) and by helping them access social support (see pp. 156–157), could enhance the effectiveness and cost-effectiveness of health care systems. Social support can also play an important role in recovery, including recovery from surgery: those who feel more supported need less medication and are discharged earlier (Krohne & Slangen 2005). Those with more social support are more likely to take care of their health and so require less professional health care. Social support may be especially important to women's health.

Complementary therapies (see pp. 146–147) are increasingly popular because patients believe the health benefits are worth paying for. Since the effectiveness of some treatments (e.g. homeopathy) cannot be explained by evidence or research-based theory, they are often regarded as capitalizing on placebo effects. Placebo effects (see pp. 92–93) demonstrate that apparently inert substances impact on physiological processes and generate positive health-related outcomes such as bronchodilation or pain relief (Stewart-Williams, 2004). Moreover, we know that adherence to placebo treatments generates greater health benefit (Epstein, 1984), indicating that adherence itself (apart from the effects of medication) has health benefits. Findings such as these indicate that people's perceptions and expectations about their health, symptoms and treatments strongly affect their health and well-being (Di Blasi et al., 2000).

The biopsychosocial model

- People's social context and interpersonal relationships and their perceptions, beliefs and expectations are important factors in the maintenance of health, the development of illness, help-seeking behaviour and responses to treatment.

- The model encourages doctors and health professionals to be aware of these factors and to practise more sensitively and effectively at individual, family, community and national levels.

Pregnancy and childbirth

This textbook appropriately starts at the beginning of life, at birth. It is also appropriate to use one of the most natural life events as an introduction to the behavioural sciences. The birth of humans differs from births in other mammals in our social construction of the event. Social behaviour is guided by institutions and customs, not merely by instinctual needs, and perhaps nothing illustrates this basic sociological principle better than the sheer diversity of human practices at the time of childbirth, and their responsiveness to historically changing influences. In other words, where and how and in whose presence a woman gives birth differ from one social setting to another. Human societies everywhere prescribe certain rituals and restrictions to pregnant and labouring women. For example, the place of delivery is often prescribed, be it a special village hut or a special obstetric hospital.

Pregnancy and childbirth are important life events that are often influenced by doctors. Every medical student is required to attend a certain number of deliveries. Doctors may be directly involved, in providing antenatal or postnatal care or attending the birth, or more indirectly through the provision of infertility treatment or birth control methods, or as back-up for midwives in case something unexpected happens during a normal delivery.

The nature of pregnancy and childbirth

There are two major contrasting views on the nature of pregnancy and childbirth (Table 1). One argues that these are normal events in most women's life cycle. This is often referred to as the *psychosocial* model. It is estimated that some 85% of all babies will be born without any problems and without the presence of a special birth attendant. Many of the risks in childbirth can be predicted and, consequently, pregnant women most at risk can be selected for a hospital delivery in a specialist obstetric hospital. The remainder of pregnant women can opt for a less specialist setting such as a delivery in a community hospital or a home delivery. A proponent of this view is Tew (1990), who discovered, to her own surprise whilst preparing epidemiological exercises for medical students in Nottingham, that routine statistics did not support the widely accepted view that increased hospitalization of birth had caused the decline in mortality of mothers and their babies.

Secondly, the view most commonly held in nearly all western societies is that pregnancy and particularly labour are risky events, where things could go wrong. This is referred to as the *biomedical* model. Childbirth

is, therefore, potentially pathological. Since we do not know what will happen to an individual pregnant woman, each one is best advised to deliver her baby in the safest possible environment. The specialist obstetric hospital with its high-technology screening equipment supervised by obstetricians is regarded as the safest place to give birth. In short, pregnancy and childbirth are only safe in retrospect. Consequently, the majority of deliveries occur in hospital. Figure 1 contrasts the percentage of home births in the Netherlands with Scotland, where Scotland reflects the trend in most industrialized countries.

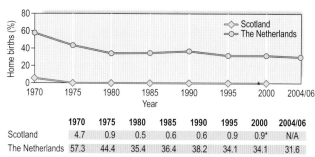

	1970	1975	1980	1985	1990	1995	2000	2004/06
Scotland	4.7	0.9	0.5	0.6	0.6	0.9	0.9*	N/A
The Netherlands	57.3	44.4	35.4	36.4	38.2	34.1	34.1	31.6

*1999

Fig. 1 Percentage of births outwith hospital in Scotland and the Netherlands (data sources: Common Services Agency (Scotland); Central Bureau voor de Statistiek (The Netherlands))

Place of delivery

Maternity services in the 1990s in the UK moved through a period of significant change in which the need of the woman to be centrally involved in her care was given greater emphasis. This represented a change from the previous 60 years, when the trend was towards more hospital deliveries. For example, an official report published in 1959 recommended that 70% of all births should take place in hospital, while a similar report in 1970 recommended 100% hospital deliveries on the grounds of safety. Political opinion changed in the late 1980s towards more choice for women, and consequently more deliveries outside obstetric units. The Winterton report (1992) moved away from total hospitalization: 'The policy of encouraging all women to give birth in hospital cannot be justified on grounds of safety.'

Birth attendant

The two views of childbirth also differ regarding who is the desired attendant at birth. If one holds the view that pregnancy and childbirth are only safe in retrospect, then the only acceptable birth attendant is the obstetrician, a specialist, just in case something goes wrong. If one holds the view that childbirth is a normal part in the life cycle of most women, then the most desirable birth attendant is the expert in normal deliveries, the midwife or the GP. Throughout history midwives have been, and continue to be, the major health care attendants at the birthing process. Over the past three centuries in most industrialized countries female midwives have slowly lost control over childbirth to male doctors.

Table 1 **Models of childbirth**		
	Model	
	Psychosocial	**Biomedical**
Emphasis	Childbirth normal/natural until pathology occurs	Childbirth only normal in retrospect
	Normality	Risk
	Social support	Risk reduction
	Woman = active	Woman = passive
	Health	Illness
	Individual	Statistical

Pregnancy is often a time of great expectations and excitement relating to the birth and parenthood. Women in modern western society have, on average, only two babies in their lifetime. At the same time, as obstetricians and/or midwives might attend deliveries many times a week or even a day, their expectations are considerably different from those of the expecting mother, and not only because the baby is not their own. Their priorities can be guided by medical requirements, hospital policies or availability of resources. Such differences can easily lead to misunderstanding and dissatisfaction by the new parents (especially if the parties have not been able to get to know each other). Considering the role and status of health professionals (see pp. 158–159), it is more likely that the mother is disappointed than the birth attendant.

What does being pregnant and giving birth mean for:

- a midwife?
- an obstetrician?
- a pregnant woman?
- her partner/husband?

Case study

The Dutch example

The Netherlands is the only industrialized country where the proportion of all deliveries taking place outwith specialist hospitals is substantial. Every year approximately one-third of all deliveries take place in Dutch homes. The UK and the Netherlands are neighbouring countries with fairly similar levels of health care provision and a similar quality of specialist obstetric care; perinatal mortality rates do not differ substantially between the two countries. (Perinatal mortality rate refers to the number of stillbirths (after 28 weeks' gestation) plus the number of deaths occurring in the first 7 days after the delivery, divided by all live births and stillbirths.) Other outcome indicators suggest that the Dutch programme is superior.

A number of factors have been suggested for this difference in the organization of maternity care:

- Pregnant women in the Netherlands are not regarded as patients, unless something goes wrong or the delivery is expected to be difficult for previously assessed reasons.
- Practical help is provided in the form of maternity home care assistants, who look after the mother and newborn baby at home for up to 8 days following the birth. They wash the baby, give advice on feeding, look after other children in the household, walk the dog, etc.
- In case of low-risk pregnancies, the fee for a GP will be reimbursed only if there is no practising midwife in the area, and only in instances of high-risk pregnancies will the fee of an obstetrician be reimbursed.
- Midwives are trained to be independent and autonomous practitioners. They are not trained as nurses first, but attend a separate 4-year midwifery course. The importance of independent training is, firstly, that nurses are trained to deal with illness and disease, whereas midwives are trained to deal with normal childbirth; and, secondly, that the hierarchical relationship between nurses and doctors tends to play a part in the medical decision-making process.
- Most midwives are practising as independent practitioners in the community, similar to most dentists in the UK. As private entrepreneurs they have to be more consumer-friendly to attract customers.
- All major political parties agree that the midwife is the obvious person to provide maternity care, and that deliveries should preferably take place at home.

One could, of course, argue that the UK and the Netherlands are different countries and therefore not comparable. However, the populations in these two neighbouring countries are not too different in terms of national income, the physiology of the average woman, life expectancy and many other socioeconomic indicators. Although the funding of health care is different, the organization of service provision and the quality of medical care are fairly similar. For example, the majority of all deliveries in the UK and the Netherlands are attended by midwives. In fact, one can turn the question of comparability round and ask, for example: Why is the proportion of home births equally low in the UK, Germany and the USA, while their organization of health care in general, and of maternity care in particular, is so different?

Breast-feeding

Pregnancy is a time when many parents are particularly interested in health matters and is an opportunity to promote health information. Breast-feeding has many health benefits and the World Health Organization (2002) recommends that wherever possible infants should be fed exclusively on breast milk for the first 6 months. Initiation rates are low (only 71% in England and 63% in Scotland in 2000), and closely related to educational levels. This contrasts with breast-feeding rates of about 98% in Scandinavia. Young mothers in low-income groups and who have fewer years of education are least likely to initiate and to continue breast-feeding. Health professionals and peers can effectively support breast-feeding mothers to continue to breast-feed (Sikorski et al., 2003).

Pregnancy can be regarded as a 'normal state of health' in that it occurs without serious problems to most women in their lifetime. Pregnancy can also be seen as an 'illness' in that many women, for example, have morning sickness, experience a slowing-down in physical functioning, seek medical care and/or deliver in hospital. How do you regard pregnancy and childbirth, and why?

Pregnancy and childbirth

- Biological events are never purely biological but always partly socially constructed.
- Where, how and in whose presence a woman gives birth differs from one culture to another.
- There are two different perspectives: (1) pregnancy is a normal event in most women's lives; and (2) childbirth is a risky event and only normal in retrospect.
- Pregnant women and health professionals are likely to see the birth differently.
- Different ways of organizing health care can have profound effects on professionals and health service users.

Reproductive issues

Reproductive events are primarily viewed as the onset of menstruation, conception, abortion, pregnancy, miscarriage, childbirth and menopause. Although predominantly focused on physical changes in women, these events involve many issues that affect both men and women, such as sexual dysfunction and infertility. Reproductive issues raise unique and strong ethical dilemmas such as at what point terminating a pregnancy is still morally defensible; the rights of donor parents and children of donors; and the use of in vitro fertilization (IVF) for pregnancy in women over the age of 60.

Biopsychosocial approach

An important point is that all these events can be viewed from different perspectives: biomedical, psychological, social and cultural. These perspectives affect our understanding and treatment of disorders. For example, a biomedical perspective would see PMS as caused by fluctuations and imbalances in hormones associated with the menstrual cycle. Treatment would therefore involve pharmacological methods to counteract hormonal imbalances or influence mood. A psychological perspective of PMS might examine how women's patterns of behaving and thinking contribute to worsening mood around menstruation, such as noticing particular triggers and maladaptive responses. Treatment might involve identifying and changing maladaptive thinking or behaviour, and finding coping strategies to help women respond in a more adaptive way. A social perspective of PMS might examine women's sociodemographic circumstances and levels of support; or cultural expectations and narratives about PMS. This might lead to treatment providing practical or emotional support to women during critical times.

It should be apparent that none of these perspectives on its own offers adequate explanation or treatment of PMS. Therefore current medical education and practice are based on a *biopsychosocial approach*, which considers all the perspectives outlined above and leads to a more informed and holistic approach to treatment.

Menstruation

The effect of the menstrual cycle on a wide range of behaviours has been studied with varying results. For example, research has shown that during the fertile phase of the menstrual cycle women prefer men who are taller, have a more masculine face and a masculine body and display more sexual competitiveness (Little et al., 2007). However, this is usually only the case when women are asked to rate or choose men for short-term relationships, not long-term relationships.

The menstrual cycle is also associated with physical and psychological symptoms just before menstruation, such as irritability, depression, labile mood, abdominal bloating and weight gain, which are commonly referred to as PMS. PMS is most common in women aged between 25 and 35 and is reported by up to 30% of women. For up to 8% of women these symptoms are very severe and affect their personal relationships, work and social functioning. This is referred to as premenstrual dysphoric disorder (PMDD). Women with a history of depression are more likely to suffer from PMDD, and PMDD is associated with poor overall health (Johnson, 2004). This makes it important to examine, in each case, whether PMDD symptoms are being caused by the menstrual cycle, or whether existing psychological problems are being made worse by the menstrual cycle.

Infertility

Conceiving a child is not always straightforward and around one in eight couples will seek help for infertility – defined as failure to conceive after 1 year of regular intercourse without contraception. Infertility is rated as more stressful than divorce, and women consistently report increased negative emotions, with 25% having clinically relevant depression scores. Sexuality and relationships are also affected, with women reporting less satisfaction, interest, spontaneity and pleasure during sex.

IVF has variable success rates, ranging from 33% for the first cycle in women under 30 to 6% in women over 40. Repeated failure can lead to depression, guilt, anger and sadness, with depression scores worse in women than men. The coping strategies couples use are important. Problem-focused or active strategies, such as seeking counselling, are associated with better well-being after IVF. Avoidance coping strategies, like use of alcohol, are associated with poorer psychological outcomes.

Pregnancy and childbirth

Pregnancy and birth are a time of great physical and psychosocial transition. Exposure to teratogens in pregnancy, such as alcohol, nicotine and maternal infection, can lead to a range of adverse outcomes. Psychosocial factors such as stress in pregnancy are also associated with poor outcomes like premature birth and low birth weight. Ultrasound studies have demonstrated variable effects of maternal stress on fetal behaviour (Van den Bergh et al., 2005; see Case study).

Miscarriage and stillbirth

Approximately one in five pregnancies ends in miscarriage. While often thought of as a lesser event than stillbirth, miscarriage can be distressing to women. Between 10 and 50% of women report symptoms of depression up to 1 year after miscarriage (Lok & Neugebauer, 2007). The experience of miscarriage can also be traumatic, and up to a quarter of women may show symptoms of posttraumatic stress disorder (PTSD) immediately after miscarriage, with 7% still showing symptoms 4 months later (Engelhard et al., 2001).

Around five babies in 1000 are stillborn (after 24 weeks' gestation) in the UK. In the majority of cases the reason for death is unexplained. Studies unanimously find this is an intensely painful loss for parents, with 20–30% of women having clinically relevant symptoms of depression during the first year and 33% of parents having marital difficulties after the loss. Current medical practice offers parents a chance to see and hold their dead infants on the premise that it will help the grieving process. However, the evidence for this is inconsistent and some research suggests that, although parents appreciate doing this, they may have poorer mental health in the long term.

Childbirth

The greatest change in childbirth in recent years has been type of delivery. Caesarean deliveries in the UK have risen from under 3% in the 1950s to 22% in 2002 as shown in Figure 1.

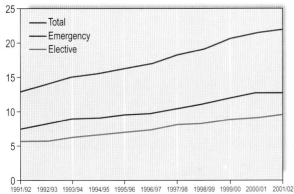

Fig. 1 Percentage of births by caesarean in National Health Service hospitals in England 1991–2002 (from Office for National Statistics 2004, with permission)

The reason for this rise is not clear. One suggestion is that more women are requesting caesarean sections. However, an Australian study found that only 6.4% of pregnant women wanted a caesarean delivery and most of these women had obstetric reasons for requesting this (Gamble & Creedy, 2001). In the UK nearly 60% of caesareans are performed as emergency deliveries, suggesting the rise in caesarean sections is either due to increased complications during delivery or an increased tendency for doctors to carry out caesareans rather than continue with a non-operative birth.

The transition to parenthood and postnatal well-being

The transition to parenthood is associated with a decline in the couple's relationship and with particular psychological problems. Potential problems include 'baby blues', postnatal depression, PTSD, puerperal psychosis and bonding disorders. 'Baby blues' are a brief period of emotional lability in the first week after birth, possibly linked to large fluctuations in hormones. Postnatal depression occurs in 10–15% of women and is associated with a history of psychological problems, anxiety or depression in pregnancy, difficult sociodemographic circumstances and low support. More rarely, up to 2% of women develop PTSD following traumatic birth, which is associated with birth factors such as low control, poor support and operative delivery. Most women with PTSD also develop depression. Puerperal psychosis occurs in only 0.1% of women but is a severe disorder in which mother and baby are at high risk and usually require hospitalization. Women with a personal or family history of psychosis or bipolar disorder are more likely to develop puerperal psychosis.

One of the main issues with postnatal psychological problems is whether they are present before the birth. For example, women with depression in pregnancy are more likely to have postnatal depression. Research suggests the prevalence of depression during pregnancy is the same or higher than depression after birth. This has led some people to question whether the notion of 'postnatal' psychological disorders is appropriate. It may be that pregnancy, birth and adjusting to parenthood exacerbate or initiate a wide range of mental health problems, as do other stressful events like bereavement.

Menopause

Menopause is defined as the last menstrual period, which happens on average around the age of 50 (range 45–55 years). During the menopause the majority of women in western cultures experience symptoms such as hot flushes, night sweats, loss of libido, irritability, problems with skin or hair, vaginal dryness and headaches. In terms of mental health, there is no consistent evidence for poor psychological well-being during this period. A biomedical perspective would see menopause as caused by a hormonal deficiency. Treatment would therefore be using HRT to replace the missing hormone, oestrogen. However, research suggests there is little association between menopausal status and psychological symptoms. In contrast, a sociocultural perspective would view the menopause as a natural process, where symptoms or experiences are culturally constructed. Thus any distress would be due to negative stereotypes or attitudes about menopause and ageing, and the coincidence of the menopause with significant role changes in women's lives. In cultures where menopause increases prestige for women, such as India and Native American Indians, much lower levels of symptoms are reported. In western cultures it has been found that concurrent stressful events are important predictors of women's well-being during menopause. Stress may also influence the production of hormones, having a physiological effect on women's experience. Therefore, as mentioned at the beginning of this chapter, a biopsychosocial approach provides a better understanding.

STOP THINK
- How would postnatal depression be explained from a biological, psychological, social and cultural point of view? What implications does this have for treatment?
- Talk to someone who has PMS. What symptoms does she report? Are these symptoms mainly physical or psychological? What does she attribute her symptoms to, and how might this be influenced by cultural beliefs?

Case study

In a study of the effect of stress and emotion during pregnancy on the fetus, DiPietro et al. (2002) asked 52 pregnant women about their emotions, daily stress, hassles and uplifts during pregnancy and examined whether this was associated with fetal heart rate, heart rate variability and movement. They found that fetuses were more active in women who reported intense emotions, stress and hassles during pregnancy. In contrast, women who reported their pregnancy to be uplifting had less active fetuses. Later in pregnancy, fetal heart rate was also affected when women reported intense emotions and pregnancy-related hassles. These findings are consistent with the majority of research in this area and researchers are subsequently looking at the role of maternal stress hormones in fetal development.

Reproductive issues

- Reproductive issues cover a wide variety of issues, events and illnesses that are relevant to men and women.
- Pregnancy, birth and becoming a parent is a time of great transition and adjustment and is associated with strain on a couple's relationship and psychological problems.
- It is important to see reproductive issues in a biomedical, psychological, social and cultural context and take a *biopsychosocial* approach.
- Many symptoms associated with the menstrual cycle and menopause are more highly associated with psychosocial and cultural factors than physical factors.

Development in early infancy

Psychological research with infants has taught us a great deal about the remarkable physical, cognitive, social and emotional development that takes place in the first 2 years of life. This spread will discuss key issues relating to: (1) the assessment of infant behaviour in the days and weeks following birth; (2) the early development of communication in the first year of life; (3) the emotional attachments between infants and their mothers (or other caregivers); and (4) the consequences of maternal mental health problems for infant development. Research on these topics shows us how important it is to see infants within the context of their relationships with their caregivers.

Neonatal assessment

Infants are born with reflexes and behaviours that enable them to respond to the world and develop rapidly. For example, in the first few days after birth babies are able to imitate facial expressions, selectively respond to humans or human-like objects and rapidly develop a preference for characteristics associated with their carers.

A variety of physiological and observational methods have been developed to assess aspects of development and behaviour in the first few months after birth, such as visual acuity, auditory assessments, stress immune responses, temperament, learning and attention. Advances in ultrasound have also enabled researchers to examine prenatal fetal development as a precursor of neonatal development.

A widely used measure of early neonatal development is the Brazelton Neonatal Behavioral Assessment Scale, which measures behavioural and reflex responses and is used to assess 10 areas of sensory, motor, emotional and physical development at birth and during the first 2 months of life. After 1 month, development can be measured by the Bayley Scales of Infant and Toddler Development, which are appropriate for infants up to 42 months old. These scales involve specific interactions with the infant through play to assess cognitive, motor and language development, as well as two parent questionnaires to assess social–emotional development and adaptive behaviour.

The advantages of these kinds of measures of neonatal development are that they help us to build a detailed profile of infants' functioning, identify developmental delays or difficulties and recommend appropriate interventions. They are also helpful for understanding how particular psychosocial circumstances, such as drug use in pregnancy or maternal depression (see section on maternal mental health, below), may be associated with delayed development.

Communication in the first year

Careful studies of infants' interactions with other people have revealed the extensive growth in communicative skills during the first year of life. Although it is not until around 12 months of age that infants produce their first words, they start cooing (vowel-like sounds, such as 'oo') and babbling (consonant–vowel combinations such as 'bababa') much earlier. Furthermore, infants show they can understand some words from as young as 6 months of age (e.g. Tincoff & Jusczyk, 1999).

In order to understand the building blocks of language development in infancy, we need to look at more than the comprehension and production of spoken language. Infants' earliest experiences provide them with opportunities to learn about turn-taking, and to use and respond to emotional expressions. For example, activities such as nappy-changing, breast-feeding and bathing often involve 'dialogues' where the baby and the caregiver respond to each other's sounds, gestures and facial expressions. Research has demonstrated that infants in the first year of life can interpret others' emotional expressions and use them to guide their own behaviour (see Case study).

A particularly important aspect of early communication is *joint attention*, a state where both the infant and the mother are focusing on the same object or event. Between 9 and 15 months, babies develop an increasingly refined ability to follow the gaze of an adult, and also to initiate and direct joint attention by using gestures such as pointing (Carpenter et al., 1998; Fig. 1). Psychologists have shown that infants can use gestures to direct caregivers' attention to an interesting sight or object (e.g. pointing to a dog), as well as to get caregivers to do something (e.g. pointing to ask for a toy). Caregivers often respond enthusiastically to these gestures, providing verbal labels (e.g. 'Oh yes, what a lovely doggy!') that contribute to the infants' language development.

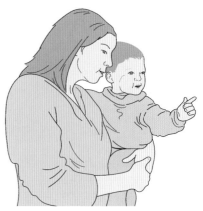

Fig. 1 Pointing.

Infant–caregiver attachment

The great strides made by infants in their communicative skills take place within emotionally intense relationships, or *attachments*, formed with their mothers (or other primary caregivers) during the first 2 years of life.

Some early theories of infant–caregiver attachment focused mainly on feeding as the key factor in the development of strong bonds between infants and caregivers, but psychologists now view this as simplistic. John Bowlby's (1969) ethological theory suggests that attachment has an evolutionary basis, involving inbuilt signals from the infant (crying, smiling, grasping, etc.) that elicit caregiving responses from the mother. Studying the emergence of this attachment has given us a fascinating insight into infants' social lives.

In the first few months of life, infants become increasingly able to differentiate between their mothers and other, unfamiliar individuals in terms of how they look, sound and smell. But it is not until around 6–8 months that infants begin to show the key features of attachment to their mothers or other primary caregivers. These include a desire to maintain physical closeness to the caregivers, and distress upon separation from them. As babies begin to crawl and explore the world around them, the caregiver becomes an important secure base. The distress that infants display when separated from their caregivers tends to increase into the second year of life, but then starts to decline as the infants develop into more self-aware, independent toddlers.

Importantly, the nature of the attachment relationship can differ widely from one family to another. Mary Ainsworth's (1978) pioneering work observing infants' interactions with their mothers demonstrated that, whereas most attachments showed the qualities described above, others did not: some 12-month-olds seemed to have little interest in maintaining proximity to their mothers and were untroubled by separation, whereas others were extremely clingy with their mothers and were so distressed by separation that they could not even be comforted by their mothers upon reunion. Research has shown that these kinds of differences relate to features of the infant (e.g. temperamental characteristics such as irritability), as well as to qualities of the care received from the mother (e.g. the sensitivity and responsiveness shown towards the infant).

Case study

In one famous series of studies, Sorce et al. (1985) showed that 12-month-old infants clearly pay attention to their mothers' facial expressions in ambiguous situations. The studies made use of the so-called visual cliff apparatus – a Plexiglas table with a 'shallow' side created by placing a patterned material immediately beneath the tabletop and a 'deep' side created by placing the patterned material some distance beneath the tabletop. Infants were placed on the shallow side and were encouraged to approach an attractive toy placed on the deep side. As most infants approached the 'cliff' separating the shallow and deep sides, they looked to their mothers for guidance (Fig. 2). In one of the studies reported by Sorce et al., 14 of 19 infants who saw their mothers posing a happy expression went on to cross the deep side. But out of the 17 infants whose mothers posed a fearful expression, not one ventured across the cliff, highlighting their sensitivity to caregivers' facial expressions as a source of information about the world.

Fig. 2 An infant on the 'visual cliff'.

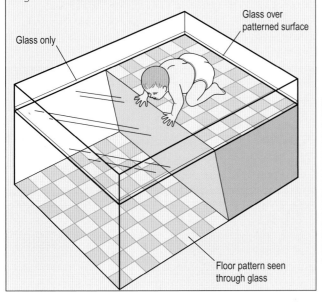

Glass over patterned surface

Glass only

Floor pattern seen through glass

Effects of maternal mental health problems

Maternal mental health has a variety of effects on infant and child development. A considerable amount of evidence shows that maternal depression is associated with poor cognitive and emotional development in the first 2 years of infant development (Murray & Cooper, 1997). This may be due to the impact of postnatal depression on the quality of the interaction between the mother and infant. For example, one study found that impaired cognitive development in babies at 18 months was predicted by features such as mothers' insensitivity to their baby's experience and their failure to communicate actively with their baby (Murray et al., 1996). The effect of postnatal depression on later child development is less clear, although there is some evidence that children of depressed mothers, particularly boys, have more behavioural difficulties (Sinclair & Murray, 1998).

An exciting and relatively new area of research examines the effects of stress and mental health during pregnancy, as a precursor to early infant development. This research suggests that stress in pregnancy is associated with a range of adverse infant outcomes, such as an increased risk of hyperactivity, anxiety, and delayed language and cognitive development (Talge et al., 2007). In line with this, Diego et al. (2005) found that babies of mothers who were depressed in pregnancy were more likely to cry, fuss and show signs of stress than those of women who were not depressed or women who were only depressed after birth.

Finally, it is important to remember that infant development needs to be examined in the context of the whole family. For example, a recent study of over 10 000 children found that even after controlling for maternal depression, paternal depression was associated with poor emotional and behavioural outcomes in children aged 3½ years (Ramchandani et al., 2005).

STOP THINK
- Compare the reactions of a 2-month-old infant and a 12-month-old infant to separation from their mother (or other primary caregiver). How do they differ and why?
- Observe a parent with a baby under the age of 1 year and note how they communicate with each other. Pay attention not just to words and sounds, but also to facial expressions, gestures and turn-taking.

Development in early infancy

- Neonatal behavioural assessment can be used to screen for early developmental problems.
- Infants learn to communicate with their caregivers through vocalizations, gestures and turn-taking before they produce their first word.
- Infants form intense emotional relationships with their primary caregivers during the first year of life, with significant increases in proximity-seeking and separation distress between 6 and 12 months of age.
- Mothers' mental health problems can have significant consequences for the early cognitive, social and emotional development of their infants.

Childhood and child health

Childhood is a process of transition from vulnerability and high dependence towards autonomy. The risk of serious ill health interfering in this process has been significantly reduced in most affluent countries, but there is still a disproportionate excess of deaths and morbidity amongst the children of poorer families.

Children's health

Relatively few children in affluent countries now die between the ages of 1 and 14 years. Improvements in children's mortality occurred rapidly between 1870 and 1950 (Fig. 1), largely as a result of improvements in economic circumstances, living conditions, sanitation and nutrition leading to a decline in mortality from infectious and environmental disease. Since the 1950s, deaths in childhood have continued to decline steadily, though the UK still has an under-5-year-old mortality rate that is higher than most other European countries, possibly reflecting the greater levels of income inequality in the UK (Collison et al., 2007). Greater national wealth, immunization, fertility control, medical advances and greater access to health services have also contributed to improvements in children's health. However, deaths and emergency admissions to hospital for unintentional injuries (accidents) remain a cause for concern, and the decline in serious infectious diseases in children in affluent countries (see pp. 158–159) has also meant that congenital disorders and cancers have become relatively more predominant, (see pp. 110–111).

Minor ill health is common in children and is mostly managed within the family, with the frequency of consultations with a doctor reducing as the child gets older (see pp. 88–89, 100–101).

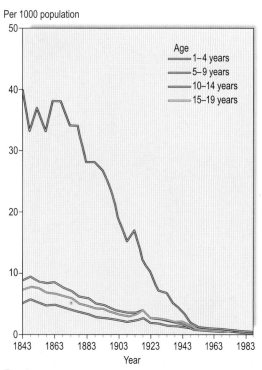

Per 1000 population

Age
— 1–4 years
— 5–9 years
— 10–14 years
— 15–19 years

Fig. 1 Trend in mortality under 20 years 1841–45 to 1986–90, England and Wales. (adapted from Woodroffe et al., 1993)

Psychological health and behavioural problems

The prevalence of mental health disorders in the UK in 2004 increases from about 5% in children aged 5–16 who live in more affluent households to 13% (girls) and 18% (boys) in households with a gross weekly income of under £100 per week (Office for National Statistics 2007).

There is evidence that adverse family factors, such as a marriage with low mutual support, are related to behavioural problems in children aged 3 years, and to the onset of behavioural problems when older. However, patterns of problem behaviour, such as sleep disturbance, challenging behaviour and temper tantrums, do not always disappear if stress factors are reduced. Counselling and psychotherapy approaches to behaviour problems would suggest that learned patterns of behaviour are often deeply internalized in the subconscious and may be difficult to change (see pp. 22–23, 132–135). Furthermore, neglect and abuse of children are known predictors of depression and emotional/behavioural problems later in life for both men and women.

Single mothers are particularly at risk of financial hardship and depression (Brown & Moran, 1997), and both poverty and maternal depression are associated with greater risk of childhood accidents. Brown & Davison (1978) suggest that a depressed mother pays less attention to, and takes less interest in, her child. In order to attract her attention, the child behaves more aggressively or problematically, but she withdraws further, which elicits even more extreme behaviour, leading to the increased risk of an accident arising from the child's behaviour and her lack of supervision. However, care should be taken to avoid blaming the mother and increasing her feelings of guilt and low self-esteem.

Unintentional injury (accidents)

The phrase 'unintentional injury' is currently preferred to 'accident' in order to make the point that most accidents are preventable. Although the rate for childhood deaths from unintentional injury in the UK has been falling, they are a major cause of death. Like most causes of death in children, they are strongly associated with deprivation (Fig. 2), and the gap between the least-deprived quintile and the most-deprived quintile has increased over the last 3 years. The picture is similar for emergency admissions to hospital for unintentional injury.

Under the age of 5 years, most accidents occur in the home, with fires being the most common cause of death, and falls being the most common cause of injury. From 5 years onwards, most childhood accidental deaths occur on the roads as pedestrians, though the number of road traffic accidents has fallen slightly despite an increase in the volume of traffic. Children from social class V are more than four times as likely to die as pedestrians than children in social class I. Although mortality from injury has also declined in all social classes, the differential in mortality for children aged 0–15 years in social classes IV and V has increased relative to children in classes I and II (see pp. 44–45).

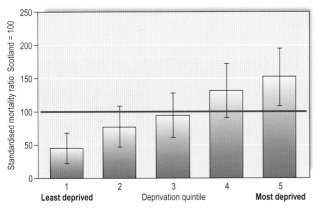

Fig. 2 Mortality from unintentional injury, children aged under 15 years of age by deprivation quintile, year ending 31 December, 2001–2005 (adapted from General Registers Office for Scotland).

Factors which help to explain these social class association are:

- Low income associated with:
  - Small, overcrowded and poorly designed homes leading to higher risk of falls or burns/scalds
  - Older and less safe equipment: cookers, fires, wiring, furniture, windows, bunk beds
  - Lack of safety equipment: stair gates, guards, smoke alarms
  - Less space to play inside, so play outside (at younger age)
  - Live near unprotected roads, particularly fast arterial roads
  - Inadequate play facilities
  - Difficulty supervising children in high-rise blocks
  - Poor local nursery facilities
  - Depression

Studies of children's ability to comprehend danger suggest that children younger than 7 years of age can be taught that something specific is dangerous, but they are unable to generalize from this understanding. For example, being told not to touch the fire in the lounge will not be related to fires elsewhere. Furthermore, younger children do not have the ability to interpret traffic speed or distance until about the age of 11, and are easily distracted.

Risk of specific cause of accidental death and injury varies by sex and age. At all ages, boys are more likely than girls to die (see pp. 46–47) from an accident or to have an accidental injury, with road traffic accidents accounting for an increasing proportion of accidents involving boys as they get older.

Three types of explanation have been suggested:

1. Boys are subjected to more 'rough and tumble' play and risk-taking than girls.
2. Parents are more likely to supervise girls than boys.
3. Boys are more accident-prone because they are encouraged to be more active.

STOP THINK
- Attempts to educate parents about the risks of accidents and to encourage them to take more responsibility for supervision leads to victim-blaming, and to feelings of guilt and defensive anger. Can you think of a more appropriate childhood accident prevention policy?

Respiratory illness

On average, a child aged 5 years will have from six to eight respiratory illnesses per year. These illnesses account for about 80% of consultations with general practitioners by this age group, which is about five times the frequency of consultation for other common conditions. About 30% of all consultations for children aged 11 years are for respiratory disease.

As with accidents, there is a strong relationship between social class and respiratory illness. Dampness in houses is a significant predictor of the incidence and severity of respiratory illness in children, even when allowing for cigarette smoking (see pp. 54–55). In contrast, whilst the incidence and prevalence of asthma have been increasing in the UK in recent years, making it the most common chronic disease in children, there appears to be no clear relationship between asthma and social class.

Poverty, illness and child development

Children in households with low incomes are more likely to experience ill health, and to spend more time absent from school. This in turn can affect their chances of performing well at school and consequently lead to reduced employment opportunities and to poorer health in later life.

In recent years, policy attention has focused on promoting parental support. Research into the provision of emotional, social and financial support has found that, in the short term, such interventions improve parental self-esteem and lower rates of childhood behavioural problems and injury (Patterson et al. 2002). In 2007 the UK introduced an American model of intensive nurse–family partnership (Cabinet Office, 2007) and we now await the results of a long-term follow up.

Case study

In a study of a Glasgow housing estate, Roberts et al. (1993) found that mothers saw accidents as just one element of their generally risky, insecure lives. They pointed to defects in the design and upkeep of their environment that contributed to the high accident rate: balconies with gaps that small children could fall through, poor kitchen design, inappropriate electrical wiring and switching, inadequate thermostatic control of immersion heaters, dangerous window design and inadequate locks, inadequate play facilities, inadequately protected roads and repair work, broken glass left by glaziers, inadequate rubbish stores and refuse collection.

The researchers concluded that only a small minority of parents were irresponsible and that professionals and contractors were often responsible for not admitting to design faults and putting them right.

Childhood and child health

- The health of children in affluent countries has improved considerably over the last 100 years.
- These improvements have largely arisen from improvements in sanitation and standards of living.
- Accidents, and particularly pedestrian accidents, are the major cause of death in children.
- Respiratory illness is the major cause of morbidity in children.
- Both accidents and respiratory illness are strongly related to social class and poverty.

Adolescence

Adolescence describes a period of transition between childhood and full adult roles. In some cultures this follows rapidly after puberty and sometimes involves a formal initiation rite but, in western societies like the UK, many people in their mid-20s have still not taken on all adult responsibilities. For example, they may still not have left home, are unlikely to have children and may have several shorter long-term relationships and jobs rather than a sole marriage or career. The ages at which different adult activities are permitted vary. Thus, adolescents are expected to behave in some ways like adults and in other ways like children. Parents and children often disagree about which roles are appropriate at a given age. Since the 1950s there has also been increasing identification of 'youth' as a distinct and positively valued life phase, which has changed rapidly (Table 1).

The physical changes of puberty are important but the psychological changes are caused by the difficulties of adolescent roles. Adolescents have near-adult intellectual abilities (although not necessarily adult knowledge or experience) and soon acquire adult physical abilities. Neurological development continues into young adulthood and it has been suggested that adolescents' cognitions and hence behaviours tend to be more impulsive and less risk-averse than adults because of this delay in brain development (Steinberg, 2007). Adolescents also have to cope with important emotional, sexual and moral developmental issues. Parents and children can often disagree about which behaviours are appropriate and at what age. The influential theorist Eric Erikson (1968) described adolescence as a time of forming adult identity.

Two sources of strain are:

1. Having to choose and adjust to adult roles. Many adolescents experiment with a variety of roles and behaviours before settling down with what suits them. This experimentation often includes activities which seem extreme to adults; for example, youth fashions often offend older sensibilities.
2. Disputes over rights and responsibilities. Adolescents often complain that adults expect them to have adult responsibilities without adult freedoms: to be responsible enough to baby-sit, but not responsible enough to choose when to have sex. Adults often feel the opposite, that adolescents expect adult freedoms without adult responsibilities: to be free to choose what time to come in, but not to be willing to help with housework.

Despite these strains, most adolescents have a fairly untroubled time and get on relatively well with their parents

Table 1 **Life for young people today has changed compared to 40 years ago**	
More	**Less**
Celebrate diversity	Marriage
Brands	Permanent jobs
Travel	Local community
Virtual and networked interactions	Social class
Text messaging	Left–right politics
Serial monogamy	Physical activity
Body decoration and body concerns	Perceived safety and security
Reality TV	
Recreational drug use	

and Table 2 shows how parenting styles can affect children. Most adolescents' interests and aspirations are similar to adults'. For example, West et al. (1990) found that the most popular leisure activities for 18-year-olds were watching TV, listening to music and reading – hardly rebellious activities! Furthermore 78% of them had always been in work or education. However, about 20% of adolescents experience problems (Coleman & Hendry, 1999). Many troubled adolescents abuse drugs or alcohol, engage in some criminal activities, may do poorly or drop out of school and are likely to be depressed or unhappy. They are also likely to engage in behaviour inappropriate for their age, although not considered a problem for older people. Both sexual intercourse and drinking alcohol are considered age-inappropriate for people under 14 (note this is not just a legal definition, but a social norm). For most, this is a temporary phase lasting a few years, but some troubled adolescents become adults with problems. Early intervention can help some adolescents, but there is also a risk of labelling someone as mentally ill, drug-addicted or delinquent, actually making problems worse (see pp. 60–61).

The two most common social psychological explanations of risk-taking in adolescents are that they have a sense of invulnerability and that they do not think in abstract ways about the future consequences of their own actions. More sociological explanations have suggested that risk-taking behaviour is a part of some youth subcultures that provide identity and meaning within a larger or dominant adult culture that is seen as irrelevant, unrewarding (or even punitive) and meaningless to their experience and life chances.

Table 2 **Effects of combined parenting styles on adolescent development**		
Two dimensions of parenting style	**Hostile** Cold, neglects or ignores child's needs, uses punishment to control behaviour	**Loving** Warm, accepts child's needs, attends to child, uses praise to control behaviour
Authoritarian Makes strict, rigid unrealistic demands on child's behaviour	Parent is consistently strict and punishing Some parents may be physically or sexually abusive Adolescent develops internalized anger: neuroses, depression or anxiety, suicide attempts	This extreme combination is unlikely because rigid demands require ignoring child's needs In less extreme form, the child may become an 'overachiever' in an unsuccessful effort to please the parent
Authoritative Has clear expectations for behaviour but these are flexible, realistic and negotiable	This combination of styles is unlikely because hostility precludes clear flexible expectations	Parent provides good guidance The ideal combination, likely to lead to a well-adjusted adult
Permissive Makes few demands on behaviour and provides few guidelines for child	Parent largely ignores child's behaviour and punishes inconsistently Some parents may be physically or sexually abusive Adolescent develops externalized anger: acting-out behaviour, delinquency, drug abuse	Parent treats child too much as an equal: child is 'spoiled' Major role conflicts, less extreme acting-out behaviour Child forced to 'be the parent'

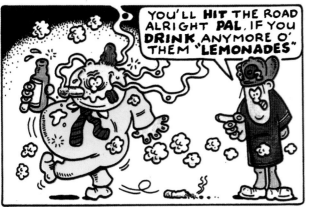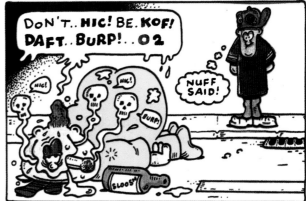

Fig. 1 Health education information designed for young people is now widely available. (Cartoon referring to 'alcopops', with permission from the Health Education Board for Scotland, from O₂ issue 3, 1994.)

STOP THINK Are you an adolescent? Your first response may be no, yet as a student you probably experience role conflict when you are told to take responsibility for your own learning while having the curriculum imposed on you. You have probably also experienced the strain and uncertainty of having to cope with practical and emotional matters on your own.

Are there activities which are still not appropriate for people of your age? Consider or discuss with classmates what age is too young for the following activities:

- Sexual intercourse
- Living with a sexual partner
- Marriage
- Having a child
- Having a credit card
- Taking a bank loan
- Drinking alcohol
- Smoking cannabis
- Moving out of your parents' house
- Buying your own home
- Studying medicine

Youth is perceived as a time of resilience when a young body can cope with overindulgence: young people will take exercise more because of concerns about attractiveness than for health reasons. Even a simple review of the health statistics tends to support this. With the exception of accidents for boys, young people are generally much healthier than older people, and there is no class gradient in health at age 15 years (West et al., 1990).

Health care needs of adolescents

Adolescents are a special target for prevention and health promotion programmes (Fig. 1). Drug abuse, alcohol abuse (including accidents while intoxicated) and suicide are among the leading causes of death in adolescents. Adolescents may also have special health concerns related to their rapid physical development, including concerns about their sexual development, acne, allergies, fatigue, headaches, and concerns about body size, diet and exercise. Many adolescents are somewhat uncomfortable about their bodies and they may find aspects of health care exceptionally embarrassing.

The provision of health care for adolescents can be problematic as they do not fit easily into child or adult services.

Case study

Jane is 14 and comes on her own to your practice asking for the morning-after pill because she has had unprotected sex. At first she says that this was with a boy she had just met. When you do not judge this and ask her whether she has had sex before, she tells you that really it was her steady boyfriend, who is 18; she has been having sex with him about twice a week for about 3 months. They have been using the withdrawal method, but it 'went wrong'. She says he will not use condoms and she is reluctant to because she says birth control is against her religion. She seems very happy with their relationship. She is very afraid of her parents' reaction if they find out she has a steady boyfriend, never mind that he is older and having unlawful, and unprotected, sex with an under-16-year-old. This case poses you the following ethical problems:

- You have a legal obligation to disclose harm to a minor. Is unprotected sexual intercourse with an 18-year-old such harm?

- You are not supposed to provide medical treatment to someone under 16 without parental consent.

- Is it ethical to persuade someone who is against it to use contraception?

- You are supposed to respect patient confidentiality.
  What do you discuss with Jane, and what do you do?

Adolescence

- Adolescence is a period of transition between child and adult roles.
- Strain can occur when there is conflict over appropriate roles and behaviours.
- Most adolescents are fairly untroubled.
- About 20% go through a period of delinquency or problem behaviour.
- Morbidity and mortality rates are low, and they make little use of health care facilities.
- Special health problems are substance abuse, risky sexual behaviour, depression and suicide.

Adulthood and middle age

As young people mature into adults, their health behaviour changes. They may become less likely to take risks when they have responsibilities and may no longer perceive themselves as invincible.

Most children long to be grown up, and grown-ups are seen as having rights and privileges that are strongly desired by children (see pp. 10–11). However, they do not always recognize the accompanying responsibilities of adulthood. Young adults grapple with problems of budgeting, relationships, demands of work and study.

Health is probably better in early adulthood than at any other time of life. As people get older they may begin to worry about the negative consequences of ageing. This realization may not be inevitable and may occur at different ages for different people, or, indeed, for men and women. At some point the anticipation of the next birthday may be tinged with apprehension about the ageing process.

The ages between 17 and 40 years are often described as early adulthood and, until relatively recently, would be regarded as the prime of life. Individuals and society emphasize growth and development on each birthday. In the UK, the 18th birthday is seen as being culturally important. Other important milestones may be the legal age of consent to sexual intercourse, drinking alcohol in pubs or voting. It is also a healthy time of life and young adults are the age group that are least likely to consult doctors apart from health related to reproduction (see pp. 4–5).

Marriage and civil partnerships

During adulthood most people will form a relationship with the opposite sex. Family patterns are rapidly changing. Many couples cohabit, though most (76% of women and 71% of men) expect to marry. In 2006 24% of children were living in one-parent families in the UK (Fig. 1) – more than triple the number from 1972 (Office for National Statistics 2007). Homosexual partnerships are becoming increasingly accepted in our society. Civil partnerships give the same rights to homosexual couples as heterosexual couples. There were over 15 000 civil partnerships between December 2005 and September 2006, 60% of which were male couples.

There is considerable evidence that men benefit from marriage in terms of physical and mental health, but for women, being married can have disadvantages. Being single, widowed or divorced is associated with lower rates of depression in women than it is in men. Blaxter (1987) found that men living with a spouse had lower illness scores than men living alone, but for women there was no difference. The protective effect of marriage for men could be linked to social support. However in 2006 58% of young women and 39% of young men aged 20–24 in England lived with their partners – an increase of 8% since 1991 (Office for National Statistics, 2007).

Although marriage appears to be good for men's health, men suffer more severely from loss of their wives by bereavement or breakdown of marriage, and they are more likely to suffer from a range of health problems.

Patients who consult with physical symptoms may be having marital problems, and sometimes these can disrupt their medical treatment. These may involve depression associated with childbirth or sexual problems, or major health and social problems if the wife has been physically abused. A marital separation may be followed by depression and would certainly impede recovery from illness or surgery. Knowledge of the psychology of relationships can help us understand the context of change in health and illness.

In 2005 7 million people in the UK lived alone, an increase from 3 million in 1987 (Office for National Statistics, 2007). This has had an impact on the demand for single-person accommodation and has implications for care of older people (see pp. 16–18).

Single women were traditionally viewed negatively by society. Women may lack confidence in their ability to survive by themselves, but with increasing education and career opportunities this may be changing. The maintenance of our identity comes from others, and our feelings of self-worth may be closely linked to the emotional support received in a relationship. However, being single and independent may be advantageous to some women compared with being a traditional wife, and it may be easier for them to avoid emotional and sexual complications.

If a single or widowed woman is ill there may be practical problems. Women often earn less than men and they may not have employment that has generous sick-pay arrangements. The absence of a partner at home may make convalescence difficult. Of course, health is also related to socioeconomic status, which may have stronger effects than marital status (see pp. 44–45).

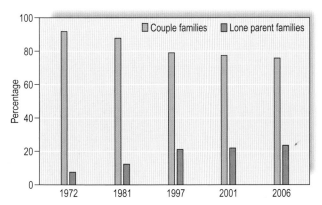

Fig. 1 Changes in the percentage of children living in one-parent families in the UK between 1972 and 2006 (from Office for National Statistics 2007, with permission).

Transitions

One perspective on ageing has been given by Erik Erikson (1902–1994). His theory suggests that middle age is a time of conflict between generativity (guiding the next generation) and stagnation (concern with one's own needs). Middle age will be associated with different patterns of health and illness, and assessment of middle-aged patients may have to include their relationship with their own increasingly ageing parents as well as their dependent teenage children.

Men are sometimes said to go through a 'mid-life crisis'. Half of the men in a study of 40 men aged between 37 and 41 years identified a period of uncertainty, anxiety and change (Levinson et al., 1978). They saw mid-life as a last chance to achieve goals but others saw mid-life as a dead end, and life as pointless. Men at this stage also become aware of changing physical strength and vigour. Yet the years between maturity and the beginning of old age may be regarded as the prime of life, and a time when many men are at the peak of their careers and are still in good physical health. For these people illness is unexpected and may be perceived as being 'unfair'. It may also be seen as being a failure of medical care or as a result of an unhealthy lifestyle.

Preventive health in adulthood

The time perspective of young adults may be limited to the demands of their jobs, marriage and bringing up families, but in middle age people may make positive plans for retirement. As people enter middle age they may increasingly focus on preventive health measures and may begin to prepare for retirement. At this time there may be an intense interest in health, shown by joining clubs or fitness programmes and attending for screening. Stressful events may occur with relative frequency in mid-adulthood and there has been much interest in the link between coping with stress and heart disease in middle age (see pp. 126–127). If elderly parents die or suffer chronic illness when their offspring are middle-aged, this may focus attention on illness (and health).

Youth and beauty are culturally associated and the association is perpetuated by media images. A youthful physical appearance is a source of power for women, although men's power depends on wealth and occupation. This has been described as the double standard of ageing. The Association of Graceful Ageing, Health and Moral Attractiveness, developed in the 1920s, illustrates the anxieties that are reflected in the belief that a healthy middle age will somehow postpone the ageing process. Physical attractiveness bears little relationship to health in reality. Those who are physically attractive may be assumed to be healthy, even though they are not.

There are noticeable changes in physical appearance with increasing age, such as greying hair and loss of skin elasticity. In an ageist society these become negative attributes and generate a vast cosmetic industry. However, greying hair and cragginess of features in men may denote increasing maturity and competence.

Child-rearing may dominate the ages between 20 and 45 and much of the contact between adults and the medical profession may be about the health of the children. Parents may consult their general practitioner with their child frequently, and this will allow a relationship to develop. This may be valuable when they become older and more likely to be ill themselves.

Health changes and age

Increasing life expectancy has not necessarily led to an increase in years of good health. Between 1981 and 2002 the number of years spent in poor health in the UK rose from 6.4 to 8.8 for men and from 10.1 to 10.6 for women (Fig. 2). The menopause has been held to be responsible for the increase in women's psychological problems in middle age but the evidence for a causal relationship is weak (see pp. 6–7).

The best predictor of psychological well-being in older people is physical well-being. The best predictor of physical well-being is material deprivation (Gannon, 2000).

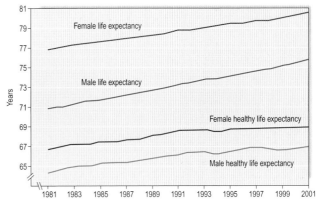

Fig. 2 Changes in life and healthy life expectancy from 1981 to 2001 in the UK (from Office for National Statistics 2007, with permission).

Sensory abilities progressively decline in adulthood. People's sight deteriorates and a sure sign of reaching middle age is when newspapers are read at arm's length. Sometimes patients at outpatient clinics or admitted to hospital may not carry reading glasses with them, and may not be able to read simple instructions or consent forms.

Hearing also declines slowly but there is little loss of psychomotor skills during middle age. On the plus side, knowledge, confidence and maturity increase with age and as yet are still valued by society. As medical technology increases we are likely to live longer, so the mid-age adult should have many healthy and productive years before an extended third age in retirement.

Case study

Forty-year-old Mr Harris and his wife (a part-time care assistant) have three children at school, four parents living and an elderly grandmother of 90. Mr Harris lost his job as a printer when his firm was modernized. How would you expect him to view middle age? His wife is concerned about the health of her father, who is a heavy smoker. She is grieving for the loss of her younger sister who died of breast cancer. How would you expect her to view middle age?

STOP THINK

- At what age do you think adults consider concealing their age?

- Why should there be a double standard for ageing for men and women? Is it changing?

Adulthood and middle age

- The age of entry to adulthood is usually considered as being about 18 years, but there are differences in social, cultural and psychological milestones.

- Marriage is more beneficial for health in men than in women. Marital problems may affect health.

- In middle age, adults become increasingly interested in preventive health.

- Adults spend much time in parenting in middle age and their main contact with the medical profession may be through their children, or their elderly parents.

- Physical events such as the menopause and changes in sensory abilities signal the ageing process, but are not directly related to loss of function in middle age.

Social aspects of ageing

There is a widespread view that ageing is an inevitable process of physical and psychological decline produced by biological change. In this biomedical view (see pp. 2–4), ageing is seen rather mechanistically as a result of the increase in life expectancy. The solutions proposed to the 'problem of ageing' tend, therefore, to be medical. Ageing, however, is a lifelong process involving an interaction between biological, psychological and social factors. Therefore care for older people must involve these three dimensions.

Social scientists acknowledge biological ageing, but highlight it must be understood in terms of the social environment. Thus, ageing can be described as a *relational experience*: that is, changes taking place in the body alter our relationships with other people. For example, a statutory retirement age changes people's status in personal and public spheres, but there is no biological reason for retirement at 65. Ageing into old age is a gradual process that varies from individual to individual. There is no single or universal answer to the question: when does old age begin?

Ageism

Ageism, or prejudice against people simply because they are old, may be indicative of fear of old age in contemporary society (Bytheway, 1995). This fear is associated with the belief that chronological age inevitably results in mental and physical decline. Jerrome (1992) studied old people's clubs and concluded that old age should be defined as a 'state of feeling and behaving' (p. 130) rather than a chronological state. She observed that older people work hard to cope with the ageing of their bodies and often turn physical ageing into a personal challenge. Involvement in club activities helps them explore the meaning of growing older and negotiate the point at which it is socially acceptable to acknowledge frailty or illness and withdraw from social activities. Talking about illness is not, therefore, a self-pitying preoccupation, but a social process through which older people come to understand changes in their roles and decide how they should behave: 'One cannot be ill by oneself and know that one is ill' (p. 101) – feelings and experiences have to be tested out with others.

The ageing body and the self

A better understanding of ageing as a personal experience grounded in social relationships requires more information about the relationships that older people experience in everyday life. Language, for example, has an important part to play. Coupland and colleagues (1991) show how age identities are shaped in sequences of talk. References to ageing and old age by both younger and older women do not necessarily indicate the older women's experience of ageing, but reflects assumptions that older people are preoccupied with old age. Aspects of age-related speech include the disclosure of chronological age, references to time passing, and a self-association with the past and recognition of social change over time. Age identity is a fluid process that varies according to time, place and the people involved.

Older people may retain an image of themselves as younger. This leads to a disjunction between how people experience themselves and their body, so that the self may be experienced as a kind of 'ageless' or youthful prisoner inside an ageing body. The ageing body and face act as a

kind of mask disguising the inner sense of personal selfhood or identity (Hepworth, 1995; Biggs, 1999). The relationship between the body and the self is therefore complicated by perceptions of the body and the value placed upon it. People who value their youth and beauty may be much unhappier with their bodies as they grow older than those who value the inner self more. The latter may find physical ageing less burdensome and an opportunity for personal development. It is therefore important to find out how people perceive their bodies as they grow older as well as looking for information about biological change.

Perhaps the reason why health care professionals think all old people are infirm and ill is that they encounter this group most frequently. However, acknowledging that older people may not think of themselves as 'older' may help understand their feelings and behaviour. It also cautions us against stereotyping older patients.

The ageing mind

It is commonly believed that old people are incapable of learning new things, depressed and that intelligence declines with age. At one time there appeared to be a substantial body of evidence showing that intelligence declines with age (see pp. 32–33). However, longitudinal studies (Schaie, 1996) showed that when the same individuals were tested over time, there was very little change in intelligence scores (Fig. 1).

Does the ability to learn decline with age? It seems to take older people longer to search their memory stores to retrieve information. Therefore, doctors should give older patients more time to 'find' the answers to questions. Filling the silence with other questions can lead to a breakdown in communication (see pp. 96–97).

Older and younger subjects differ in the ability to filter out irrelevant information, the 'cocktail party' effect. When young people go to a party they have little difficulty filtering out the irrelevant conversations around them. Older people find this difficult. Studies involve asking subjects to listen to headphones in which one message is played to the left ear and a different one to the right. The subject is asked to follow only one message (so-called dichotic listening experiments). As people age, more and more information from the 'wrong' ear appears in the test (Stuart-Hamilton, 1994).

These findings are relevant to the practice of medicine:

- When taking a history or explaining something to an older patient ensure that there are as few distracting and irrelevant noises about as possible; patients find it stressful to have to struggle to listen to and concentrate on one particular conversation.
- It is not uncommon for middle-aged patients to ask GPs to have their hearing tested or for wax to be removed. Testing often reveals no wax and little decrement in the acuity of the patient's hearing. The patient goes away frustrated and still convinced that he or she is going deaf. Explanation of this 'central processing' phenomenon usually provides reassurance.

Alzheimer's disease

Alzheimer's disease has been described as the loss of self. Sabat & Harré (1992) divide the self into two parts: self i and selves ii. Self i is the personal singularity indicated by the use of

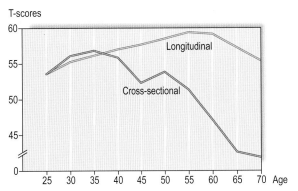

Fig. 1 Findings from cross-sectional and longitudinal studies of intelligence and age.

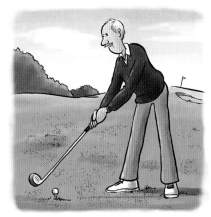

Fig. 2 The experience and image of ageing is changing.

expressions such as 'I', 'me' and 'mine', which is made possible by the structure of language. The 'I' is the sense of personal identity we all possess. Selves ii is the social aspect of identity and this is made up of the ensemble of social selves that is displayed during our relationships with other people. Selves ii require the collaboration of other people in recognizing our various social identities. These are the selves that are socially presented: public expressions of a type of character drawn from a 'local repertoire' (p. 452). For example, we may present different identities as 'student' and 'friend' or 'daughter'.

Sociological studies of dementia suggest that the process may be more than simple loss of capabilities due to physical changes. Kitwood (1997: 31) developed a person-centred approach to understanding dementia, suggesting that the changes that are observable tend to result not only from biomedical factors, but are also related to loss of resources, including social support for the self. Biomedical change is, therefore, aggravated by changes in the responses of other people to the sufferer when they withdraw the social support he or she needs to continue maintaining a social self. Thus, social support and interaction are also factors in the development and manifestation of dementia. Kitwood (1997) argued that 'those who are well supported only very rarely suggest that their relative has acquired a different personality or "disappeared". Perhaps they have found ways of maintaining relationships and communication and can deal more accurately with their own feelings of loss and bewilderment.'

Ageing and social change

Increased life expectancy and reductions in the birth rate are resulting in a situation where people aged over 50 years will no longer be a minority group in industrialized countries. This change will not necessarily result in an increased burden of older people (Coleman et al., 1993), because the evidence is that many older people continue to make an active contribution to social life. As politicians recognize the votes to be won in the age group, it may affect policy proposals about health care facilities that favour older people. For example, the Netherlands saw the emergence of the 'old folks' party in politics. The role of grandparents as babysitters and debates about increasing the retirement age are good examples of active roles of older people.

Demographic change means that the traditional models of the roles of older people in society are no longer relevant. The experience of ageing is changing and becoming more diverse as societies become more complex, and new models

and images of ageing have to be created (Fig. 2). Hence it is no longer acceptable to regard life after the age of 50 as a period of decline into old age. Care provision is not just a matter of looking after the body, but must, therefore, change to ensure the continuity of personal identity and individual independence in later life.

Case study

The writer Linda Grant (1998) provides a detailed and moving account of the effects of Alzheimer's disease on the 'self' of her mother Rose (who suffered from Alzheimer's) and on herself. She discusses in vivid detail Rose's gradually developing sense of confusion as a threat to her mother's sense of identity. Rose sometimes seemed to be aware of the changes taking place in her ability to control her presentation of self, on the occasions when she would show she was 'ashamed, embarrassed and afraid of [the] response [of other people]. She had cut herself off because she could no longer manage the skills she needed to be in company ... "I cringe inside when someone tells me I'm repeating myself," she said once, in a rare acknowledgment'.

The experince persuaded Grant that individuals do not have a fixed identity through their lives, but throughout their lives experience a range of selves.

STOP THINK ■ 'You're only as old as you feel!' How does this relate to the old people you know, perhaps your grandparents or other relatives or family friends?

Social aspects of ageing

■ Biological ageing occurs in social environments.

■ Ageing is a relational process.

■ Physical and mental decline are not inevitable in later life.

■ As people grow older they work to maintain their own sense of personal identity.

■ People may experience the self as 'younger' than the body.

■ Alzheimer's disease does not necessarily mean the loss of self.

■ New models of ageing and old age are emerging to replace traditional beliefs and attitudes.

Bereavement

In the course of their careers, doctors will often have to care for people who are coming to terms with the loss of someone through death. The process occurring after the death, during which individuals learn to adjust to the loss, is known as bereavement. Grief can be described as the emotional response to that loss, while mourning refers to the expression of grief (Stroebe & Stroebe, 1987). The bereavement period can provide the opportunity for doctors to assess the needs of the surviving spouse or family, and to intervene where appropriate with relevant back-up and services. This is important because studies show that bereaved people can have higher levels of morbidity and mortality than non-bereaved people (Parkes, 1996).

Determinants of grief

Many factors can affect the way in which someone reacts to being bereaved. These may precede the bereavement, for example, a childhood experience, a previous life crisis like divorce or mental illness, or the nature of the relationship between the bereaved person and the deceased. The reaction may also be influenced by the bereaved person's present circumstances, for example, his or her age, sex, religion, type of personality or even cultural background. Reactions may also be determined by the circumstances of bereaved people after the death, for example, the amount of support they have, and other stresses in their life, such as young children. Such determinants have been referred to as the antecedent (previous experience), concurrent (present circumstances) and subsequent determinants of grief (Parkes, 1996).

Cultural and religious beliefs affect how people display grief and feel they should behave during bereavement. Strict rules govern the preparation of the body after death and the rituals associated with burial and mourning among different ethnic groups (Firth, 2001) (see pp. 130–131).

The mourning process

In the same way that the dying process has been described as a series of stages (Kubler-Ross, 1970, see pp. 130–131), the process of mourning has similarly been defined as a series of phases or stages that must be passed through before grief can be resolved The initial phase of numbness gradually gives way to feelings of pining, yearning and searching, as the bereaved person seeks to recover what has been lost. When the intensity of this second phase diminishes, it is replaced by feelings of depression, disorganization and despair when it becomes apparent that the loss is irretrievable. Finally, the bereaved person moves to a phase of recovery and reorganization when s/he begins to adjust to a new way of life without the deceased (Parkes, 1975; Bowlby, 1998). Worden (1991) describes the process as a series of tasks that must be worked through. He describes these as accepting the reality of the loss, working through the pain, adjusting to an environment in which the deceased is missing and moving on with life. Although these stage and phase theories can be a useful way of beginning to understand the complexity of the grief process, they are not intended to be prescriptive. Individual reactions will vary and may not conform to a specific pattern, i.e. a bereaved person may not pass through these stages sequentially.

More recently, the Dual Process model suggests that bereaved people move between confronting grief (loss-oriented behaviour) and avoiding grief (restoration-oriented behaviour) (Stroebe & Schut 1999). This and other newer models advocate that the bereaved do not return to the way they were before the death as the stage models may have implied but adapt to a new way of living which incorporates a continuing bond with the dead person (Klass et al., 1996; Walter, 1999).

Normal grief

Normal grief reactions can include a range of different feelings, moods, symptoms and behaviours. Worden (1991) has classified examples of these under four headings. These are illustrated in Figure 1.

Risk factors

Faulkner (1995) suggests that the reaction to loss may not be normal if:

- A difficult relationship with the deceased existed before the death, for example, the bereaved person may have been overly dependent on the dead person, or disliked him or her.
- The death has been violent (e.g. murder) or sudden or unexplained (e.g. suicide).
- The nature of the bereaved's involvement in the death has been unsatisfactory, for example, the bereaved person may not have had time to say goodbye, may not have visited the person before the death or may not have been present at the death.
- The bereaved person has previously experienced difficult losses, for example, divorce or mutilating surgery (Faulkner, 1995).

Atypical grief

Abnormal or complicated grief reactions occur when bereaved individuals are unable for some reason

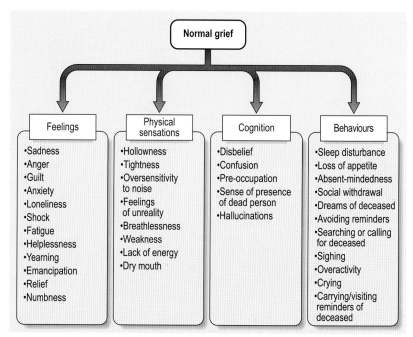

Fig. 1 A typology of normal grief (from Worden, 1991, with permission).

to express or work through their grief, which prevents their recovery from the loss and adaptation to life without the deceased. These reactions can be excessive and prolonged, or absent and short-lived. Such reactions can be classified as delayed or absent, chronic, masked or exaggerated grief.

Delayed or absent grief

The bereaved person is unable to mourn the loss. This may be conscious, when the bereaved person's situation makes it difficult for him or her to grieve freely, for example, in the case of a mother who carries on normally for the sake of her children. It can also be unconscious, when the bereaved person does not believe that the death has occurred, for example, when there has been no definite confirmation, as in the case of soldiers missing during a war. This may be called absent grief (Faulkner, 1995). Delayed grief reactions are often triggered by other losses occurring a long time after the death, e.g. a later divorce or other unrelated loss (Worden, 1991).

Chronic grief

The bereaved continues to experience the immediate pain of the loss months or even years later. That person is therefore unable to move on in the grieving process and adapt to life without the deceased. Usually chronic grief reactions occur in people who have had ambivalent relationships with the deceased (Parkes, 1975).

Masked grief

The grief reaction is masked by the development of physical or somatic symptoms that appear to the bereaved to be unassociated with the loss. Often these are physical symptoms that replicate those experienced by the deceased and these commonly appear on the anniversaries of the loss (Worden, 1991).

Exaggerated grief

The grief reaction is excessive and intense. In these cases the bereaved's experience may develop into a serious psychiatric illness, e.g. clinical depression or an acute anxiety state (Worden, 1991).

Disenfranchised grief

Persons may react to other losses or illnesses in the same way as they would to a bereavement through death, for example, reaction to a cancer diagnosis (see pp. 98–99), amputation, miscarriage, stillbirth, physical dependence, divorce, unemployment or even relocation to a new town or city. With these losses the grief experienced and exhibited by the person may be as intense and as debilitating as grief expressed at a death. However, the grief may not be acknowledged or sanctioned by others, making it difficult for the bereaved to grieve openly or gain support (Doka, 2002). For these reasons health professionals may miss or fail to appreciate the extent of a person's distress. This may mean that the person experiencing the loss is not offered the help he or she needs to come to terms with it.

Bereavement care

The amount of support available for the bereaved varies greatly according to the setting where patients and their relatives are cared for. Doctors working in general hospitals may not have the time or resources to follow up carers during bereavement. Often this is done by general

practitioners or community nurses, who are able to visit the bereaved at home. Not every bereaved person will want or need professional support at this time. The majority rely on family and friends or find their own ways of coping. In cases where the grief reaction is problematic, the doctor should recognize his or her limitations and summon the help of someone who is specially trained in bereavement counselling. In extreme cases, it may also be necessary to refer the person on to a clinical psychologist or psychiatrist (see pp. 132–133, 136–137).

Case study

Ethel was a 61-year-old woman whose husband Jack had died 6 months earlier after a sudden heart attack. At around the same time her youngest daughter, Ruth, had left home to start a university course in a city about 30 miles away from where they lived. Her two elder children were both married and living abroad. Previously a lively woman, with many and varied interests, Ethel had shared most of these with her husband as they both enjoyed early retirement. Lately, however, Ethel had become withdrawn and morose, and seemed to have lost all interest in anything. She had stopped going to the clubs of which she was a member and preferred instead to spend her days looking at old family photos or going through her husband's belongings, which she refused to part with. She constantly phoned her daughter in tears and said she did not want to carry on living without her husband. As a result Ruth felt guilty at having left her mother to cope alone, and at a loss to know what help to give her. Eventually, Ruth asked the family general practitioner for help. She suggested that Ruth phone a local voluntary bereavement counselling service. After a few visits from a trained counsellor, Ethel began to come to terms with her husband's death. Although she knew that her life would no longer be the same without her lifetime partner, she realized that she had to make a new beginning for her own and her family's sake. Ruth was relieved that her mother was now able to resume some of the hobbies she used to enjoy, and her own life at university became happier.

STOP THINK
- Write down the factors you think might have influenced the way Ethel reacted to Jack's death.
- Think about how you would cope with Ethel if you were Ruth.
- Think about the counsellor's task in helping Ethel through the grief (see pp. 132–133).

Bereavement

- Bereavement refers to the situation of someone who has experienced the loss of a loved one and grief is the emotional response to the loss.
- Normal grief can be described as a series of stages individuals must work through until they adapt to life without the deceased.
- The way people react to a loss will depend on their past experiences and present circumstances.

Personality and health

We can see similarities in how people act as well as clear differences. Scientists have been describing these similarities and differences for centuries and the concept of personality is an important part of current psychological research. Reliable measures of personality have been found to predict performance and health. Such research has important applications. For example, many businesses now use personality profiling as part of their selection procedures so that they can employ people who have predictable social skills and behaviour patterns. Similarly, if someone behaves out of character, we should look for causes that might be related to health, such as drug abuse, the onset of dementia or a breakdown in a relationship.

Below we focus on some of the implications of research into personality for health and health care.

Personality and context

Behaviour is shaped by social roles as well as by personality differences. If you look around a lecture theatre, most people are acting in a very similar manner. This is true of many social situations. The roles people occupy within social situations determine, to a large extent, how they behave. Yet there are differences. For example, whereas two lecturers may both deliver the same lecture, the manner in which they do this is likely to be shaped by their different personalities. Moreover, these differences become more evident in less structured social situations. Thus while social contexts shape behaviour, we can still identify stable individual differences in how people behave.

Traits

Traits are clusters of individual differences in emotion and behaviour observed between people and across situations (Stone & McCrae, 2007). Trait theories can be used to predict differences in behaviour and health between individuals. Cattell (1971), Eysenck (1967) and others used factor analysis (a statistical technique that investigates correlations between variables, and identifies clusters of association which suggest an underlying structure) to identify key factors shaping personality.

Much recent research on personality has focused on five broad personality traits: openness to experience (or intellect), conscientiousness, extroversion, agreeableness, neuroticism (also referred to as emotional stability and negative affect) (Fig. 1). This group of five traits is known as the big five or OCEAN model of personality and research indicates that the big five traits may determine the extent to which people engage in general clusters of health-related behaviours like substance

 STOP THINK Does personality change over time? Are these changes in underlying personality or changes in how people learn to cope with familiar situations?

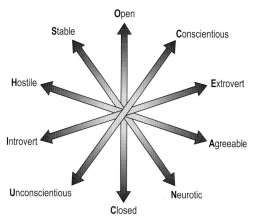

Fig. 1 OCEAN dimensions of personality (from McCrae & Costa, 1987, with permission).

use risk behaviours such as smoking (Booth-Kewley & Vickers, 1994).

Openness (O)
Openness refers to the tendency to welcome new ideas and to be curious about new ways of looking at everyday reality. It is associated with intellectual curiosity, intelligence and creativity. High O scorers may be more likely to appreciate the arts and be engaged in intellectual work but may be more easily bored. Low scorers prefer familiarity and some types of work focusing on routine and procedure may be better suited to those with low O scores. There is little evidence linking O scores to health.

Conscientiousness (C)
Highly conscientious individuals are more organized, careful, dependable, self-disciplined and achievement-oriented than those low in conscientiousness (McCrae & Costa, 1987). High C scores are associated with a greater use of problem-focused and support-seeking in the face of life challenges. Longitudinal data suggest that childhood C also predicts longevity, with high C children living an additional 2 years compared to low C children (Friedman et al., 1993). This may be because high C individuals are more likely to engage in health-protective action such as exercising and screening attendance and also less likely to risk their health by smoking (Booth-Kewley & Vickers, 1994).

Extroversion (E)
Extroverts (those scoring high on extroversion) tend to be energetic, outgoing, socially engaging and assertive. They are sensation-seekers and welcome new challenges but get bored easily. By contrast introverts (who have low E scores) show the opposite pattern of behaviour. Extroversion is associated with better psychological well-being and better physical health. For example, extroverts tend to suffer less from coronary heart disease, ulcers, asthma and arthritis (Booth-Kewley & Vickers, 1994).

Agreeableness (A)
People high in agreeableness are more concerned with social harmony and value getting along with others. They tend to be friendly, considerate and helpful and have a

trusting and optimistic view of others. Consequently, high A scorers tend to be better liked and have greater social support. This is likely to help them deal more effectively with stressful experiences. By contrast, those scoring low on A tend to distrust others and be less friendly and cooperative. Therefore, A has been seen as the opposite of hostility, which has been found to be associated with coronary heart disease (see Case study).

Neuroticism (N)

People high in neuroticism experience negative emotions including anxiety, fear, anger and guilt more often and more intensely. They report worrying a lot and getting upset more easily than others. In addition, they report experiencing more and more intense symptoms of illness (McCrae & Costa, 1987). High N people may be more affected by stress (see pp. 126–127) and experience less social support. They may also be more likely to consume more alcohol and to smoke. However, research relating N to objective measures of health has found few associations (Watson & Pennebaker, 1989). Thus N is strongly related to symptom-reporting but not to illness itself. This emphasizes the importance of controlling for the effects of N when using symptom reports as outcome measures.

Pessimists die younger

Another important trait found to relate to health is the tendency to be pessimistic about explaining why bad outcomes occur. Such explanations can be classified along three dimensions: (1) whether they are internal or external (e.g. was it my fault or a result of my environment?); (2) whether they are stable or unstable over time (e.g. was this caused by my ability or physique or just bad luck?); and (3) whether they are global, referring to many events or specific to a particular event (e.g. my personality means this type of thing will always happen to me, or it was just a one-off in

this situation). Pessimists tend to explain bad events as due to internal, stable and global causes (Peterson et al., 1988). For example, pessimists might believe that they contracted an illness because they are always susceptible to illness, whereas optimists might believe that they became ill because of an unusually stressful period. This different pattern of explanation strongly affects expectations about the future.

A pessimistic explanatory style is bad for your health. Peterson et al. (1988) found that explanatory style measured in men at the age of 25 predicted health as assessed by doctors at both 45 and 60 years. Similarly, Danner et al. (2001) found that examination of what young nuns had written about themselves when they entered the church predicted their longevity. Those who included most positive emotions in their writing (e.g. happiness, pride, love) lived on average 10 years longer than those who included fewest positive emotions.

How do individual differences affect health?

The tendency to react in an anxious manner or to distrust others may have direct and immediate effects on our endocrine, immunological or cardiovascular systems and over time consistently strong reactions may lead to differential physical wear and tear on bodily systems. At the same time, such reactions may lead people to make different behavioural choices. A person low on C and high on N may prioritize immediate stress reduction while someone with the opposite characteristics may plan more carefully for the future and so better avoid accidents and health damage. We vary across a range of traits. Someone may be high N, high C and high A while someone else is pessimistic but mid C and A. It is likely that the effects of personality on health are most evident for small groups which show more extreme scores on these traits.

Case study

Does type A behaviour matter?

The idea of type A behaviour originated in observations by two cardiologists, Meyer Friedman and Ray Rosenman, who noticed that many patients with heart disease spoke quickly and appeared agitated (Friedman & Rosenman, 1974). The behaviour pattern includes a competitive drive, aggression, chronic impatience and a sense of time urgency. The Western Collaborative Group Study examined risk factors for coronary heart disease (CHD) in a sample of over 3000 healthy middle-aged men for more than 27 years. Initial results suggested that type A behaviour was an important risk factor for CHD. However, later results from this study and others cast doubt on the importance of type A behaviour and, in a meta-analysis of available findings, Matthews (1988) concluded that it was not type A as such but one particular aspect of this behaviour pattern, namely hostility, that predicted CHD. This finding has been confirmed by subsequent studies and the consensus is that there is little or no relationship between type A and CHD but that there is a clear link between hostility (distrust of and aggressiveness towards others) and CHD. How much more likely hostile people are to develop heart problems is less clear, with some studies suggesting that this may be a minor risk factor (Myrtek, 2001). This research over three decades shows how theory develops as measurement improves and larger prospective data sets can be combined in meta-analyses. For example, the evidence suggests that measuring type A using a structured interview revealed hostile elements more effectively than self-report measures so these measurements of type A were associated with CHD whereas others were not.

Personality and health

- People's tendencies to behave in similar ways across situations can be reliably measured.
- Much research has focused on the big five or OCEAN model of personality.
- High C scores predict better health probably because they are associated with health-protective action.
- Hostility (low A) is associated with coronary heart disease.
- High N scores are related to symptom-reporting but not to illness itself.
- High E is associated with better psychological well-being and better physical health.
- A pessimistic explanatory style has also been found to predict poorer health.

Understanding learning

Learning is not just about acquiring facts or knowledge. Social skills, beliefs and values are also learned. We learn how to respond emotionally, how to recognize symptoms and, as children, we learn appropriate (and inappropriate) ways of behaving (Fig. 1). If we understand how behaviour is learned we may be able to change it. We may wish to change to a healthier lifestyle, to learn how to monitor our own glucose levels or to overcome a phobia. Understanding learning has been of central concern to psychologists, and the source of much debate (Eysenck, 1996).

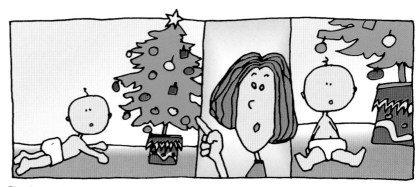

Fig. 1 If an infant approaches the Christmas tree decorations it will be restrained: this will decrease the frequency of approach. In practice punishment is a very poor way of changing behaviour and often it arouses emotional responses. What does the baby do when it is not allowed to touch the tree (or approach medical equipment)?

Learning can be defined as a relatively permanent change in behaviour. Behaviourist theories of learning assume that there are laws of learning that are fundamental to all animals, and that humans are no different in this respect. Behaviourism suggests that learning results from stimulus–response associations. A stimulus can be any change, such as the sight of food or a moving ball. A response is a reflex action such as salivation, or a muscular response such as catching the ball. Of course much learning is cognitive – such as the acquisition of knowledge and concepts that is taking place as you read this book. Research into adult learning has informed medical teaching and the way in which you are taught is likely to differ from the experience of senior medical staff. It is recognized that adults learn in different ways from children so you may find a very different approach to learning from your school experience.

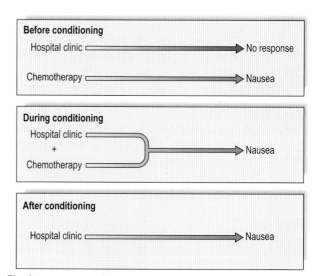

Fig. 2 Classical conditioning applied to nausea and chemotherapy.

Theoretical background

Operant conditioning

A kind of learning, known as operant conditioning, was described by an American psychologist, B.F. Skinner. In operant conditioning, the likelihood of a response occurring again is increased if the behaviour is followed by reinforcement. Thus, the behaviour is controlled by its consequences. The principles of operant conditioning have been established through experimentation on animals such as rats and pigeons, as well as humans (Table 1).

If a goal results from an accurate kick, then the motor responses leading up to the kick will be reinforced. In this case the reinforcement would be in the form of satisfaction and approval by the team and fans. Success in walking following an amputation would be rewarded internally by feelings of mastery and enhanced self-efficacy, and externally by the approval of others. Praise (especially from medical staff) can be a very powerful reinforcer.

Classical conditioning

Operant conditioning is contrasted with classical conditioning described by a physiologist, I. Pavlov. In classical conditioning an initially neutral stimulus becomes associated with an involuntary response by its association with a previously conditioned stimulus. Pavlov worked with dogs, who naturally salivate at the sight of food. After pairing a bell with the food, the dogs learned to salivate at the sound of the bell alone. These principles were later tested with human emotional responses.

Watson & Raynor (1920) used classical conditioning to produce a phobia in a 9-month-old child known as Little Albert. Before the experiment the child had no fear of white rats but was frightened by loud noises. In the experiment the loud noise was paired with the presence of a white rat. After six pairings Albert showed a fear response in the presence of the white rat alone. Fear had now become a response conditioned to the previously neutral stimulus of the white

Table 1 **Principles of operant conditioning**			
Principle	**Definition**	**Effect on behaviour**	**Example**
Positive reinforcement	Provides positive, pleasant consequences	Increases probability that the response will occur again	Verbal praise in rehabilitation
Negative reinforcement	Removes unpleasant conditions	Increases probability that response will occur again	Adjusting gait to avoid pain in walking
Punishment	Removes a positive reinforcer or applies an aversive stimulus	Decreases the probability that response will occur again	Vomiting after eating poisonous fungi
Extinction	Removes positive reinforcer	Decreases the probability that response will occur again	Ignoring tantrums in waiting room
Shaping	Reinforces successive approximations to the one required	Gradually increases approximation to desired behaviour	Teaching someone with a learning disability how to feed him- or herself

rat. Moreover the fear generalized to other furry animals. White rats and loud noises are not an everyday occurrence but white coats may be associated with painful injections. The fear of pain may become associated with the white coat (and its wearer) and generalize to white coats worn by any staff.

Some patients may develop conditioned responses to the sight or smell of hospitals. If hospital treatment has been associated with nausea, as, for example, in the case of chemotherapy for cancer, the mere sight or smell of hospital can induce nausea or even vomiting (Fig. 2).

In practice, both operant conditioning and classical conditioning probably occur in many learning situations. Food elicits salivation but also acts as a reinforcer.

Observational learning

This model suggests that behaviour patterns can be learned by watching other people's behaviour. Many clinical skills are learned in this way. Both voluntary and involuntary responses can be learned by modelling.

- What has been your experience of problem-based learning? Did you select your medical school on the basis of having or not having this approach? What about your colleagues?
- What reinforcements do you think would be appropriate for medical staff to use in a hospital setting?
- If someone is on a medically advised weight-reducing diet, success will be reinforced by praise from doctors, family and friends. Why is this not an effective reinforcer and why is it so hard to resist eating crisps and chocolate?
- If playing a fruit machine (or the National Lottery) gave too few prizes, people would soon stop playing. Why?

Children who were going to be admitted to hospital were shown a film of an unstressed child going into hospital, undergoing surgery and going home. Compared with others who were shown an unrelated film these children showed less anxiety both before and after the operation (Saile et al., 1988). The closer in age and sex the model was to themselves, the more imitation took place. However, the films may have reduced the anxiety of the parents as much as the children so that the child had a very powerful model

of an unanxious parent to imitate as well! In the same way, anxiety or embarrassment shown by a doctor will be quickly picked up and learned by a patient. Doctors and medical staff are powerful models.

Systematic desensitization

Systematic desensitization or graded exposure would treat a phobia such as Albert's learned fear of furry animals by gradually exposing the person to the feared object while replacing the anxiety with a relaxed condition. This can be achieved by reassurance or relaxation training. In a diabetic outpatient clinic someone with a needle phobia might be treated by such methods so that he or she can tolerate injections. Initially this might be done by imagination alone, by visualizing the object, and once this is achieved without fear, the syringe could be introduced in the form of a picture. Later it might be shown in vivo, firstly at a distance and then gradually brought nearer (see pp. 112–113).

Cognitive-behavioural therapy tries to alter behaviour by undoing the learning of maladaptive behaviour and by learning new behaviour patterns (pp. 136–137). It is based on theories of classical and operant conditioning.

Principles of learning have also been used in theories that enhance coping with stress, such as rational emotive behaviour theory and biofeedback.

E-learning

Learning by using modern information technology gives learners control over the content, learning sequence, pace of learning, time and a choice of media. Research shows that this is at least as effective as traditional instructor-led lectures (Ruiz et al., 2006). Faculty staff may become facilitators of learning and assessors of competency rather than imparters of information. This will mean a radical role change (see pp. 164–165).

Learning factual material

Medical students find that they have to learn and recall difficult material (see pp. 28–29). Various strategies have been proposed to help this. Mnemonics can be associations of two words or letters, or a word and a visual image. Rehearsal can establish words in long-term memory, and this is most effective if they are organized. Many students make lists or mind maps of a topic.

You will find that much of your course uses self-directed learning and this is thought to promote learning skills and team-working as well as factual knowledge. Problem-based learning has also been adopted by many medical schools.

Case study

Night-waking in children can be a problem for both child and parents. An otherwise healthy and happy 2-year-old child woke up regularly at night, and early in the morning. His parents were becoming exhausted because of broken sleep; they were becoming irritable with each other and their work was suffering.

The parents were asked to monitor their behaviour when the child woke up. They described how they gave the child a drink, read him a story and sometimes took him into their own bed to settle him. It was pointed out that these were acting as reinforcers, as well as the drink filling his bladder, causing soaking nappies in the morning.

The parents then left him to cry for longer before responding and gave him minimal attention in the night. Reinforcers were given for sleeping through the night such as giving cuddles and toys in his own bed, not the parents'. Within a few weeks the broken nights were fewer and the child's behaviour was further reinforced by having happy, rested parents.

Understanding learning

- Learning is a relatively stable change in behaviour and may occur by operant conditioning, classical conditioning or observationally.
- Operant conditioning has been used to change health behaviour and is based on principles of reinforcement, punishment, extinction and shaping.
- Principles of learning have been used in behaviour therapy to modify undesired behaviour patterns.
- Theories of adult learning have influenced current medical teaching.

Perception

Why do we perceive what we do? How does the brain process information so that what we see or hear is what we create, not what is actually 'out there'? This spread shows how perception is not a passive process, but is active, creating and constructing our world. Whereas sensation (the stimulus which impacts upon the sense organs) provides the raw data about the environment, it is perception which provides meaning.

The main emphasis in this spread will be on visual perception, but these points also apply to other types of perception such as auditory, olfactory or tactile perception.

The main features of perception

- Perception is knowledge-based and partly learned. Early works of art show that artists (and young children) have to learn about perspective; likewise, your perception of pathological signs on a slide under a microscope improves with medical education.
- Perception is inferential. When we see part of an object, like the top half of a person sitting at a table, we perceive this as a 'whole' person, not half a person. A lot of what we perceive is effectively guesswork, which can have dangerous consequences.
- It is categorical. We tend to categorize what we see, so that a variety of clinical signs are perceived as a disease in a patient, even though they may not in fact be related.
- Perception is relational. What we perceive as small or large depends on context. A 2-cm flesh wound on a thigh is seen as less serious than the same size of wound on a finger.
- Perception is adaptive. We tend to perceive significant things better than insignificant things. For example, we notice a car which is moving more than we notice a stationary vehicle: this is more important for our survival.

What are illusions, and why are we subject to them?

Illusions demonstrate how creative a process perception is, because the stimuli are ambiguous, or presented in a context which distorts our perception. Figure 1 illustrates this.

We are subject to illusions, not because we are unintelligent or not paying attention, but because the brain interprets reality in the light of our prior experience. This is important because different people perceive things differently, and not necessarily because one is wrong and one is right.

(a) Ponzo

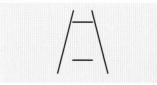

(b) Muller–Lyer

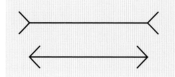

Fig. 1 In these two figures, the sets of horizontal lines are the same length, but we see them as differing lengths according to the rest of the drawing.

How do we recognize what is perceived?

Recognition is organizing what is perceived into something meaningful by using past experience. A number of theories exist to explain this:

- Bottom-up processing. The perceptual system is assumed to analyse a stimulus into a set of features and then the brain matches it to other sets already existing in the brain. If a match occurs, then there is recognition. In examining a rash, a general practitioner takes note of the shape, type, size, colour and distribution of spots on the skin, then matches them to previous cases of measles that s/he has seen, or the colour illustration and description of measles that s/he has seen in a textbook.
- Top-down processing. The context creates expectancy and sets up what is known as *perceptual set*. We 'see' what we expect, or want to see, and recognition occurs. For example, the general practitioner learns from the patient that s/he has been in contact with someone suffering from German measles. This creates an expectancy, and a perceptual set

STOP THINK ■ What factors may help to explain why one 45-year-old man perceives his symptoms of dyspepsia as severe and serious, whereas another similarly aged man perceives them as trivial? (see pp. 90–91)

when examining the patient's rash. It can sometimes lead to misdiagnosis when the expectancy is strong.

- Both mechanisms together. In trying to read a page of poor handwriting we may use both processes: puzzling out what each letter looks like, as well as guessing meaning from the context. Figure 2 shows how you do this, demonstrating how easy it is for our perception (diagnoses) to be mistaken.

What does this squiggle mean?

Analysis of features alone will not tell you.

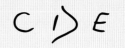

Context is also needed.

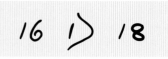

Fig. 2 Interpretation in context.

How do we influence perception?

We control our perception by paying attention to different aspects of our environment. Attention is the directing and focusing of perception. It may be:

- Selective. We attend more to stimuli that are changing, repeated, intense and personally meaningful. Certain words catch our attention, for example our names, words connected with significant interests, or important concerns such as words like 'sex'.
- Divided or focused. Our ability to divide attention is limited, although it can be improved with practice. It is easier to divide attention if two

different types of stimuli are used. For example, you can probably look at pictures and listen to music simultaneously, but it is hard to read and listen to someone talking at the same time.

■ Negatively affected by stress and fatigue. When we are tired, or when there are more demands being placed upon us than there are resources to meet those demands, our attention may decrease. This can have disastrous results. Tired doctors are more likely to make errors because they are no longer able to pay full attention to all the details of a particular set of diagnostic signs.

The relevance of the psychology of perception to medicine

The brain is an active component of the perceptual process. Brain damage will result in perceptual distortion, hence an early indicator of organic damage may be perceptual disturbance.

There is often no such thing as the 'correct' way to perceive something: perceptions vary because the perceptual process is a creative one. Most of the time we do not notice this, but sometimes the differences are critical. A pathologist may carry out a postmortem examination, with an assumption about the cause of death. It may lead him or her to seek, identify and report an incomplete set of evidence. A second pathologist may discover another, highly significant sign which can change the course of the police inquiry completely.

We are prone to see what the context indicates we should see. Given ambiguous cues we 'recognize' things according to our expectations.

Attention can be divided, with practice. When you start to acquire a skill (e.g. taking blood from a patient) it is almost impossible to do anything else at the same time, such as talking reassuringly to the patient. In time, however, the skill of attending to both aspects of the patient encounter simultaneously can be learned.

Social perception

Past experience

We may be influenced by our previous experience when making a diagnosis (see Case study). Our perception may also be influenced by our past

Case study

We see what we expect to see

A junior doctor, just starting in obstetrics and gynaecology, admitted a pregnant woman late one afternoon who was complaining of stomach pains. The doctor had herself been in hospital on and off during her pregnancy with a series of minor complaints. She carried out a physical examination, as well as asking for an account of the patient's symptoms, and then recommended bed rest. A second junior doctor was covering the ward at night and was asked to check the patient. His cousin had recently been admitted for an ectopic pregnancy. He immediately suggested an ultrasound scan, although the scanning unit was closed for the night. As a result, a life-threatening ectopic pregnancy was detected, and a successful operation was immediately carried out.

experience. For example, we tend to be more positive towards physically attractive people. In studies of social perception people were asked to choose the company with whom they would prefer to watch television. Most expressed a preference for people who were not physically disabled. In many cases this may be due simply to a lack of experience with disabled people. Congenital deformities may at first seem distressing but as you become familiar with such patients you will find that the deformity becomes less distressing and less pertinent. In a sense you no longer 'see' the deformity. Instead you are able to see past it to the person within.

Cognitive constructs

Our impression of people depends on how we perceive and think about them; these are known as our cognitive constructs. These include our perception of their sociability, likeability and intelligence, which depend both on the context and the people. You will use different constructs when forming impressions of people that you meet at a party from those that you use when seeing patients in an outpatient clinic. Sometimes we make errors in assuming that the behaviour of hospital patients is because of their personality rather than the situation of being ill in hospital (see pp. 102–103). On the other hand you may also attribute a patient's behaviour to having a particular disease rather than the fact that he/she really does behave in that manner.

Schemas

We have many expectations of other people's behaviour. These are called schemas. For example, students expect certain standards of behaviour from

their lecturers and doctors expect certain behaviour patterns from their patients. Schemas influence what we see even if the behaviour has not occurred. The diagnostic process may involve schemas. When you make inferences you may fill in the gaps about the relationship between symptoms. You use schemas in order to do this. The trouble is, you can make inferences which are in fact not true. For example, you may assume that a patient from a certain part of the country will have certain characteristics which may not be the case, or you might assume that because someone is of a particular sex that individual will behave in certain ways. We also have schemas about ourselves, called self schemas. Through life we gain information about ourselves and this may influence our selective perception. We often see ourselves in a more positive way than others do.

Patients have schemas too. Anxious patients may believe that they are unable to cope. Depressed patients may have negative self schemas in which they view themselves as inadequate, hopeless and worthless. These schemas influence what they see, think, feel and do. Patients who are depressed will be much less able to solve day-to-day problems than other people because they do not believe themselves capable of doing so, and in a sense, their predictions about themselves are fulfilled.

Perception

■ Perception is an active, creative process.

■ Perception depends on the brain's ability to interpret the senses.

■ Attention is part of the perceptual process, and it too can be affected by a variety of psychological factors such as previous experience, motivation, and fatigue.

Emotions

Emotions are transient, internal experiences involving sensations, feelings and changes in bodily arousal; they connect us to thoughts and images and influence how we react to and communicate with others. Most people distinguish between the meaning, or *valence* (positive or negative) and *intensity* of emotional experience, but psychological researchers have yet to come up with a universally accepted classification system. For example, joy (close to happiness or pleasure), excitement, anger, sadness, fear and embarrassment would be included in most people's emotional lexicon, but are pity, awe or pride classifiable as emotions? Moreover, some emotions (regret versus fear) require more sophisticated representations of reality than others.

Universals in how emotions are identified and classified

Emotions (or affective responses) organize various forms of *action readiness*. Their impact is also mediated by an awareness of internal feelings and an ability to reflect on them. Panskepp (1998) distinguished four distinct neural circuits underlying common emotions:

1. A foraging–expectancy–curiosity–investigatory network
2. An anger–rage network
3. An anxiety–fear network
4. A separation–distress–sorrow–anguish–panic network

The perception of basic emotions in others' faces may be biologically determined, rather than learned. This was first suggested by Darwin in 1872, but only systematically studied later. Ekman (1993) proposed that six primary emotions could be recognized from the same facial expressions across cultures: (1) fear; (2) anger; (3) disgust; (4) sadness; (5) enjoyment or happiness; and (6) surprise. Evidence supports the universality of the first five. When 70% or more of one cultural group judge a picture of facial expression to be one of these emotions, a similar percentage in other cultural groups will make the same judgement. We know too that the whole body transmits cues even when we adopt a 'poker' face! We cannot consciously control these signals.

Moods last longer and are not as reactive as emotions (Gross, 1998).

Controversy: what comes first: arousal, perception or identification of emotion?

That emotions involve physiological changes in the body is not disputed, but the nature of that relationship has been the topic of debate over centuries. In the late 19th century, James (1884) and Lange independently proposed that we experience emotion (e.g. fear) after perceptual events (e.g. I have just been told I must undergo major surgery) and subsequent physiological changes (e.g. heightened sympathetic arousal; see pp. 126–127). However, the James–Lange theory could not explain emotions reported by people with spinal injuries blocking physiological feedback to the brain. Two physiologists, Cannon (1931) and Baird, subsequently argued that, whereas heart pounding corresponds with fear, one does not cause the other: they represent two outcomes of the same (or parallel) processes. Later Schachter (1964) proposed his two-factor theory, arguing that whereas physiological changes appear to be necessary for emotion, the nature of

the emotional experience depends on how these changes are interpreted (e.g. how a person interprets the situation in which his or her heart is pounding). So different situations will determine whether a person experiences joy or anger or fear. Finally, while there is no doubt that many important emotional responses and behaviours arise from their cognitive interpretation, a growing number of psychologists believe that there may be different *kinds* of emotional response: some may occur instantly, *prior* to any cognitive processing and outside conscious awareness (Zajonc, 1998). Figure 1 portrays both direct (faster) and indirect (i.e. slower, cortical-mediated) routes by which emotion-related information can affect behaviour.

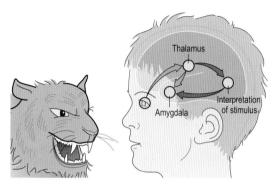

Fig. 1 Faster (green arrows) and slower (red arrows) activation of the fear response.

Emotions as internal messages

Emotions represent a distinct system by which we process information from the environment, separate from, but parallel to, the logical, linear processes associated with language and rational thinking. This system offers a faster channel for processing information when it has personal or high significance for us, or signals that a discrepancy exists between current perceptions and what we expected (Scherer, 1984). Emotions give us energy, and tell us whether to approach or avoid situations. Some of the pathways carrying emotional information end at subcortical centres (e.g. the amygdala), permitting a faster response than would ordinarily occur if processing required cortical processing *first*. A variety of neurotransmitters and hormones (e.g. adrenaline, noradrenaline, dopamine, oxytocin) are involved in generating arousal, regulating emotional states and activating behaviours. There is some evidence that particular neurochemical patterns may distinguish positive and negative emotional states (Greenfield, 2000).

Clinical findings indicate that emotion-related information needs to be fully 'digested'. For example, if a person consciously or unconsciously tried to limit his or her awareness of difficult feelings (e.g. because they are painful or confusing), over time the arousal associated with the 'blocked' emotions can contribute to physical symptoms, as well as chronic states of depression or anxiety. Chronic states of anxiety (resulting in high sympathetic arousal) have been known to lead to breakdowns in physiological systems (see pp. 126–127).

Emotion as social communication

Even subtle emotions influence social expectations and our relationships, informing others about our responses to them (Fig. 2). They also tell us about our own needs in

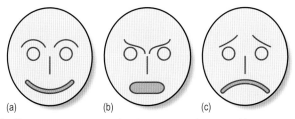

Fig. 2 Universally recognized facial expressions of emotion. (a) Happy, (b) angry, (c) sad.

relationships, as a kind of internal feedback (e.g. anger when we feel our intentions or goals are threatened by others; surprise when people act in unpredicted ways). Different cultures have different display rules (that is, what is socially acceptable in terms of the expression of emotion) and there are differences in these rules as they apply to gender and power relationships (e.g. crying might be appropriate at a wedding or funeral in one culture, but not in another).

The relationship between emotions and anxiety

Autonomic arousal underlies the experience and expression of all emotion. Emotional arousal needs regulation. Feeling too much emotion (even joy or excitement) may overwhelm and create anxiety. Coping strategies were initially divided into problem-focused (i.e. strategies that aim to solve the problem) and emotion-focused categories (i.e. strategies that decrease negative emotion). Initial findings suggested that emotion-focused coping strategies were less adaptive, but this is now believed to represent an oversimplified view. Seeking comfort, safety or advice from social resources, or *self-soothing* when confused or frightened, is an adaptive response in many situations (Stanton et al., 1994).

Regulatory processes may be automatic or deliberate. Individuals may choose to worry repetitively, for example, as focusing attention on particular thoughts – even unpleasant ones – may help limit the person's awareness of other emotional reactions (e.g. conflicting feelings, fear of the unknown). Emotional dysregulation (both overregulation and underregulation) is implicated in many examples of psychopathology, including mood and anxiety disorders, and addictive disorders (Williams et al., 1997), as well as somatic disorders like irritable bowel syndrome, fibromyalgia, chronic pain syndrome (Montoya et al., 2005). Chronic emotional dysregulation can endanger health in both direct and indirect ways. For example, people who feel unhappy may be less concerned about health risks associated with smoking, drinking or drug-taking (see pp. 80–85).

Health care professional–patient communications

When breaking bad news, the emotional state of *both* health care professionals and patients affects their perception of messages sent and received (see pp. 98–99). Patients worried about their condition may feel afraid of what they are about to hear, and not take in the message – even when the news is good! Patients may be embarrassed about their bodies, and their lack of health knowledge; they may experience some humiliation if their lack of understanding is highlighted. They may not even be aware of feeling intimidated by a doctor's powerful social position, but later wonder why they didn't ask more questions, or request changes to their treatment.

Such emotional responses – and their impact on the person – will influence whether a patient decides to consult (see pp. 88–89), and whether, and how, the individual adheres to health advice after consultations. Consequently, it can be helpful to introduce information in a way that minimizes strong emotional responses without misleading patients.

STOP THINK Imagine you are told you need to be admitted to hospital for major surgery. List some of the emotions you might experience. Think about how you might respond to these emotional experiences. What kind of support would be helpful to you?

Case study

George is recovering from a myocardial infarction in hospital. A nurse notices he is upset and talks to him. He begins to explain some of his worries and the nurse says: 'Don't worry about those things now – you just relax and get well'. He talks to a doctor who says, 'There's no need for you to be worried. Everything will be fine'. Although both clinicians want to help he feels somewhat rejected and isolated because he has no one to talk to about his feelings. This may affect his decision to enter into a rehabilitation programme and his recovery. A more helpful response from the clinicians would be to acknowledge George's upset and allow him to talk through his worries.

Emotions

- Emotions involve physiological arousal and cognitive interpretation. They often evoke fast responses to something unexpected, or highly positively or negatively valued.

- Facial expressions of certain basic emotions are recognized across many cultures, but cultures also have their own 'display rules'.

- Disconnecting from emotional experiencing is disconnecting from important information, and can contribute to the development of symptoms of psychological distress or physical illness.

- People can experience positive emotion even when they are upset or stressed. This may be important to effective coping.

- Emotional management of consultations is crucial to patients' responses to doctors and, therefore, to the effectiveness of consultations.

Memory problems

We are all familiar with lapses of memory – not being able to put a name to a face; forgetting to keep an appointment; and poor recall during an exam. Psychologists have learned a great deal about the process of memory in the past 100 years through both laboratory-based experiments and by studying patients with brain damage resulting in unique forms of memory loss. Although a very simplified view, Figure 1 is a useful summary of a widely held basic model of memory. Items are initially held in a short-term store and whether they become permanently represented in a long-term memory (LTM) store will depend on a host of factors such as how important and interesting they are, and whether we engage in active rehearsal strategies to encode items into permanent or LTM. There are also many different divisions of LTM, in particular a distinction between *declarative* and *procedural* memory (i.e. between memory for facts and autobiographical episodes and memory for skills and other cognitive operations).

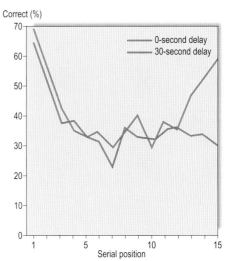

Fig. 2 The recency effect and short-term storage.

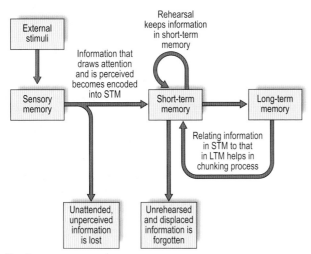

Fig. 1 Memory: short-term and long-term storage. STM, short-term memory; LTM, long-term memory.

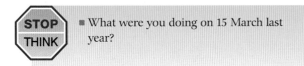

STOP THINK ■ What were you doing on 15 March last year?

Stages of memory

If we listen to a list of unrelated words read out to us, and then are required to recall the words immediately, items presented either first or last are better remembered than those in the middle. This better recall for the more recent items is because we are retrieving them directly from the short-term memory store. If we were to delay recall of the word list by 30 seconds, then this recency effect disappears (Fig. 2).

Even items which do successfully enter into LTM may not be recalled when we need them but much later are recalled. This illustrates the problem of *retrieval*, rather like a book which has been stored in a library: if we lose the catalogue slip, then the book is very difficult to find. This problem of memory loss is clearly very different to being unable to locate the book because it was never stored correctly in the first place. A good practical illustration of this distinction is the

difference between testing your knowledge about anatomy by *recall* ('describe the structure of the brain') and *recognition* ('which of the following is part of the limbic system?'). Multiple-choice exam questions have already carried out the retrieval part of remembering, leaving only the recognition component to be necessary.

When we are consider the problems of forgetting and the poor memory of head-injured and elderly patients, and we are trying to devise methods to aid recall, we need to have clear ideas about the stage at which the process is disturbed. Is it the initial learning which is defective or do those with poor memories simply forget more quickly?

How much can we remember?

Realizing that we have seen a film previously, but only about 10 minutes before its end, or revisiting a childhood home and having a flood of forgotten memories are powerful experiences which may tempt us into thinking that we do indeed store all events, and given the right conditions could retrieve such memories. Although there are well-documented cases of people with exceptional memories (one fascinating account, *The Mind of a Mnemonist*, is provided by the Russian neuropsychologist Luria (1969)), there is no scientific evidence to support this 'videotape' view of memory. To acquire permanent representation in memory we need to organize the new material and establish connections with the existing LTM store. Hence the use of mnemonic techniques which rely on devices such as learning a list of items in relation to an easily remembered rhyme, or first-letter mnemonics such as Richard Of York Gave Battle In Vain for the colours of the visible spectrum. Memory tricks like this should not be scoffed at and have proved useful in helping elderly patients remember people's names.

Helping patients to remember better

When patients have been asked to recall what they have been told during a consultation, they have been found to forget almost half. Memory for medical advice as opposed to diagnostic information can be particularly poor, especially in the case of highly anxious or elderly patients. Statements made early in the consultation are more likely to enter LTM (the primacy effect) and those at the end are remembered better initially but then tend to be forgotten (the recency effect). General or abstract statements are more difficult to remember than more specific concrete suggestions. Researchers have concluded that patient recall is aided by following some simple rules:

- Give the most important information early in any set of instructions.
- Stress the importance of relevant items (e.g. by repetition).
- Use explicit categorization under simple headings (e.g. I will tell you what is wrong … what treatment you will need … what you can do to help yourself).
- Make advice specific, detailed and concrete rather than general and abstract.

Memory after traumatic brain injury

Memory problems often follow accidental trauma from a closed head injury. In their most dramatic form, the patient may be unable to recall not only the events leading up to the accident, but for many years prior to that. This memory loss extending backwards in time is known as retrograde amnesia, as distinct from the inability to form new memories, which is known as anterograde amnesia. Such patients may well report themselves as 10 years younger than they are, and be unable to recall all the events of those 10 years, such as marriage, birth of children and employment. At the same time, they will repeatedly need to be told why they are in hospital and the names of the nurses and doctors caring for them. Eventually these years of memory loss will be recovered, indicating that the problem was difficulty of retrieval, but they may be left with enduring deficits of memory which may be secondary to attentional or concentration difficulties. The exact nature of the deficit will require extensive testing by a neuropsychologist. A collection of essays dealing with the effects of brain damage is Oliver Sacks' book *The Man who Mistook his Wife for a Hat* (1986).

■ How would you set about establishing the extent of retrograde amnesia in a patient for whom you have no autobiographical information?

Organic amnesia

Permanent memory loss is a serious problem necessitating continuous care of such patients. These instances of organic amnesia may be due to long-term alcohol abuse and development of Korsakoff's syndrome; to the brain damage from viral encephalitis; or to other surgical interventions. In cases where the memory loss is primary and not secondary to other cognitive deficits, patients are likely to have suffered damage to components of the limbic system, with the hippocampus being a key structure (see Case study).

Brain imaging

Brain imaging techniques such as functional magnetic resonance imaging allow researchers to examine directly the parts of the brain involved in cognitive processes. In the last decade there have been several important discoveries relevant to understanding memory mechanisms, and which also demonstrate the considerable plasticity of the brain with

respect to function. Animal studies have long implicated the hippocampus as playing a particular role in spatial memory, and this has also been shown to apply to humans in a particularly interesting study of London taxi drivers performed by Maguire et al. (1998). The researchers studied taxi drivers qualified in the 'knowledge' – a 2-year acquisition of street locations and one-way systems in London. Comparing taxi drivers and a control group of casual drivers they found differences in the cellular density of the left and right hippocampus, with the posterior hippocampus having a larger volume on both sides for the taxi drivers whereas in the control group the anterior hippocampus was larger. The researchers found a positive correlation between years of experience in the job and volume of the right posterior hippocampus and a negative correlation for the anterior hippocampus. This strongly suggests the changes are acquired as a result of the experience of taxi driving and the spatial maps formed as a result. There are clear implications here for rehabilitation suggesting that a similar environment-related plasticity is possible in other regions of the brain.

■ Can you recall the moment you first encountered a younger sibling? Your first day at school? Why do such memories endure?

Case study

HM is an engineering worker who, in 1953, in his late 20s was operated upon in an experimental procedure intended to relieve his epileptic seizures. The operation involved a radical bilateral medial temporal lobe resection, destroying the anterior two-thirds of the hippocampus, as well as the uncus and amygdala. It was successful in alleviating the epileptic symptoms, but left HM with profound memory impairment. Although he can remember events and facts he acquired up to 2 years before his operation, he can remember essentially nothing that has occurred since. He does not know what he had for lunch an hour ago, how he came to be where he is now, where he has left objects used recently or that he has used them. He reads the same magazines over and over again. He has learned neither the names of doctors and psychologists who have worked with him for decades nor the route to the house he moved to a few years after his surgery. Yet despite such difficulties he is not intellectually impaired. His language comprehension and production and conversational skills are normal, he can reason competently and do mental arithmetic. His IQ measured in 1962 was an above-average 117 – higher than the 104 measured presurgery in 1953. This neurological dissociation supports the idea that the temporary retention of information in working memory and the permanent storage of new information depend on different brain mechanisms (for a lengthier account of HM's problems, see Hilts, 1995).

Memory problems

- The distinction between registration, retrieval, recall and recognition processes in memory is clear.
- Different kinds of memory mechanisms underlie short-term memory and LTM, as shown by the serial position effect and the nature of the amnesic syndrome in brain-damaged patients.
- Improving memory recall by means of mnemonic aids is especially useful for unconnected items and events.

How does sexuality develop?

Sexual identity and behaviour are fundamental in the development of the person and the relevant influences are diverse and complex. The nature of sexuality is such that it has an important effect on health and well-being, and in turn is strongly influenced by these factors.

Gender identity

Biological influences

Gender identity (whether you feel male or female) usually coincides with sexual identity indicated by chromosomes, hormones and sexual organs, but this is not always the case. Biological indices can occasionally be abnormal so that gender may be ambiguous or contradictory. Also some women and men feel they are in the wrong biological body (transsexual), and might decide to undergo a sex change operation, which can be very stressful both psychologically, as it affects the notion of identity (who we are) and socially, as it upsets our common-sense notion of gender/sex as a fixed entity.

The sex chromosomes determined at conception, and the subsequent hormonal activity in the fetus, set the pattern for development of the internal and external sex organs and the sexual differentiation of the brain. There are exceptions. For example, abnormal chromosomes may give rise to a definite gender identity, but altered sexual organs and atypical social and sexual behaviour or a fetus with normal chromosomes may be exposed to unusual levels of hormones in utero. Some mothers given progestogens to prevent abortion had daughters who developed genital abnormalities, and atypical sexual and social behaviour.

Cultural factors

During puberty, gender identity becomes linked to sexual activity. There is often a period of sexual experimentation before individuals feel confident of their orientation. In the development of homosexual orientation, there is some evidence for a genetic factor: monozygotic twins show higher concordance than dizygotic twins, but cultural factors and individual learning experiences will also determine attraction to a partner.

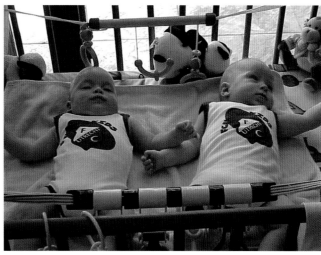

Fig. 1 Girls or boys? Two babies in gender-neutral outfits.

Social and cultural influences

Psychological influences on gender start at birth, where in the UK traditionally we dress baby boys in blue and girls in pink. Also our interactions are determined by the perceived sex of the baby, which we often only notice when babies are dressed non-gender-specifically (Fig. 1). We have expectations of boys and girls from a very young age, which may include playing more 'rough and tumble' games with boys, and more talking and cuddling with girls. This process quickly extends to peers, school and the media. It is thought that a core gender identity is fixed by about the age of 4 years.

Cultural pressures may delay the acceptance of sexual identity, since in many societies variations from the norm are not accepted. It may take a long period of adjustment and considerable courage to 'come out', accepting one's own sexuality and letting others know. Fear of one's sexuality being discovered may lead to secretive or reclusive lifestyles, and can be the source of enormous distress. Social norms are changing: witness the changes in the media's (see pp. 52–53) portrayal of sex and sexuality in, for example, documentaries, soap operas and discussion shows over the past decades.

The development of sexual activity

Although some sexual behaviour (genital play and stimulation) is seen in infants, the level of activity rises before puberty and this takes the form of sexual play with other children or solitary genital stimulation (masturbation). Peers are the major source of knowledge about sexual behaviour.

The age at which sexual intercourse first takes place varies not only from culture to culture, but also across time and according to class. A UK study in the early 1990s indicated that average age of first intercourse has fallen in the last 40 years from 21 to 17 (Table 1). More recently, an increasing proportion of young people have sexual intercourse before they are 16 (Wight et al., 2000) and studies have found that sexual intercourse before the age of 16 is often regretted. In the 1960s, surveys in Europe showed that sexual activity including intercourse took place at an earlier age in working-class males and females than amongst the middle classes. By the 1970s, the differences were disappearing.

The most common pattern of long-term sexual partnership is heterosexual monogamy. Although in many societies polygamy is part of religious and cultural structures, in practice many men do not take more than one wife at a time, through lack of availability or resources. Worldwide, the pattern of human attachment is often serial monogamy (one partner after another) rather than lifelong monogamy. The high rates of divorce in the industrialized world are one example of this.

Sexual activity continues through adulthood into old age (see pp. 16–17). While the sexual behaviour of young

Table 1	Age at first sexual intercourse by age at interview				
	Women			Men	
Age at interview (years)	Median age at first intercourse (years)	% (No.) reporting first intercourse before age 16		Median age at first intercourse (years)	% (No.) reporting first intercourse before age 16
16–19	17	18.7 (182/971)		17	27.6 (228/827)
20–24	17	14.7 (184/251)		17	23.8 (271/1137)
25–29	18	10.0 (152/1519)		17	23.8 (268/1126)
30–34	18	8.6 (116/1349)		17	23.2 (235/1012)
35–39	18	5.8 (73/1261)		18	18.4 (181/982)
40–44	19	4.3 (55/1277)		18	14.5 (150/1042)
45–49	20	3.4 (37/1071)		18	13.9 (115/827)
50–54	20	1.4 (13/933)		18	8.9 (61/684)
55–59	21	0.8 (6/716)		20	5.8 (35/603)

Analysis was based on weighted data.
Data from Wellings et al. (1995).

Case study

A 29-year-old woman came to see her family doctor because of infertility. Karen stopped the contraceptive pill 2 years ago but had not conceived. She was well, and reported no relationship difficulties. Her 34-year-old husband, Chris, was a marketing manager on a short-term contract.

Before referral to the infertility clinic, the doctor asked to see each partner separately. Both said that the frequency of sexual intercourse was low. Karen assumed that this was due to her husband's tiredness through overwork and did not want to put pressure on him. Chris acknowledged that he was very anxious about work, had resumed heavier drinking again with a recurrence of gastritis and was experiencing erectile difficulties. Afraid of impotence, he did not initiate sex, but wished that Karen would do so sometimes. He was too embarrassed to say this to her.

Instead of referral for infertility, they went to a sexual problems clinic. There was a ban on intercourse at first to take the pressure off both. With the therapist as intermediary, they began to communicate honestly about their own worries and expectations of sex. Chris was given advice on anxiety management and drinking less. In their homework non-threatening goals were set for increasing sexual activity, which included Karen taking the initiative sometimes. By the fourth session, Chris was drinking less, and the frequency of intercourse had increased to two or three times per week. Karen conceived 7 months later.

STOP THINK

■ Transvestism (most commonly males dressing in female clothing) has always taken place in many societies, either as entertainment for others or in secret. Many cross-dressers have no wish to change their sexual identity but get pleasure from cross-dressing. Sexual excitement is sometimes involved, but cross-dressing is also done in private to comfort the individual and to relieve stress. What does this say about society's sex role stereotypes and expectations of men?

How does sexuality develop?

■ Sexual development is influenced by biological, social and cultural factors.

■ Difficulties can arise in sexual function, compatibility, fertility and psychosocial function, or as a result of sexually transmitted disease.

■ Medical and psychological disorders can interfere with sexual function.

■ Sexual problems can be effectively treated by medical or surgical interventions, or by counselling (e.g. behavioural psychotherapy).

adults and those in middle age is discussed, and forms the subject of films and plays, the needs of older people are seldom portrayed. Sexual interest continues in this age group, although functioning changes; for example, in postmenopausal women, reduced oestrogen may cause thinning and dryness in the vagina, making intercourse more painful. In men, ageing is associated with increased time to achieve an erection, longer refractory periods and increased need for tactile rather than psychic stimuli. For men these changes are most marked after the age of 70 or so. It may be difficult for older people to discuss sexual problems with a doctor because their interest in sex is sometimes seen as inappropriate.

Sexual problems

Sexual difficulties can arise through problems in functioning (e.g. erectile difficulties in the male, or failure to achieve orgasm in the female); incompatibility (differences in appetite or style of sexual activity); problems of fertility (inability to conceive, or fear of conception); psychosocial problems arising through sexual behaviour (e.g. problems of sexual identity or problems with the law); and sexually transmitted infections (see pp. 108–109). A number of medical conditions give rise to sexual problems. Most common among these are multiple sclerosis, cardiovascular disease, diabetes, epilepsy and renal disease. A person who is dependent on alcohol is also likely to experience sexual problems, and there are prescribed drugs that carry loss of interest, or problems in functioning, as unwanted secondary effects. For example, drugs given to reduce blood pressure may cause erectile and ejaculatory difficulties in men. Psychological factors, especially anxiety and depression, frequently affect sexual interest and performance (see pp. 112–115).

Sexual problems arising from condition treatment may be overlooked by doctors through their own embarrassment or that of their patients. Yet many sexual problems can be effectively treated by a combination of approaches: medical intervention (e.g. changing a drug (e.g. Viagra), the use of hormones), surgical interventions (e.g. vascular surgery) or counselling (see pp. 132–135).

Intelligence

Intelligence has been described as the ability to: learn from everyday experience; think rationally; solve problems; act purposively and engage in abstract reasoning. Assumptions about intelligence may affect how we treat others and, for a very small minority of people, their intelligence limits their capacity for self-care.

'Intelligence' is a value-laden term. No one wants to be categorized as unintelligent and stereotyping patients or students as 'intelligent' or 'unintelligent' has consequences for how they are treated. When someone is perceived to be unintelligent people may think it is not worth explaining things to them, resulting in communication breakdown, loss of confidence and uninformed decision-making. This can be especially problematic when we want to encourage self-management and adherence amongst patients (see pp. 94–95). Consequently, health professionals should be cautious about making inferences about their patients' intelligence.

What do intelligence tests measure?

Intelligence tests are designed to assess how well a person will be able to learn or acquire skills in the future and depend, to some extent, on prior experience and learning. Intelligence tests have been designed to identify individual differences in general reasoning abilities while other aptitude tests, such as tests of musical ability, focus on particular abilities.

Psychologists have distinguished between *crystallized* and *fluid* intelligence. Crystallized intelligence is based on skills and knowledge learnt within particular cultures. Fluid intelligence is the capacity to reason and solve problems. Fluid intelligence enables us to learn from experience. Tests that measure abstraction and generalization primarily assess fluid intelligence. For example, the Raven Progressive Matrices test involves a series of pattern-matching problems. Carpenter et al. (1990) examined the reasoning required by this test. They concluded that the test measures the ability to infer abstract relationships and patterns from data and assesses the capacity to decompose problems into subtasks and hold multiple subtasks in mind simultaneously.

Tests that assess vocabulary, general knowledge and scholastic attainment provide information about crystallized intelligence. For example, the Wechsler Adult Intelligence Scale (WAIS) has 11 subscales. Six of these combine to generate a *verbal intelligence* score: (1) information; (2) comprehension; (3) arithmetic; (4) similarities; (5) digit span; and (6) vocabulary. The other five allow calculation of a *performance* score: (1) digit symbol; (2) picture completion; (3) block design; (4) picture arrangement; and (5) object assembly. Tests in this measure of intelligence draw on culture-specific learning, assessing crystallized as well as fluid intelligence. For example, 'What is the capital of Spain?' (comprehension) and 'How are a comb and a brush alike?' (similarities). A children's version of the test (the Wechsler Intelligence Scale for Children: WISC) is used to assess performance and progress at school.

Intelligence tests are often scored so that the average (or mean) score is 100 and the standard deviation is 15. This means that 68% of the population have scores, or intelligence quotients (IQs), between 85 and 115 and 95% score between 70 and 130. A score of 148 is required to become a member of MENSA, a society that only admits those with an exceptionally high IQ, and people scoring less than 70 (2 standard deviations below the mean) may have learning disabilities and need special help in school and with everyday living.

Scores on intelligence tests tend to be stable. Successive test scores correlate highly and children's scores, e.g. at age 6, predict adult scores, e.g. at 18 ($r = 0.8$), although an individual's score may change over time. Children's scores also predict performance at school and the number of years they stay at school ($r = 0.5$–0.55). However, other determinants are also important. IQ scores can predict various measures of job performance such as supervisor ratings and samples of job performance but other characteristics such as interpersonal skills, particular knowledge and aspects of personality are probably of equal or greater importance to job performance. Task-specific assessment is usually required to make accurate predictions about how someone will perform on job-related tasks or aspects of everyday living.

Thurstone (1938) proposed that intelligence consisted of seven distinct mental abilities. Guilford (1967) considered 120 separate mental abilities and Gardner (2001) has suggested that as well as linguistic, logical/mathematical and spatial intelligence (measured in tests like the WAIS), we should also consider musical, body-kinetic, interpersonal and intrapersonal intelligence. Gardner later added naturalist intelligence and considered defining and measuring spiritual and existential intelligence. Thus, rather than thinking of intelligence as a single dimension, we may be better able to understand differences in people's abilities by investigating a range of distinct intelligences.

Is intelligence genetically determined?

Performance on intelligence tests is affected by many factors. Those with closer genetic relationships tend to have more similar scores. The correlation between the IQ scores of monozygotic (MZ) twins brought up in the same family is 0.9 whereas the correlation for MZ reared apart is 0.7–0.8. By contrast, the correlation between genetically unrelated children reared together in adoptive families ranges from 0.0 to 0.2. This does not mean that performance on intelligence tests cannot be changed. One of the mechanisms by which genetic make-up affects performance is through the selection of environments that enhance particular skills. If the environment and available learning experiences change then so will performance, including intelligence test performance (see Neisser et al., 1996). In this context it is interesting to note that children's IQ scores correlate better at 18 years than at 6 years old with their parents' IQ, suggesting that shared learning experiences may contribute to this correlation.

Group differences on intelligence scores

Most intelligence tests have been standardized for sex; that is, items producing different scores for men and women have been eliminated. Consequently, it is unsurprising that, in general, men and women tend to have equal intelligence scores. Differences have been found between other groups such as black and white Americans, with the white mean being about 10 points higher. A range of explanations has been proposed for this difference. Most controversially, it has been suggested that there may be differences in the black and white gene pools that confer a different range of intellectual abilities. This explanation is problematic if other factors affecting performance are unequal between the two groups. By analogy, imagine two plants with the same genetic make-up planted in soil that is either rich or poor in nutrients. The plants will grow to different heights even though height is genetically determined. If the environment relevant to intelligence test performance differs, on average, for black and white Americans then group performance might differ, even if the two populations share the same intelligence-relevant genes. A larger proportion of black Americans live in poverty, which is associated with poor nutrition, less adequate parenting and a lack of intellectual resources and stimulation during development. In addition, only one generation ago, black Americans did not have equal civil rights (in relation to voting, schooling etc.) and continue to suffer discrimination (Neisser et al., 1996). Can we assume that the environment (analogous to the soil) is the same for both black and white Americans? Another explanation for group differences is that intelligence tests draw on particular cultural experiences so that people brought up in a different culture are disadvantaged.

Health and intelligence

In 1997 Whalley & Deary (2001) traced more than 2000 children born in Aberdeen in 1921. Mental ability scores based on childhood tests converted into IQ scores were found to be positively related to survival to age 76 years in both women and men. Overcrowding in the person's school catchment area, estimated from the 1931 UK census, was weakly related to death. Such data suggests that intelligence scores are related to mortality. However, intelligence scores and socioeconomic status (SES) are also correlated. For example, the correlation between one's parents' SES and one's own IQ is about 0.33. Mortality and morbidity rates are inversely related to SES.

A number of environmental factors can affect intelligence and health. For example, malnutrition, exposure to lead and antenatal exposure to alcohol are all associated with lower IQ scores. Associations between lower IQ and antenatal exposure to aspirin and antibiotics have also been reported (Zigler & Valentine, 1979).

Are we getting more intelligent?

Yes! This is known as the Flynn (1987) effect. Average scores on intelligence tests have increased over time. Interestingly, the largest gains are on tests focusing on fluid intelligence. For example, Raven's Matrices IQ scores in the Netherlands increased by 21 points between 1952 and 1982. This implies that if we transported a person with an average IQ today back in time by 70 years that person would be regarded as exceptionally intelligent (e.g. scoring up to 149). By comparison, US WAIS scores, which reflect crystallized as well as fluid intelligence, have risen by about 3 points per decade. Similar effects have been observed in other countries and these effects are typically larger than IQ differences between groups. The Flynn (1987) effect may be due to better schooling and in a more visually sophisticated and information-rich culture; they might also be related to improved nutrition. For example, Colom et al. (2005) found that increases in the IQ scores of Spanish children over time were primarily due to improvements at the lower end of the distribution (see also Colom & Garcia-Lopez, 2003). Alternatively, as Flynn (1987) suggests, these gains may mean that intelligence tests measure a particular type of problem-solving ability that may not have important implications for cultural development and achievement.

Does intelligence decline with age?

Yes and no. Fluid intelligence declines with age but, as we get older, we also get wiser. On many tests of intelligence, especially those of crystallized intelligence, IQ increases with age, peaking around the mid-50s. Older people, including those in their 80s, can draw upon knowledge built up over their lives. Younger people may outperform older people on tests focusing on fluid intelligence, especially when these are timed tests. The best predictor of an older person's IQ score is likely to be his or her IQ score when younger.

Can we boost intelligence?

During Project Head Start, a series of preschool schemes run in the USA in the 1960s, children were provided with extra teaching and play opportunities designed to enhance the intellectual content of their environment. Participating children in such schemes had higher intelligence test scores than similar children not involved. However, once the schemes ended, these differences tended to fade and disappear by age 11–12. However, children taking part were less likely to be assigned to special education, less likely to be held back in school and less likely to leave school than matched children who did not have extra preschool input (Neisser et al., 1996).

Intelligence

- Intelligence can be defined as the ability to learn from everyday experience and to think rationally.
- Psychologists distinguish between fluid and crystallized intelligence.
- 68% of the population have IQs between 85 and 115.
- People with closer genetic relationships tend to have similar IQs.
- Average group differences in IQ are not helpful in predicting an individual's intelligence.
- IQ is associated with mortality, but both are associated with socioeconomic status.
- Average scores on intelligence tests have increased over time (the Flynn effect).
- Older people do better than younger people on tests of intelligence that draw on their experience.

Development of thinking

Do children simply know less than adults or do children and adults think in qualitatively different ways? For example, are children just as capable as adults of understanding why they are ill or why they should take their medication, if they are presented with the relevant information? Or do children under a certain age lack the necessary concepts to make sense of such explanations? Questions like these are addressed by psychological research into cognitive development, which investigates age-related changes in intellectual abilities.

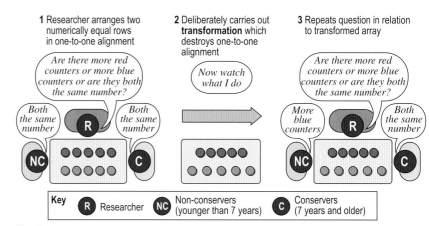

Fig. 1 Conservation of number task.

Differing views of cognitive development

Jean Piaget (1896–1980) revolutionized the study of cognitive development by arguing that young children do not just know less than older children and adults, but view the world in radically different ways. For example, Piaget argued that, until the age of about 7 years, children are not able to reason logically and lack fundamental concepts in areas such as number and causality.

Most researchers agree with Piaget's general claims that:

- Cognitive development is influenced by an interaction between biological and environmental factors.
- Children play an active role in acquiring knowledge.
- Children's thinking is sometimes qualitatively different from adults'.

On the other hand, many researchers (e.g. Donaldson, 1978) have challenged certain aspects of Piaget's views and have argued that he has tended to underestimate:

- Young children's conceptual understanding.
- The influence of contextual factors.
- The extent to which children's performance depends on their familiarity with the specific content of reasoning tasks.

To illustrate these differing views, we will consider two aspects of cognitive development: understanding of number and of causality.

Understanding of number

To investigate children's ability to reason about numerical relationships, Piaget used tasks like the one in Figure 1. He found that children younger than about 7 years typically changed their answer when the question was repeated after the transformation, and he described these children as *non-conservers*. In contrast, children of about 7 years and upwards typically succeeded on the task and were therefore classed as *conservers*. Piaget interpreted young children's failure to conserve as being symptomatic of their inability to reason logically: they lack an understanding of general principles, such as that the number of objects in a set is independent of their spatial arrangement.

However, other researchers have found that young children's performance on conservation tasks can be improved by modifying the way the task is presented. For example, when the transformation was carried out by a 'naughty teddy' character who likes to 'mess up games', many more 4–6-year-old children responded correctly than when the transformation was carried out deliberately by the researcher (Donaldson, 1978). In interpreting this finding, Donaldson argues that the deliberate nature of the transformation in Piaget's version of the task misleads children into inferring that it is relevant to the question which follows it, and thus into misinterpreting the question as referring to length. This type of reasoning is characteristic of what Donaldson terms embedded thinking, in which the child actively attempts to make sense of the total situation by attending to non-verbal cues as well as to what is said and by making inferences about other people's intentions. Young children, according to Donaldson, are capable of reasoning logically, but they are most likely to demonstrate this in contexts where they can exploit their understanding of human purposes and where non-verbal cues support the spoken message.

Understanding of causality

With respect to children's understanding of causality (Donaldson & Elliot, 1990), Piaget argued that until the age of about 7 years children show:
- An inability to distinguish between causes and effects.
- A tendency to 'psychologize' by inappropriately explaining physical phenomena in terms of human motives.

For example, when they were asked to complete sentences, they tended to reverse the order of the cause and effect, as in: That man fell off his bicycle because… he broke his leg. Also, when Piaget interviewed children about the causes of various phenomena, they gave explanations which were not simply incorrect but were of the wrong type, in that they tended to explain physical phenomena in psychological terms, for example: Why do the clouds move across the sky? Because they want to.

However, the phenomena which Piaget asked children to explain were ones for which information about causal mechanisms was not directly accessible to them, so it may be that they psychologized as a last resort. Several studies have shown that when children are presented with demonstrations of physical phenomena involving familiar principles (e.g. that an object will fall if a supporting object is removed), even 3-year-olds tend to give explanations in terms of physical causes. Similarly, when they are explaining events with which they are directly involved, children as young as 3 years show an ability to distinguish appropriately between causes and effects. Thus, it appears that young children do have a basic understanding of causality, but their ability to apply their understanding depends on the context and on their knowledge of specific causal phenomena.

Understanding of illness

How do these findings and arguments relate to children's understanding of illness? Some researchers have argued that children's developing understanding of illness is consistent with Piaget's account of the development of causal reasoning (Table 1). It is important to be aware of the types of explanations of illness that may be given by children at particular stages of development, since this can be helpful in alleviating misunderstandings and anxieties. For example, young children who believe that all illnesses are caught through contagion or contamination may be anxious about coming into contact with children with non-infectious illnesses, such as epilepsy or leukaemia. On the other hand, the typical stages may not represent the limits of children's ability to understand explanations of illness. Since most young children do not receive much tuition about the causes of illness, the typical stages may partly reflect what they have had the opportunity to learn. For example, most childhood

Table 1	**Developmental changes in understanding of causes of illness**	
Approximate age	**Explanations of illness**
4–7 years	Contagion: illness caused by proximity to ill people or to particular objects
	Illness viewed as punishment for own misbehaviour
7–11 years	Contamination: illness caused by physical contact with ill person
	Illness caused by germs
Over 11 years	Internalization: processes (e.g. swallowing, inhaling) through which external causes influence internal bodily processes
	Psychological factors can influence physiological processes
	Multiple, interacting causes

Based on studies by Bibace & Walsh (1980); Kister & Patterson (1980).

illnesses are infectious so it is perhaps hardly surprising that young children sometimes overgeneralize the concepts of contagion and contamination.

More recent research indicates that the 'typical' stages may under-estimate both the complexity of children's understanding of illness and the extent to which it is influenced by knowledge about specific illnesses (Myant & Williams, 2005). Findings from an intervention study show that children's understanding of illness can be improved by listening to stories containing factual information about illnesses and discussing these with their peers, although the intervention was not effective for all children (Williams & Binnie, 2002).

Similarly, the case study suggests that children's understanding of medical phenomena may be influenced by their personal experience. However, other research indicates that the extent of children's medical experience (duration of illness, frequency of hospitalization) does not affect their understanding of the causes of illness (Kury & Rodrigue, 1995). Therefore, in order to communicate effectively with children about health and illness, health care professionals need to be careful neither to overestimate the knowledge of children with prior medical experience, nor to underestimate the extent to which children's understanding could potentially be enhanced by presenting explanations geared to their individual cognitive levels. (For further discussion of clinical applications see Rushforth, 1999.)

 ■ What would you do or say to help a 4-year-old child who was worried about catching appendicitis from the child in the next bed?

Case study

Children's understanding of their blood

When a 3-year-old girl with leukaemia joined a playgroup, the staff were concerned about how to explain her illness to the other children, and a group of researchers decided to investigate this topic (Eiser et al., 1993). They interviewed healthy 3- and 4-year-old children about their knowledge and experiences of blood, and then gave the children an explanation of the functions of different types of blood cells, illustrating their explanation with drawings. Although on the whole the children had difficulty understanding the explanation, the children who showed most understanding were those who had mentioned a personal experience involving blood.

The researchers also interviewed the 3-year-old girl with leukaemia. In the course of her treatment, she had received more extensive and more frequently repeated explanations about blood than the healthy children had, and these explanations obviously had clear personal relevance to her. Her knowledge of the structure and function of blood was found to be much more advanced than that of the healthy children: 'she knew that blood... is full of red cells which make new blood, white cells which fight infection, and platelets which stop bleeding'. 'Sometimes the platelets don't come and then you keep bleeding.' About the leukaemia, she said that she was 'full of bad cells – they just come' (Eiser et al., 1993, p. 535).

Although this explanation includes some misunderstandings and some of the phrases may be simple repetitions of adults' speech without full understanding, and although we do not know how typical the explanation is of other 3-year-olds who are receiving treatment, it is nevertheless extremely impressive for such a young child and it suggests that young children's ability to understand explanations of illness may be much greater than has often been supposed.

Development of thinking

- Young children do not simply know less than older children and adults: they sometimes think in qualitatively different ways.

- Piaget's view that these differences reflect an inability in children younger than 7 years to reason logically and to understand fundamental concepts (such as those of number and causality) has been challenged.

- Young children's cognitive abilities depend not only on their underlying concepts but also on the context in which tasks are presented.

- Children are most likely to understand explanations which:
  - Take account of their existing level of understanding.
  - Are linked to their own experiences and immediate concerns.
  - Are presented with appropriate non-verbal contextual support.

Understanding groups

The effectiveness of medical staff depends on team work. No doctor works completely alone. So, if doctors are going to be effective they need to know how best to work with and in groups. Research shows that groups produce more effective solutions than the sum of individuals working on their own. Groups can also have negative effects, which can be controlled, if understood. For example, groups can often pressurize us to behave in ways we wouldn't do if we were on our own. Finally, groups influence our social and personal identity. Becoming medical students, and eventually joining the medical profession, results in more changes in people than just occupational category: they become different people, with different identification, interests and loyalties. Being aware of the power of groups is an important part of professional training.

What are groups?

Groups are essential and pervasive. Each of us belongs to many groups of different kinds. It has been estimated that we each have membership of about 100 groups, ranging from our family, our nationality, or our professional group, to the gang of personal friends. A group can be defined as consisting of three or more people who interact with each other, have shared goals and relationships and have mutually agreed ways of doing things and a shared identity.

Features of groups

Conformity

In groups we all tend to be conformists. Most people will conform to group opinion, despite having private reservations. Conformity is sometimes seen as negative: for example, it can be as a result of real or imagined pressures. Not surprisingly, as a medical student, you will tend to agree with a group of consultants about a diagnosis, even if you disagree privately. Yet perhaps you know something important they don't, having had time to talk to the patient alone. The more we want to belong to a group, or feel involved, the more we conform. A conformist might also be defined as a person who has managed to avoid being defined as a deviant. Conformity can be important and valuable; to an extent we all conform when we learn professional skills. We do as others do when we learn to become a competent professional, but there may be negative influences, as for example when we fail to challenge an incorrect but popular opinion.

There are three underlying dynamics of conformity:

1. Normative pressures – be like others to get rewards or avoid punishment.
2. Informational pressures – group provides useful information.
3. Intergroup pressures – we may support our group versus other groups, as we may see them as threatening to our group.

These pressures are especially acute when we are being monitored or when it's not clear what's going on, like when we join a new group.

Obedience

Most people obey authority. In one well-known psychological experiment, carried out by Milgram (1963), subjects were asked by a respectable-looking experimenter to administer electric shocks to volunteers. The prediction was that 1/1000 would obey. However, in fact two-thirds did as requested. (The shocks were not in fact real!)

Factors which influence the likelihood of obedience are not only similar to those affecting conformity, but also include the perceived benefit of obeying the person in authority.

Many human systems depend upon obedience of authority, e.g. the armed services. To some extent hospital medicine relies on obedience to authority to ensure that there is a clear and appropriate understanding of responsibility for patients. If consultants are ultimately responsible for patient care, they must be able to trust that junior medical staff will carry out instructions. Automatic obedience, however, is not wise. Occasionally, senior staff make errors in their instructions, and young doctors need to think critically as they work, and be courageous enough to question a wrong decision.

Deviance

Groups do not easily tolerate people who do not conform. Dissenters:

- Are normally unpopular, because they threaten the cohesiveness of the group and challenge its opinions.
- Are likely to be rejected by the group because they are threatening and produce feelings of discomfort for others.
- Are usually seen as particularly valuable by the group if won over.
- Need one another to survive the hurt of rejection by a group, possibly by setting up a new group of their own.
- Offer alternative and new solutions, which paradoxically may be vital for the group's long-term survival.
- Challenge the group to explore, elaborate and justify its position.

It is not comfortable being a dissenter, but dissenters are often important in the long run, and may therefore need protection and support.

Structure

Groups consisting of people who are very similar to each other are called homogeneous groups. These groups often get on well together, and quickly establish working practice. However, they may be poor at innovating or dealing with difficult problems. Groups with many different types are known as heterogeneous. These often take time to settle down, and may experience conflict, but may be able to generate better solutions in the long run – rather like dissenters do.

Groups which function well have both social and task aspects; that is, there is a social, interpersonal aspect to the group as well as its formal, stated objective or task. A group which only completes tasks may seem efficient, but it engenders little loyalty and does not survive long (Fig. 1). Paying attention to people's social needs as well as tasks is therefore important.

Intergroup conflict

Sometimes groups conflict with one another. Intergroup conflict is very common and occurs between rival football clubs, different schools, National Health Service professional groups and nations. Although

STOP THINK

■ Consider groups in places where you have been, for example, in a tutorial or work group. Most groups or teams tend to show the above features, especially if the team has worked together for a long time. You may also have noticed that group members tend to do different things to keep the team functioning (Fig. 1). Also, different people tend to behave fairly consistently in one group, but may also behave differently in another group.
■ Which one are you? You may well have noticed that your role changes depending on what group you are in. Why?

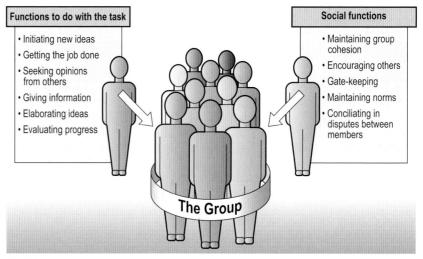

Functions to do with the task
• Initiating new ideas
• Getting the job done
• Seeking opinions from others
• Giving information
• Elaborating ideas
• Evaluating progress

Social functions
• Maintaining group cohesion
• Encouraging others
• Gate-keeping
• Maintaining norms
• Conciliating in disputes between members

The Group

Fig. 1 Typical roles in a group.

competition may be healthy, if it escalates, conflict can lead to serious disputes, even war, and eventually genocide. This can happen when one group thinks itself so superior to another that even total annihilation of the other group eventually becomes legitimate. This stems from all the above features of groups. 'In-groups' and 'out-groups' are formed where the 'in-group' feels good about itself and simultaneously superior to, but persecuted by, the 'out-group'. Perhaps the 'out-group' consists of deviants who were rejected by the 'in-group' because they would not or could not conform. Alternatively they may have disobeyed the leader of the 'in-group', or be different in some way, for example, by racial origin or sex.

One notable feature of intergroup conflict is stereotyping, whereby members of the 'out-group' are lumped together and seen as bad, weak or aggressive, or as possessing admired but feared characteristics such as intelligence, cunning or sexuality. Individual differences between people are minimized: hence all white people are seen as mean, all women as petty, all football supporters as hooligans, and so on.

Group therapy

Therapy is often carried out in groups. Obviously if many people can be helped by one trained professional, instead of individual half-hour sessions, this has economic benefits. Membership of groups has also been shown to have psychological benefits. Support from other people may come from self-help groups (see pp. 142–143) but more formal groups may also be set up in hospital or general practice.

Group therapies may take one of four basic approaches or a combination that may be pragmatically chosen on the basis of the composition of the group. Firstly, the *analytical* approach might analyse motives for the group members' behaviour to encourage insight in the members and hence to encourage change. Secondly, an *interpersonal* approach might provide an opportunity for social learning where people can learn from each other how to cope with a particular condition. Thirdly, an *experiential* approach might generate emotional experiences, which it is hoped will resolve emotional difficulties. Fourthly, a *didactic* approach might impart new information and teach new skills.

The evidence for the benefits of group therapy compared with individual therapy is positive. For example, membership of a group increases the chances of stopping smoking, and membership of cardiac rehabilitation provides social support, which increases the likelihood of adhering to a programme. These effects may be partly due to conformity.

Case study

Intergroup conflict

The medical staff of a large inner-city general practice decided to establish an asthma clinic in order to respond to the increasing numbers of patients coming to the surgery for help. Part of the strategy of the clinic included the assessment of patients within their own home environments, which would be carried out by the community staff in the practice. The medical staff then announced the plan to the health visitors and district nurses, without consulting them about the feasibility of the assessment procedures. Some nurses tried to carry out the assessments as requested, while others declared the whole strategy to be unworkable given other time constraints. One of the nurses who was eager to implement the strategy was criticized heavily by the others, and soon afterwards gave in her notice. Some of the medical staff felt some sympathy for the nurses and suggested that the plan had been implemented too hastily, but they were accused by the others of being behind the times. Each group of staff considered the other group to be thoughtless, unprofessional, selfish and lazy. The atmosphere in the practice became unpleasant and hostile, so that even the patients began to notice it. Only the appointment of a practice manager, who agreed to review the whole issue, allowed the situation to calm down and return to normal again.

Understanding groups

■ Groups reach better outcomes than the sum of individuals working on their own.

■ Groups encourage conformity and give us a sense of belonging.

■ Groups may punish non-conformers by making them feel odd, unwanted and rejected.

■ Groups can be a force for good, encouraging support, patriotism, team work, loyalty and identity.

■ Intergroup conflicts also underlie most forms of industrial dispute, religious and political rivalry, war and even genocide.

Concepts of health, illness and disease

Health and illness are concepts that relate to social and moral values as much as they relate to disease. Medicine is particularly concerned with identifying and treating diseases: this model of disease is called *biomedicine*, drawing as it does on medical sciences with an emphasis on biological abnormality. Biological abnormalities are not found for all diseases (e.g. some mental illness), and biomedicine is only one way of looking at the ill health that people experience. Health and illness are also rooted in everyday experience so it is also important to understand how people feel when they are ill, and what their own interpretations of their symptoms are (Radley, 1994). In this way, health care can be provided more sensitively, doctors can get a fuller picture of what ails their patients and patients can be part of the process of identifying what is wrong with them and what can be done about it.

Health has also become an important concept in recent years, especially through an increasing emphasis on promoting well-being as well as preventing illness (Crawford, 1987). However, health is not easy to define. Health, illness and disease mean different things to different people. We will consider the extent to which these concepts are as much social (that is, to do with society) and personal (to do with individual experience) as they are to do with pathology.

Disease

Defining disease may at first seem to be quite straightforward. However, changes in medical knowledge may alter our understanding (e.g. many diseases are now thought to have a genetic component) and new symptoms and diseases may appear or be discovered (e.g. HIV/AIDS, myalgic encephalomyelitis). Typically, in western medicine, disease refers to pathological changes diagnosed by signs, symptoms and tests: it is considered to be objective and medically defined. Yet, as the above examples show, definitions are not fixed but change over time in the light of new knowledge and experience. Homosexuality used to be defined as a disease but is now much more socially accepted as a lifestyle choice; alcoholism used to be seen as immoral, but it is now often typified as a disease. Heart disease, although existing before the 20th century, was seldom considered a specific cause of death until this century. We are increasingly able to define disease at earlier and earlier stages, or even identify risk factors for disease. This can lead to many more people being defined as diseased, or 'at risk', even in the absence of any symptoms. So, it is possible to feel quite well but for disease to be present.

Armstrong (1994) has argued that normality plays a crucial role in how medicine defines disease. If the definition of normal relates to what is statistically normal, or an average measure, it is not always clear-cut where the normal becomes the abnormal or pathological. What is normal for one person may not be normal for another, or whole populations may display some kind of pathology which, while representing disease or risk of disease, is normal in some sense. Normality can also be seen as being socially rather than biologically defined. Here, normality is viewed more in terms of what is considered acceptable or desirable. Mental illness, for example, is very much rooted in culture, and what is considered abnormal behaviour varies across cultures. An extreme example would be the labelling of political dissidents as mentally ill, as occurred in the former Soviet Union. There are also concerns about possible overdiagnosis of mental illness amongst some ethnic minority groups, such as Afro-Caribbean men in the UK. Some disabled people challenge the medical definitions of their conditions and argue that it is society that disables them (see pp. 118–119). Disease, then, is not such a straightforward concept.

Biomedicine is only one way of understanding disease. Humoral theories, elaborated by Hippocrates, present disease as an imbalance between four humours. Echoes of such understandings are still present today, for example, in the promotion and use of cough expectorants and laxatives. Other systems of medicine, such as Indian ayurvedic medicine or Chinese medicine, also stress the importance of balance. These are complex, professionalized systems used in other cultures to explain disease (as well as health and illness) and organize health care. Patients and doctors may work within several systems of belief at any one time.

Illness

Illness is a subjective experience and as such will be defined and responded to differently by different people. How people interpret bodily experiences may have no direct relationship to the presence of a medically defined disease. People's own experience, as well as their wider knowledge, is drawn from their own culture (for example, their 'lay referral network', as well as from wider values within their society) and from other sources of knowledge – the media, including the internet, their doctors or other healers. It is important to understand people's own beliefs about health and illness as these may influence whether they seek health care, the type of health care they seek and also their reasons for seeking professional advice (see pp. 72–73).

Importantly, illness can be thought of as a moral category, especially in a society that emphasizes personal responsibility for health (Crawford, 1987). People like to think of themselves as healthy. Research, such as Cornwell's detailed study conducted in the East End of London (Cornwell, 1984), has found that many people consider that having the right attitude is important in preventing illness and maintaining good health; this attitude means that you should not 'dwell on illness'. When she first started interviewing residents in the area, she found that people produced what she termed 'public accounts'. Because of the moral imperative to be seen as healthy, people wanted to prove the legitimacy of illness by describing it as normal, real or a health problem that was not illness (Fig. 1).

As her study continued, she found that people became much more prepared to talk about a whole range of experiences that they felt had affected their health. Getting behind these 'public accounts', Cornwell found that people discussed their experience of illness as part of their everyday lives, affected by their social roles (work, domestic commitments) and

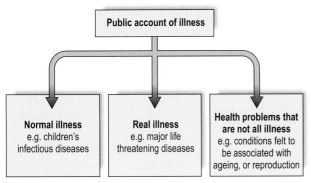

Fig. 1 Public accounts of illness (from Cornwell, 1984, with permission).

Case study

Making sense of illness

People always try to make sense of misfortune and illness is no exception to this. Research conducted by Williams (1984) identified how the diagnosis and experience of chronic illness affected people's sense of identity. People then made sense of their own illness by considering its causes within the context of their own life experiences. This helped them answer the question 'why me?' In one case study presented by Williams, a study participant, Gill, considers her arthritis to have been caused by stress – something built up over the years as well as related to specific difficult life events:

> I'm quite certain that it was stress that precipitated this...
> not simply the stress of events that happened but the stress perhaps of suppressing myself while I was a mother and wife; not 'women's libby' but there comes a time in your life when you think, you know, 'where have I got to? There's nothing left of me'.

their experience of health services. She called these 'private accounts'. Since doctors often only have a short time with their patients, it is important that they allow for the tendency of people to provide 'public accounts', and that they realize that patients' underlying concerns and worries may be much less clearly and openly expressed (see pp. 88–89).

Health

A negative view of health would define it simply as the absence of disease. However, the World Health Organization (1946) offers a more positive definition: a 'state of complete physical, social and mental well-being and not merely the absence of disease or infirmity'. Such a state may be hard to attain and, although this definition provides a good contrast to the former, narrower definition, it may still not reflect the everyday experiences of people. A range of research has shown that people may have different concepts of health. Williams (1983) found that elderly people in Aberdeen viewed health as the absence of disease, a dimension of strength and as functional fitness. Large-scale surveys and other smaller, indepth studies have found that people define themselves as healthy despite experiencing symptoms. A study of working-class women in the north-east of Scotland (Blaxter & Paterson, 1982) found that the grandmother generation (average age 51 years) had low expectations of what good health was – it was being able to carry on and being able to work, despite experiencing disease and illness. In other words, they had quite functional definitions of health, and their norms of health were low. Calnan (1987) found that middle-class women were more likely to think of health in terms of overall well-being and working-class women to have more functional definitions of health. Concepts of health will also differ across the life course. The Health and Lifestyle Survey (Blaxter 1990) found that younger men thought of health as physical fitness, whereas younger women emphasized energy and coping. In middle age the emphasis moved towards notions of mental and physical well-being, while older people stressed the ability to do things, as well as contentment and happiness (Fig. 2).

Practical application

Different groups within society and different cultures will have varied concepts of health, illness and disease. All these concepts are inherently social, and it is important to recognize this in medical practice. Doctors and patients may have different views about health, and patients may not reveal their subjective experiences in the belief that these are not important or valid. However, if medicine is to deal

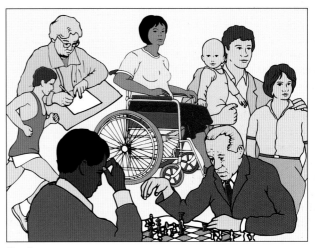

Fig. 2 Health means different things to different people as it is not just the absence of disease.

seriously with patients in the context of their family and social relationships, then listening to and understanding the patient's perspective becomes a prerequisite for good practice.

STOP THINK
- What does being healthy mean to you? What do you think it may mean to someone who is 75 years old?
- What impact might defining something as a disease have on a patient?
- Why is it important to understand the patient's own beliefs?

Concepts of health, illness and disease

- Health, illness and disease are social concepts.
- Health and illness are defined differently by different social groups.
- Individuals can perceive themselves to be healthy yet at the same time experience illness and disease.
- People initially provide 'public accounts' of their experience and concepts of illness, in contrast to more 'private accounts' as their trust in the interviewer/doctor grows.
- Medical science plays a crucial role in defining disease, but these definitions change over time.

Measuring health and illness

The measurement of health and illness has become increasingly important as doctors, health service agencies and governments try to assess the effectiveness of treatments and the performance of health services. However, measuring health and illness can be problematic.

Mortality

All births and deaths in developed, and in many developing, countries are legally required to be registered so that, together with census data, accurate counts can be made of birth and death rates, and of population change. Mortality rates, particularly infant and maternal mortality rates, are often used as proxy measures of a country's health and development (see pp. 158–159). Life expectancy also provides a summary measure of health in an area or country, and Figure 1 summarizes overall life expectancy and healthy life expectancy (Box 1) for selected countries.

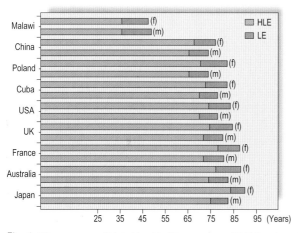

Fig. 1 Life expectancy (LE) and healthy life expectancy (HLE) for selected countries, 2005. Males and females.

Box 1 **Definition**
Healthy life expectancy: the average number of years that a person can expect to live in 'full health', taking into account 'years lived in less than full health due to disease and/or injury'. See http://www.who.int/whosis/indicators/2007HALE0/en/ for details and methods of estimation.

Crude death rates are calculated by dividing the total number of deaths by the number of people in the population. However, because older people and men are more likely to die over a given time period than younger people and women, allowance is normally made for the age and sex of the population when making comparisons between areas/countries.

Cause-specific death rates are also useful. Cause of death is entered on death certificates and then coded using the International Statistical Classification of Diseases and Health Related Problems (ICD-10). Table 1 gives details of a selection of death rates for selected countries.

Care is required in the interpretation of data like this because of different reporting procedures and fashions

Table 1 **Mortality rates**					
Country	**Infant**	**Maternal**	**Cardio**	**Cancer**	**Injuries**
Japan	3	10	106	119	39
Australia	5	6	140	127	35
France	4	17	118	142	48
UK	5	11	182	143	26
USA	7	14	188	134	47
Cuba	5	33	215	129	54
Poland	6	10	324	180	53
China	23	56	291	148	79
Malawi	78	1,800	430	150	105

Infant, mortality rate per 1000 live births; Maternal, mortality rate per 100 000 live births; Cardio, age-standardized mortality rate per 100 000 population; Cancer, age-standardized mortality rate per 100 000 population; Injuries, age-standardized mortality rate per 100 000 population. (from World Health Organization, 2008).

between countries and regions, and changes in medical knowledge and fashion over time, all of which can lead to apparent differences. Coding errors may also occur.

Standardized mortality ratios (SMRs) (Box 2) are commonly used to compare deaths for specific subgroups in a population. An SMR of 100 indicates that observed deaths equals the expected number of deaths (average mortality). An SMR > 100 indicates that observed deaths exceed expected deaths, and an SMR < 100 indicates that observed deaths are lower than expected deaths. SMRs are useful summary indicators of mortality in a subpopulation or specific social group, and social scientists have used SMRs particularly to investigate social inequalities in health (see pp. 44–45).

Box 2 **Standardized mortality ratio (SMR)**

$$SMR = \frac{number\ of\ observed\ deaths \times 100}{number\ of\ expected\ deaths^*}$$

*which would have occurred if the study population had experienced the same mortality as the reference population, allowing for age and sex differences.

Figure 2 shows that suicide between 1996 and 2002 has increased in the most deprived areas of Scotland from an SMR of < 140 to an SMR of > 160 relative to the average in Scotland (SMR = 100), whereas in areas of least deprivation it has reduced from an SMR of > 60 to an SMR of < 60.

Avoidable mortality is a relatively new measure which seeks to identify deaths which might have been avoided had

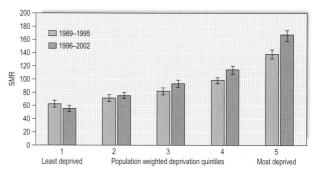

Fig. 2 Suicide standardized mortality ratios (SMRs) by population-weighted deprivation quintile, all persons aged 15 years and older, Scotland, 1989–1995 to 1996–2002 (from Platt et al., 2007, with permission).

good medical, preventive and health promotion services been available, accessible and taken up. Recent research has suggested that approximately 10% of deaths annually in Scotland might be 'avoidable'. The UK's Office for National Statistics is currently comparing different methods for calculating 'avoidable mortality' (see http://www.statistics.gov.uk/downloads/theme_health/HSQ34.pdf).

Morbidity

Although death is, generally, a certain and countable event, mortality rates do not tell us much about illness or health in a population, though 'healthy life expectancy' and 'avoidable deaths' are attempts to derive more useful mortality indicators. Illness, morbidity and health are, however, considerably more difficult to define, and hence to measure, than death.

Consultation rates with doctors are sometimes used as a proxy measure of illness in a population. Measured as the number of consultations over a defined time period in a given population, consultation rates suffer from a number of limitations. In many countries it may be difficult to define and measure the denominator population from which the consulters came. Use of a doctor is strongly influenced by availability of doctors in a particular area and psychological, social and cultural factors strongly influence people's decision to consult (see pp. 88–89), and these may change over time.

Referral rates to hospital and hospital admission rates (by diagnostic groups) provide some information on patterns and trends in morbidity, but these also vary by referrer practice, supply of hospital services and admission and discharge practice.

Disease registers, which hold details of the identity of every person diagnosed with a particular disease (e.g. cancer), its type and its treatment, provide excellent individual, longitudinal data for research, but they are expensive to set up and to maintain.

In the UK, the General Household Survey (GHS) is a national sample survey of households which, once a year, asks questions about chronic and acute illness. It is also one of the morbidity measures used to adjust for healthy life expectancy. Although the GHS provides a regular picture of ill health, the sample size makes it difficult to examine differences in morbidity at regional or district level.

A large number of self-report instruments have been developed to measure the impact of specific diseases and illness on health (Bowling, 1995a), most of which incorporate a variety of scales designed to assess the physical, psychological and social effects of the disease.

A number of instruments have also been designed to measure health and well-being more generally (Bowling, 1997). For example, the SF-36 (Box 3) has been shown to be reliable and valid (Box 4), and has become a commonly used

evaluative instrument. More recently, a shorter 12-item scale has been constructed, the SF-12, and the EuroQol group has constructed a five-item scale, the EQ-5D (see Case study).

Overall, it is important to be clear about the purpose for which measurement instruments have been designed and how this relates to their use. If using instruments in a new context or population, particularly different ethnic groups, it is important to make sure that they are valid and reliable. Care should also be taken not to assume that these instruments measure health or ill health comprehensively – they are summary indicators. Finally, care should be taken when comparing the results of studies using different instruments.

Box 4 **Reliability and validity**

An instrument is reliable if it reproduces the same results if tested twice on the same population (test–retest reliability). The instrument should also be internally consistent and interrater-reliable.

Validity relates to the extent to which an instrument actually measures what it sets out to measure. The main aspects of validity are:

- Face validity
- Content validity
- Criterion validity
- Construct validity
- Convergent
- Discriminant

Case study

Which health status instrument should I use?

A recent study of 978 Australian patients with type 2 diabetes compared the use of three health-related quality of life questionnaires, the EQ-5D, the SF-12 and the SF-36. All three measures were found to have some limitations but the EQ-5D generally performed as well as the SF-36 and, given its simplicity to use and its short time for completion, was the preferred option (Glasziou et al., 2007).

Could one instrument measure the health of people being treated for:
- Angina?
- Depression?
- Eczema?

Measuring health and illness

- Infant and maternal mortality rates and life expectancy are useful indicators of a country's overall health and development.

- Mortality rates need to be adjusted for the age and sex of the population.

- Disease-specific mortality rates can reveal trends in specific disease, but tell us little about illness or morbidity in a population.

- Measurement of morbidity ranges from measures of health service use to instruments measuring self-reported perceptions of illness and self-report measures of health, well-being and functional ability.

- Considerable care should be taken when using instruments for measuring health and when interpreting their results.

Box 3 **The SF-36 questionnaire**

The SF-36 uses 36 questions to ask about eight health attributes:
1. Limitations in physical activities because of health problems
2. Limitations in social activities because of physical or emotional problems
3. Limitations in usual role activities because of physical health problems
4. Bodily pain
5. General mental health (psychological distress and well-being)
6. Limitations in usual role activities because of emotional problems
7. Vitality (energy and fatigue)
8. General health perceptions

Changing patterns of health and illness

In the UK births and deaths are recorded by the Registrar General. The data provided on birth and death certificates are compiled by the Office of Population Censuses and Surveys, which publishes annual reports showing the incidence of disease and deaths due to specific causes and a variety of statistics relating to use of hospital and outpatient services. These reports are public documents and can be consulted in libraries and on the web.

Changes in life expectancy

Over the last century there has been a marked decline in premature death throughout the developed world. In 1888, a newborn baby girl in England and Wales had an average life expectancy of just over 40 years. By 1930, this had risen to just over 60 years, and by 1999 it had reached 80 years (Fig. 1). However, if a child survived into middle age, life expectancy even in 1888 was quite high. A 45-year-old woman in 1888 could, on average, expect to live to nearly 70 years of age, and in 1999 she had an average life expectancy of over 80 years.

The major cause of increase in life expectancy is a dramatic fall in the death rate for infants during their first year of life. In 1888 in England and Wales, out of every 1000 infants under the age of 1 year, 145 died. By 1930 this figure had been more than halved to 68 infant deaths and the rapid decline continued until the present-day rate of 5–6 infant deaths per 1000. At the beginning of the 21st century almost all newborn babies in the UK can expect to live through childhood. In many developing countries in the world, life expectancy at birth remains below 50 years of age because of high rates of infant mortality. According to McKeown (1979), the most important factor leading to changes in infant and child mortality has been a dramatic improvement in child and maternal nutrition over the past century.

Diseases that have declined

Another way to look at the changing nature of health and illness is to compare rates of death due to particular causes over the years. In order to examine the relative importance of different diseases over time, we need to take account of the fact that the population structure might also have changed over time. For example, cancers are more common in the older age groups and if the proportion of older people in the population has increased whilst the actual rate of cancer has stayed the same, we are likely to make the mistake of assuming that the rate of cancer is increasing. This could be very misleading. In order to calculate real changes in the rates of different diseases over time we can calculate what are called standardized mortality ratios (SMRs) (see pp. 40–41). These enable us to examine changes over time and consider the possible causes of these changes (Table 1). Over the past century, death rates due to nearly all causes have declined. Striking changes in death rates have occurred for tuberculosis and influenza. SMRs for tuberculosis have changed from 867 in the period 1891–1895 to four in 1986–1990; however, they are now on the increase. Similarly, SMRs for influenza have changed from 514 in 1891–1896 to seven in 1986–1990. An important improvement in health has been due to our ability to control the spread of infectious disease and fight it more effectively when we are infected.

An important debate surrounds the explanation of changing rates of infectious disease. A great deal of medical research effort has been devoted to the identification of viruses and bacilli, and to the development of vaccines

■ If you were going to practise medicine in a developing country today, what sorts of ill health would you expect to encounter and what sorts of intervention would you become involved in?

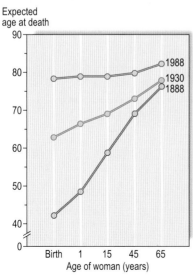

Fig. 1 Average life expectancy for a woman at different ages in 1888, 1930 and 1999 (England and Wales) (from Registrar General's Mortality Statistics, 1999, with permission).

Cause of death	1891–1895	1921–1925	1946–1950	1961–1965	1986–1990
Tuberculosis	867	393	157	20	4
Influenza	514	359	57	36	7
Digestive diseases	750	263	114	75	79
Diseases of the respiratory system	526	250	93	94	60
Diseases of the genitourinary system	309	226	113	60	35
Diseases of the skin, subcutaneous tissue, musculo-skeletal system or connective tissue	671	381	127	97	182
Malignant neo-plasms	–	–	96	103	115
Diseases of the heart	–	–	93	89	63
Cerebrovascular disease	–	100	92	95	60
Suicide	137	125	106	112	74

Table 1 **Standardized mortality ratios for selected causes of death, 1891 to 1990 in England and Wales**

From Registrar General's Mortality Statistics, with permission.

and cures during the last 100 years. For example, the tubercle bacillus was first identified in 1880. However, the introduction of the bacille Calmette–Guérin (BCG) vaccination to prevent infection did not take place until the 1950s. It can be seen from Table 1 that deaths due to tuberculosis had dropped dramatically long before the introduction of the BCG, suggesting that some other factor, such as improved nutrition, public health measures and housing conditions, or changes in the nature of the bacillus, must have contributed to the decline (McKeown, 1979) (see Fig. 1, p. 64).

Deaths due to some causes have not changed a great deal over the years. The SMRs for diseases of the heart, cerebrovascular disease and suicide have shown a steady but undramatic downward trend over the last 50 years. Although the rate for suicide has gradually declined over the years, it reached an all-time high during the years of the economic depression, 1931–1935, with an SMR of 150. The only cause of death to show an upward trend over all the years it has been recorded is malignant neoplasm or cancer. Over the last 20 years, death rates amongst women from cancer of the trachea, bronchus and breast have increased steadily, whilst amongst men death rates for cancer of the prostate have increased steadily.

■ Bearing in mind the impact of immunization on death rates from tuberculosis, speculate on how important vaccination against HIV might eventually prove to be.

Current common diseases

Although SMRs are very useful for examining trends in the rates of disease over time, if we want to know which are the most common causes of death in a population we need only examine the rates per head of population (Table 2). In 1999, deaths certified as due to disease of the circulatory system

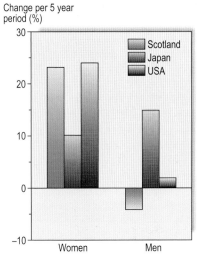

Fig. 2 Change in lung cancer incidence 1972–1987 (from Registrar General's Mortality Statistics, 1994, with permission).

accounted for 40% of all male deaths and 39% of all female deaths. Treatments for these conditions are an important area of research, and survival rates are improving. However, an understanding of the causes of heart disease and cancer remains important and they have been linked to a variety of socioeconomic, cultural and behavioural factors. Figure 2 shows recent changes in the incidence of lung cancer in Scotland, Japan and the USA. These changes may be closely linked to changes in the tendency of men and women to smoke cigarettes, which may in turn be related to cultural changes in the past 30 years.

An important consequence of increases in life expectancy and in the prevalence of diseases for which cures are unknown is that medical practice is increasingly concerned with the management of chronic ill health and the prevention of disability amongst a population whose average age is on the increase.

■ What implications do the changing patterns of mortality have for the demographic structure of the population and health care over the next 50 years?

Table 2 **Death rates per million population in England and Wales in 1974, 1991 and 1999, by cause of death**						
Cause of death	**Women**			**Men**		
	1974	1991	1999	1974	1991	1999
Diseases of the circulatory system	6118	4533	3985	6149	4570	4216
Neoplasms	2771	2833	2689	2244	2559	2439
Diseases of the respiratory system	1816	1043	1666	1458	1054	2008
Accidents. violence and poisoning	496	427	395	379	223	221
Diseases of the digestive system	292	285	373	309	361	442
Diseases of the nervous system	126	203	186	132	213	197
Diseases of the endocrine system	113	170	132	178	200	151
Mental disorders	28	145	–	47	282	–
Diseases of the genitourinary system	179	97	120	153	115	153
Diseases of the musculoskeletal system	30	44	36	83	135	99
Diseases of the blood	27	38	32	47	45	37
From Registrar General's Mortality Statistics, HMSO, 1999. Note: 1999 figures are for England only.						

Changing patterns of health and illness

■ The single factor which most accounts for our improved life expectancy at birth in the UK is that at the start of the 21st century almost all newborn babies can expect to live through childhood. This has occurred largely as a result of improvements in nutrition.

■ Over the last century infectious disease has declined dramatically. This may be a result of: (1) changes in people's susceptibility to infection; (2) changes in the nature of the biological agents; and (3) the introduction of medical treatments.

■ In 1999, diseases of the circulatory system accounted for 39% of all deaths. Malignant neoplasms accounted for 25% of all deaths.

■ Regular UK statistical bulletins concerning mortality and morbidity are on the HMSO website: www.statistics.gov.uk.

Social class and health

In clinical practice, we are particularly concerned with the health of individual patients. When clerking a patient we ask about occupation with an expectation that what we are told – bus driver, publican, lawyer, computer programmer, cleaner – will tell us something about the risks associated with work. We may also make an instant appraisal of the patient's lifestyle and material circumstances. Whilst there are significant differences between individual bus drivers and individual lawyers, there is also strong evidence that people's health is closely associated with their occupation (see pp. 56–57), their occupational group and their social class.

What is social class?

Social class is a general measure obtained by combining occupational groups roughly equivalent in terms of employment relations to form occupational classes in the UK; these can also be seen as an indirect indicator of education, income, standards of living, environment and working conditions. In 2001 the new classification, the National Statistics Socioeconomic Classification (NS-SEC) was introduced to overcome some of the drawbacks of the previously used Registrar General's (RG) classification (for example, the RG did not include people who were unemployed nor deal adequately with women's occupations). The NS-SEC is now being linked to mortality and morbidity data but as it has only been applied recently this spread relies on analyses based on the older RG classification. Other important categorizations which you may come across that use information on employment status and occupational data are socioeconomic group (SEG) and socioeconomic status (SES).

Social class and health

Over the last 100 years there have been great improvements in the health of the UK population (see pp. 40–41). However, inequalities between different sections of the population still exist; one form of increasing disparity that has received particular attention is social class inequality in health (Davey Smith et al., 2000). Death rates for the UK can be calculated for occupational classes by combining data collected on birth and death certificates with occupational data collected at the decennial census. Although reproductive and adult mortality rates for each social class have been decreasing over the last 100 years, there has, however, been an increase in the disparity in mortality rates between social classes I and II, and social classes III to V.

Figure 1 illustrates the most recently reported gradations in life expectancy at birth (see pp. 42–43) from social class I through to social class V (RG classification). Class differentials exist in each of the 14 major cause-of-death categories used in the International Classification of Diseases. When married women are classified according to their husband's occupation, similar if smaller differentials also appear. Only one cause of death for men, malignant melanoma, and four for women, including breast cancer, show a reverse trend. In general, the evidence also shows that disparities in illness, and especially chronic illness, are at least as wide as disparities in death.

These facts are not challenged; controversy lies in their interpretation and in the implications of different explanations

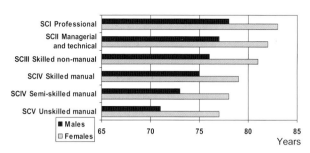

Fig. 1 Life expectancy at birth: by social class and sex, 1997–1999, England and Wales (from Coulthard et al., 2004, with permission).

for policies of preventive or corrective action. In the 1990s the influential Research Working Group on Inequalities in Health produced the Black report (Townsend et al., 1992). Four major theoretical explanations were presented, which were to become the matrix for future debate in this field.

Explanations for these relationships – the four hypotheses

Cultural/behavioural explanations

These explanations stress individual or lifestyle differences, rooted in personal characteristics and levels of education, which influence behaviour and are therefore open to alteration through health education inputs leading to changes in personal behaviour. Cultural and behavioural explanations suggest that lack of knowledge and lack of long-term goals give fewer possibilities of making maximum use of health and other services, and of taking preventive health measures (see pp. 64–65). Their main focus has been on the health-related behaviours of cigarette smoking, diet (including alcohol consumption) and lack of exercise:

- There are higher rates of smoking among manual groups, which will contribute to ill health.
- There is lower consumption of vitamin C, carotene and fibre, along with a higher dietary sodium/potassium ratio among the manual occupational classes. There are lower rates of vegetable intake, but elevated rates of the consumption of saturated fats.
- People in manual occupations take less exercise than those in non-manual groups.

Materialist or structuralist explanations

These explanations emphasize the role of economic and associated sociostructural factors, for example, the labour and housing markets, in the distribution of health and well-being. Proponents of this explanation believe that social structure is characterized by permanent social and economic inequality, which exposes individuals to different probabilities of ill health and injury:

- Poor-quality and damp housing has been shown to be associated with worse health and particularly with higher rates of respiratory disease in children (see pp. 10–11).
- Low SES, low pay and insecurity produce inadequacies in diet and dietary values.
- All-cause mortality has been shown in one study to be directly related to income, with the age-adjusted relative rate of the poorest group of subjects being twice that of the richest group. The rate increased in a stepwise fashion between these extremes (Bartley et al., 1998).

Social selection

These explanations argue that the occupational class structure is seen to act as a filter or sorter of human beings, and one of the major bases of selection is health: physical strength, vigour or agility. In this hypothesis, health determines one's social class of destination. People in better health have greater chances to ascend the social hierarchy while those with poorer health may undergo downward social mobility.

Artefact explanation

This suggests that both health and class are artificial variables produced by attempts to measure social phenomena and that, therefore, the relationship between them may itself be an artefact – an accidental effect – of little causal significance:

- Errors may be produced when two different data sets (e.g. death certificate and census data on occupation) are combined in order to calculate mortality rates for social classes.
- The failure of health inequalities to diminish in recent decades may be counterbalanced by the reduction in the proportion of the population in the poorest classes as a result of increased upward social mobility.

Developments up to and following the millennium

Following the Black report's own conclusions, research tended to favour the materialist/structural hypothesis. This was supported by the discovery of similar socioeconomic differentials in health and mortality in European countries, as well as in the USA and Australia. Although the developing consensus acknowledged the other explanations, these were given a subsidiary role. Cultural influences could be at work, but any behavioural differences in subcultures were seen to be directly related to social classes. There was also some evidence for indirect health selection, via differences in nutrition and other behaviours and attitudes, though less for direct health selection. Longitudinal studies carried out on census data tended to diminish the importance of the artefact explanation.

As the millennium approached the Acheson report (Acheson, 1998) brought the empirical findings up to date and discovered the worrying fact that social class inequalities were in fact increasing. Also around this time Wilkinson's work (1998) cast the inequalities debate in a new perspective. He did this by bringing the relational concept of relative deprivation into play. It was not so much the total amount of disposable income available to people in each social class that was important (as had been argued in the materialist explanation), but rather the scale of the differences between the social classes that was crucial (in other words, we should focus on the relationships between the classes). Large gaps between rich and poor in developed societies threatened social cohesion and produced high levels of social conflict, leading to social disintegration. These were the mechanisms that led to the development of inequalities in health.

Policy implications

Each of the above theories has practical implications as to what needs to be done to reduce social class inequalities in health. Although recent research favours a combination of materialist and behavioural approaches, where healthy or unhealthy lifestyles are seen to be linked to people's social positions, Wilkinson's ideas suggest that if we reduce income

inequality, whilst at the same time increasing various forms of social security provision, then social class inequalities in health will diminish. His policy focus, therefore, stresses the need for societies to develop good social security provisions for their citizens. Judge & Paterson (2001), however, have suggested that the most important strategy is for policies to reduce poverty, especially in families with children. The latter approach was strongly favoured by the Acheson report. Oliver et al. (2002) have argued for a more ethically and theoretically grounded reasoning in the inequalities debate. Indeed they have been highly contentious, arguing that we need to be careful, as societal resources spent in narrowing the distribution of health might lead to a reduction in the average health across our society.

Regardless of interventions at a macro level, we should also be aware of the important role doctors can play. Acheson stressed the crucial role of the National Health Service at all levels for helping to reduce inequalities in health. For example, doctors can ensure that their patients are claiming the benefits to which they are entitled.

Box 1 **Doctor's role**

- Awareness and recognition
- Open question–Do you have any money worries? Do you have any family worries? Do you get any benefits or tax credits?
- Referral to Citizens Advice Bureau or other advice services
- Fill in forms quickly and accurately

Case study

The Whitehall II studies

The Whitehall II research project of the 1980's originates from the first Whitehall study of the health of men in the Civil Service set up in the 1960s.

Work by Marmot et al. (1991) discounted the artefact explanation and minimized that related to social selection. They focused on health-related behaviours and also on financial elements. This research supports the interrelationship of causality between the materialist and the cultural–behavioural theory. Chandola et al. (2003) also produced evidence that health selection was not a primary explanation.

Bartley (2004), writing of both the Whitehall studies, stated: 'The observed patterns of health-related behaviour did differ between grades, but this only explained about a quarter of the fourfold difference in the risk of death over a seven year period'. She implies a strong link to materialist causes being supported by the results of the Whitehall II study.

Social class and health

- Mortality rates for all social classes have been falling over the last 100 years.
- However, the mortality rates for social class I have been decreasing faster than rates for social class V.
- Morbidity rates follow a similar pattern to mortality.
- The main explanations are: materialist, behavioural, social selection and artefactual.
- High rates of disparity between rich and poor in affluent countries may be a significant contributor to disparities in social class mortality rates.
- Different explanations for the relationship between social class and health imply different health, social and economic policies.

Gender and health

Gender is one of the important divisions in society along with social class and ethnicity. Gender patterns existing within wider society are reflected in medicine. Health services providers need to understand gender differences and their implications for health and health service uptake in order to provide the most appropriate and acceptable care to patients.

Gender and sex

Social scientists make the distinction between sex and gender, whereby 'sex' refers to physical and biological differences and 'gender' refers to the social definitions of how women and men should behave under certain circumstances. Society 'prescribes' how the biological sex is transformed into the social gender. Thus biological men learn to behave in a male way and to carry out male tasks. The philosopher Simone de Beauvoir (1960) summarized this transformation in the phrase: 'One is not born, but rather becomes, a woman.' Every society produces norms, rules and expectations for each gender and these differ from place to place as well as over time. Consequently, what is regarded as male behaviour in one time and place can be seen as female in another. Thus society as a whole produces women and men.

Difference in mortality and morbidity

Women live longer than men, even in the least developed countries (Fig. 1). Men are more likely to die compared with women in the same age group, from the day they are born. Table 1 clearly shows differences in Scottish perinatal mortality statistics. The rates indicate that baby boys are more likely to die than girls. This pattern is the same for any other age group in Scotland and for other industrialized countries, and many developing countries.

Morbidity statistics for Scotland (Table 1) indicate that women are more likely to have had an acute illness in the previous 2 weeks than men. This gender difference is even more profound in the over-75 age group.

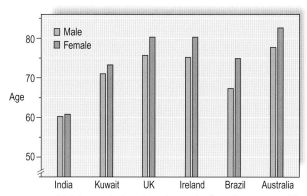

Fig. 1 Life expectancy at birth by gender for selected countries (from Department of Economic and Social Affairs, Population Division, 2006, with permission).

Table 1 Selected mortality and morbidity data for men and women, Scotland			
	Measure	Female	Male
Life expectancy at birth (2006)	Age in years	79.7	74.8
Mortality (2006)			
Perinatal mortality rate (2006)	Rate*	7.6	8.6
Intentional self harm/'suicide' (2006)	Numbers	115	427
Morbidity (2003)			
Acute illness in past 2 weeks (all ages)	%	17	15
Acute illness in past 2 weeks (age 75 and over)	%	25	18
Overweight/obese (2003)	%	57.3	64.0

*Rate per 1000 total births including stillbirths and deaths up to 7 days after birth.
From Scottish Executive (2005a), Registrar General (2007).

Gender differences in health

Some of the gender differences in mortality, especially in babies and infants, are related to 'natural' differences in biological and genetic make-up. However, as boys grow up to become men, social causes of death, especially those related to lifestyle, become more important. Men are more likely to be exposed to a hazardous environment than women, and many hazardous occupations in the UK are male-dominated, e.g. mining, fishing and construction work. Men are more likely to display more dangerous behaviour – to drink, to drive too fast, to use illegal drugs, to be involved in dangerous sports such as boxing or motor racing, or to commit suicide.

At the same time many diseases that do not in themselves kill but are often chronic and disabling affect more women than men. Approximately two-thirds of the disabled population in the UK are women, and a large proportion of that inequality is due to age difference (see below). However, not all differences between men and women

can be traced back to social factors. Some of the difference between male and female mortality and morbidity in coronary heart disease can be linked to the contraceptive pill and hormones (Committee on Health Promotion, 1996). However, men in Scotland are more likely to be overweight or obese than women.

Health service use and gender

Women are not only more likely to be ill, but also more likely to use health services. Figure 2 illustrates that American women – especially younger women – consult their primary care doctor more often for preventive care than men. This pattern generally holds for industrialized countries. Men are not only less likely to use health services, they are also more likely to delay and hence come with more serious symptoms to the consultation.

Women visit the doctor more often than men even if one ignores the consultations related to child-bearing (Miles, 1991), but the hospitalization rate is higher for men than for women, when

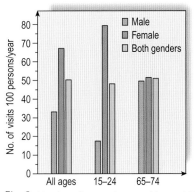

Fig. 2 Number of preventive care visits per 100 persons per year to primary care specialists by gender and selected ages, USA 2004 (from Hing et al., 2006, with permission).

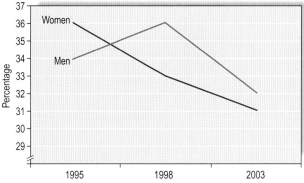

Fig. 3 Smoking prevalence in Scotland in women and men aged 16 years and over (from Scottish Executive, 2005b, with permission).

maternity and gynaecological cases are excluded (Leeson & Gray, 1978).

Differences in illness patterns of women and men will lead to different needs for health care provision. Women live longer than men, so consequently a large proportion of the elderly are female. The overwhelming majority of hip fracture patients are elderly people, hence the majority of patients with a hip fracture are female, and they are more likely to occupy a bed in an orthopaedic ward. Moreover, the uptake of health care is not only determined indirectly through morbidity, but also directly by social and cultural factors. Two main factors are highlighted below:

1. What is defined as illness in women is often a social definition instead of the purely scientific exercise of diagnosis and treatment. Childbirth, for example, helps to define women as being ill, because of their biological role (see pp. 4–5).
2. Women consult family doctors more often than men do, not only for themselves but also for their children and elderly relatives (see pp. 90–91).

The first explanation is related to the fact that all societies make assumptions about what is appropriate gender-related behaviour. This is often referred to as sexual stereotyping. One aspect of this in western cultures is that female socialization makes it more acceptable for women to adopt the 'sick role'.

One of the possible explanations is that women are less likely to be in full-time employment, therefore they are likely to lose less income than men when they take on a sick role. There is also evidence that doctors give different emphasis to the 'same' symptoms, according to gender. For example, men's 'back troubles' are regarded

more seriously, being seen as directly caused by heavy work. Women's 'back problems' are often labelled as part of general gynaecological conditions. Similarly, mental health problems in women are seen to be internally caused, and thus subject to medical intervention, whereas in men these are seen as caused by external factors. In other words, men's problems are seen to be related to what they do, and women's problems are related to what they are.

Smoking

Smoking illustrates the importance of gender for the medical profession for two quite distinct reasons (see pp. 84–85). First, smoking is the most important cause of preventable death. Secondly, patterns in smoking prevalence between men and women have been changing over the past three decades. It also shows that differences between men and women in health behaviour – in this case smoking – are not static. Fifty years ago it used to be 'normal' among men from all social classes to smoke, whilst only a small proportion of women smoked. Smoking prevalence among adults has fallen steadily since 1972. However, whilst the proportion of men who smoked regularly dropped, the proportion of female smokers increased in the same period. In the 1980s the proportion of women taking up smoking in their teenage years increased rapidly. In the 1990s the proportion of Scottish women smoking was, for the first time ever, greater than that of men (Fig. 3). The reason for this change has been sought in women's emancipation, advertising and health promotion.

Furthermore, the incidence of lung cancer is increasing among women, and this is closely related to the social changes in smoking prevalence.

Case study

M is an obstetrician who visits the family doctor because of sleeping problems. During the consultation the doctor asks him about factors that might have an influence on getting to sleep. He mentions the heavy workload in the maternity hospital, drinking a little too much in order to deal with stress and sleeplessness, the frequent quarrels with his partner for no apparent reason, having two noisy children (under 5 years) at home, and living a long distance away from his elderly parents. Do you think the family doctor would advise this patient differently if you were told that obstetrician M is a woman rather than a man?

 STOP THINK ▪ Women live longer than men but are more likely to be ill. What explanations can you give for this paradox?

 STOP THINK ▪ Why are women more likely to be resident in mental institutions than men are?

Gender and health

- ▪ At any age men are more likely to die, but women are more likely to be ill.
- ▪ Gender differences have a greater impact on health and health care than differences in biological sex.
- ▪ Women consult doctors more often than men do.
- ▪ Medical professionals have different expectations of, and ways of dealing with, male and female patients.

Ethnicity and health

It is important for health professionals to consider their roles in developing and delivering equitable health services for all ethnic groups as this population is considered one of the most ethnically diverse within the European community. Ethnic minorities in the UK are sometimes referred to as Black and minority ethnic (BME) communities.

Race, culture and ethnicity

In order to monitor whether equitable access to health care is achieved, the UK government requires NHS hospitals to record the ethnicity of all admitted patients. Ethnicity is also collected as a variable in epidemiological research. However, defining the concept of ethnicity in relation to understandings of race and culture is fraught with difficulties.

The concept of 'race' does not exist in any biologically meaningful way; genetic explanations for the differences seen in health status have long been shown to be scientifically flawed. There is more genetic variability within than between so-called racial groups, and over 99% of the genetic make-up of human beings is shared by all ethnic groups. Although there are clear differences in physical characteristics between people whose ancestry lies in different parts of the world (colour of eyes, skin or hair), these characteristics are of no major importance to health apart from certain genetic disorders such as the haemoglobinopathies, which have more to do with geographical conditions than genetics. Physical characteristics are only important when values are attached to them in a society, so that one group defines another as 'different' and assumes them to have particular behavioural characteristics because of the way they look. It is equally important to consider how health professionals perceive non-indigenes because these perceptions can cloud their judgement and affect service provision and delivery.

Culture is a set of shared beliefs, values and attitudes that guide behaviour. People identify themselves as members of a group on cultural grounds; they may share similar language, religion, lifestyle and origins and this helps them define their ethnic group. We all have ethnic identities, whether we consider ourselves to be 'Scottish', 'English', 'Bangladeshi' or any combination that describes our national, cultural and social identities. Thus the concepts of 'race', culture and ethnicity, although interrelated, have different meanings.

■ How might the various components of your ethnicity and culture relate to your experiences of health and illness?

Ethnicity is measured by asking people to assign themselves to a category, as in the 2001 census in England. This approach attempts to capture the way people think of themselves in relation to colour of skin, continent of ancestral origin and cultural background. Other questions included country of birth and religion, these data should help in the planning of services that are appropriate in relation to religious observance and diet. The notion that this classification of populations aids services planning and delivery is flawed because the inconsistencies in the categories used, e.g. skin colour, continent or country of origin, portrays different meanings and in themselves do not give accurate information to direct services, therefore perpetuates inequality. Self-classification of ethnic group, can also pose problems for those interpreting the data.

About 4 million people living in the UK consider that they are from a minority ethnic group; that is, about 7.1% of the total population (Johnson, 2003). Between 40 and 50% of this group were born in Britain. Most people from the minority ethnic groups live in inner cities, and some towns or metropolitan boroughs have become known for local concentrations of people from particular ethnic origins; Leicester greatly benefited from the settlement of migrant workers who responded to the recruitment call of the 1950s and 1960s (Narayanasamy & White, 2005). People who migrated to the UK 40 years ago have different profiles from those who came more recently. For example there is a recent movement of people from Eastern Europe. The health needs of these populations will differ greatly from those of Caribbean and Asian origin, who came to the UK 40 years previously.

Socioeconomic inequalities

Unemployment rates for most minority ethnic groups are considerably higher than those for indigenes, particularly amongst young people (see pp. 58–59). This inevitably affects health (Table 1). Although national data on average income are not routinely broken down by ethnic group, a survey by Leicester City in the mid-1990s showed evidence of lower incomes amongst people of Asian origin: the gross median weekly earnings of 'Asian' men and women were just 82% of their white counterparts. Similarly, whilst about 19% of the white population live in 'council estates and low-income areas', about 40% of Black and Indian groups, and as many as 63% of Bangladeshi and Pakistani groups, live in such areas (Johnson, 2003). However, there remain significant differences in the socioeconomic experiences of sectors of minority ethnic groups.

Diversity

Patterns of health and disease are profoundly influenced by socioeconomic, environmental, genetic and cultural factors (see pp. 42–43), and there are significant differences in patterns of disease between ethnic groups. However, the major health problems of ethnic minority communities, and, therefore, priorities for health improvement and health care, are similar to the majority population (for example, cardiovascular disease and cancers). This is important when using data on ethnicity in the planning of health services (Kai & Bhopal, 2003).

Table 1 shows that comparing deaths emphasizes differences. For example, liver cancer or tuberculosis are much more common in men from the Indian subcontinent but they account for fewer deaths. Looking at absolute number of deaths, the major fatal diseases for the minority group are similar to those of the population as a whole. Thus, although there are differences in experience of health between all ethnic groups, the major diseases of the majority are also important to minority ethnic groups.

The varied patterns in the experience of health and illness between different ethnic groups do not have a single

Table 1 **Deaths and standardized mortality ratios (SMRs)* in male immigrants from the Indian subcontinent (aged 20 years and over; total deaths = 4352)**							
By rank order of number of deaths				**By rank order of SMR**			
Cause	Number of deaths	% of total	SMR	Cause	Number of deaths	% of total	SMR
Ischaemic heart disease	1533	35.2	115	Homicide	21	0.5	341
Cerebrovascular disease	438	10.1	108	Liver and intrahepatic bile duct neoplasm	19	0.4	338
Bronchitis, emphysema and asthma	223	5.1	77	Tuberculosis	64	1.5	315
Neoplasm of the trachea, bronchus and lung	218	5.0	53	Diabetes mellitus	55	1.3	188
Total	2412	55.4	–	Total	159	3.7	–

*Standardized mortality ratios, comparing with the male population of England and Wales, which was by definition 100.
From Senior & Bhopal (1994), including data originally published by Marmot et al. (1984); reproduced with permission of BMJ Publications

Case study

Lack of services for sickle-cell disease in the UK

Sickle-cell disorders and thalassaemia are inherited disorders of red blood cells mainly affecting black and ethnic minority groups.

Services for sickle-cell disease, although improving, are lagging behind the numbers of cases arising in the UK. There is need for health professionals to update themselves with the needs (see pp. 152–153) of the population for whom they provide care.

A consultant haematologist wrote in 1990:

I was hearing that not enough money goes to research on sickle cell. It's not a disease of the white people and they don't know much about it…

Debbie (17 years) wrote:

They know that I have got the disease but they don't really know too much about it, and I don't think, this is my personal view, I don't think they're interested because it's not a white man's disease, and I mean, and I can't see them really digging into this thing to get any knowledge out of it, because it is black people, and it's black people's problem (quoted in Anionwu, 1993).

What needs to accompany education is an exploration of attitudes towards provision of appropriate services at all levels of the NHS.

explanation. Genetic inheritance contributes to the aetiology of some diseases, e.g. the prevalence of sickle-cell disorders is higher in people of African and Asian origins. However, lifestyle and cultural factors (especially smoking and diet), exposure to poor living circumstances and the stress of racism will also contribute (Nazroo, 2003). Explanations for differences in experience of health and illness that point out the impact of socioeconomic inequalities and racism are used less often by researchers, but used more often by people in minority groups themselves. It has always been a difficult thing to prove racism: it is often said that to appreciate fully what it is like to be 'Black' in a predominantly 'White' society one should try wearing the identity.

Experience of prejudice

In 1997, about 25% of white people said that they were prejudiced against minority ethnic groups, whilst between 20% and 33% of people from a range of minority ethnic groups reported being worried about being racially harassed (Coker, 2002). This fear is not unfounded; reported racist incidents in London increased from 11 050 in the year ending March 1999 to 23 345 by March 2000 (Coker, 2002).

'Racism' and 'institutional racism' have been defined as follows:

'Racism' in general terms consists of conduct or words or practices which advantage or disadvantage people because of their colour, culture or ethnic origin. In its more subtle form it is as damaging as in its overt form.

'Institutional racism' consists of the collective failure of an organization to provide an appropriate and professional service to people because of their colour, culture or ethnic origin (para 6.34) (Home Office, 1999, cited by Foster et al., 2005). Epidemiological studies that include perceptions of racism or prejudice are rare but a 3-year study in the general population in the Netherlands found higher rates of 'delusional ideation' (a suggested precursor of psychotic disorder) amongst people who reported discrimination than those who did not (Janssen et al., 2003).

Unequal provision of health care

For a range of reasons, some related to unwitting but institutional racism many health services are inappropriate to the needs of minority ethnic populations. For example, health services have been concentrated on issues that are seen by health professionals to be of special relevance to particular ethnic groups, whereas people themselves may not attach such significance to them. In the UK this led to health education on issues such as rickets or fertility control, whereas until recently haemoglobinopathy services have been largely ignored (see Case study).

The other criticism is that the methods by which health issues are brought to the attention of minority groups is often inappropriate. For example, recent policies to increase fruit and vegetable intake and decrease the proportion of fat in the diet all too frequently miss out foods often eaten by minority ethnic groups. Therefore, there is a risk that the health education message (see 78–79) does not reach (some) ethnic minority groups.

Ethnicity and health

- 'Race' does not exist in any biologically meaningful way.
- Ethnicity is a complex concept consisting of the interplay between cultures, history and language, and so on. We all belong to an 'ethnic group'.
- Ethnic minority groups are at increased risk of being poor, principally through the effects of racism and negative discrimination.
- The major diseases and health problems of most minority ethnic groups are the same as for the general population.
- There is evidence of unequal and inappropriate provision of health services for in ethnic minority groups.

Quality of life

There is no universally accepted definition of quality of life (QoL), and there are many different models used in relation to health (Bowling, 2007).

The World Health Organization (WHO) (1946) defined health as 'complete physical, mental and emotional well-being'. Thus health and health-related QoL were no longer limited to physical health and an absence of illness. In 1993, the WHO defined QoL as 'individuals' perceptions of their position of life in the context of the culture and value systems in which they live and in relation to their goals, standards and concerns' (World Health Organization division of mental health, 1993). The definition includes six domains:

1. Physical health.
2. Psychological state.
3. Levels of independence.
4. Social relationships.
5. Environmental features.
6. Spiritual concerns.

Similarly, the WHOQOL Group 1998 defined QoL as 'an individual's perceptions of their position in life taken in the context of the culture and value systems where they live in relation to their goals, expectations, standards and concerns', and they subsequently developed a standardized measure, the WHOQOL. In contrast, Calman (1984) proposed that QoL is the extent to which hopes and ambitions are matched by experience, and Bowling (1995) suggested that it relates to things people regard as most important in their lives. Certainly, QoL is a multidimensional dynamic concept that includes both positive and negative aspects of life.

Functional or subjective?

QoL used to be seen as an objective assessment of the person's functioning, whereas the current approach tries to measure QoL as an individual's perceived health status or well-being. Hence QoL is very much an individual construct (Fig. 1). Physical functioning might mean the ability to perform specific tasks or the activities of daily living and of mental functioning in performing cognitive tasks and social interactions. Individuals' own appraisal of their health status may be more influenced by the way that they perceive their relative health status

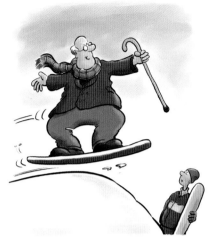

Fig. 1

and by other non-medical aspects of their lives. Health professionals may have a different perspective from the individual patient (Fig. 2).

Behavioural questions such as 'can you walk up stairs?' (functional QoL) may be easier to answer than 'does your health interfere with your enjoyment of life?' (individual or subjective perspective), but the latter may be regarded as being more important by the person. Perhaps unsurprisingly, subjective indices of QoL correlate reliably with standard measures of depression and anxiety (Muldoon et al., 1998). The expectations of QoL outcomes of medical treatment may also differ between patients and health professionals.

There is a paradox here in that patients who have significant health and functional problems do not necessarily have poor scores of QoL. People with severe disabilities may report having a good QoL despite having difficulties with activities of daily living and being socially isolated (Albrecht & Devlieger, 1999).

Assessment of quality of life

The perspectives of individuals, carers and health professionals may be very different. In a healthy state it is hard to imagine what life would be like if wheelchair-bound, or visually impaired. We can gain some insight from novels or films, but there is a qualitative aspect to QoL which may not be captured by standardized scales. Like pain, QoL may be best regarded as what patients tell us.

QoL is a dynamic construct and changes over time. People assess their health-related QoL by comparing their expectations with their experience. If expectations match experience there is no impact on QoL, but if it is worse then there is an impact. Clinical trials of efficacy of therapy often require assessment of QoL, and outcomes of therapy may depend on expectations (Alder, 2002). In the Heart and Estrogen/progestin Replacement Study (HERS) randomized controlled trial of hormone therapy (Hlatky et al., 2002) QoL was assessed on measures of physical activity, energy/fatigue and mental health. Only women who had hot flushes showed improvement on hormone therapy but all women showed a decline in scores over 3 years, apart from depression.

Quality of life in children

Children may place great importance on their perceived competence, social acceptability, athletic or sporting prowess and their physical appearance. Look at teenage magazines to see the health and social concerns of adolescents.

In a study of over 100 obese children and adolescents in California it was found that on a paediatric QoL inventory, obese children and adolescents reported significantly lower health-related QoL. There were no relationships with gender, ethnicity or socioeconomic status (Schwimmer et al., 2003). Reducing obesity in children should therefore benefit more than physical health.

Quality of life in older people

In seeking to enhance QoL in older people the medical model may suggest searching for cures and the reduction or absence of symptoms as well as increases in levels of functioning. In contrast to this, the older person may be more concerned with issues of self-identity and preservation of meaning in life. Brandstater & Greive (1994) see the gradual ageing process as leading to successive loss of control, and higher rates of depression (which may be associated with bereavement) and lower self-esteem in the context of youth and beauty being emphasized in western society. They suggest

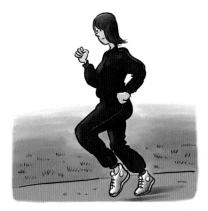

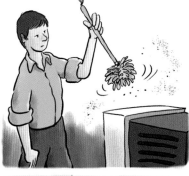

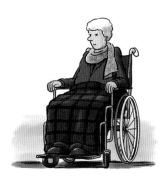

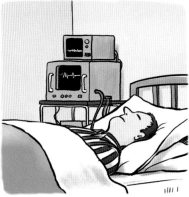

Fig. 2 Classification of state of illness. (a) No disability; (b) only light housework; (c) confined to wheelchair; (d) unconscious. (adapted from Fallowfield, 1990, with permission).

that elderly people cope by moving through stages of assimilation and accommodation. In assimilation people maintain current activities, goals and aspirations, for example, making strong efforts to maintain fitness by taking exercise, and using aids such as reading glasses to achieve their goals. As the ageing process continues, people may assimilate to the process by changing goals and aspirations which better match their abilities, that is, they may give up difficult goals or reduce their level of expectations about their level of performance.

 STOP THINK
■ At what age do you think your quality of life will be at its peak?

Quality-adjusted life year

Health economists often use a utility or decision theory approach to measuring QoL. The utility approach assesses the value that someone places on the consequences of different courses of action. For example, if chemotherapy would extend life but involve costs of treatment and side-effects, how would this be valued

against no treatment costs or side-effects but a shorter life?

The quality-adjusted life year or QALY is a measure derived from a combination of mortality, morbidity and function, with quality-of-life value or utility with increased time of survival resulting from treatment. QALYs have been used in assessing the relative value of treatments offered by national health services, e.g. by the UK National Institute for Health and Clinical Excellence.

The Oregon experiment (see pp. 154–155) is one of the best-known applications. In a study of treatment for alcohol problems the conclusions were that if a QALY was worth £30 000, motivational therapy would have a 58% chance of being more cost-effective than social therapy (UKATT research team, 2005). Considerable reservations have been expressed about the applications of this approach, as it may differ between healthy people, patients and health professionals and does not take into account expectations, previous history or the time spent in ill health (Fallowfield, 1990).

Improvement in QoL is the goal of both patients and health professionals and it is important to ensure that they understand each other when discussing treatment options.

STOP THINK
■ We can only know about someone's quality of life by what they tell us. Discuss

Quality of life

■ QoL has many different definitions.

■ Measures of functional QoL may differ from a person's individual appraisal.

■ QALY analyses require careful appraisal.

Media and health

The role of the media

The mass media are a rich source of information about all aspects of health. They are constantly presenting us with ideas about everything from the symptoms of disease or the risks of different behaviours to the validity of government health policy or the trustworthiness of the medical profession (Fig. 1). That is why so much money is now spent on trying to affect media representations, through advertising, public relations activities, media advocacy and direct health education initiatives. However, the role of the media is not straightforward. A direct impact may be evident when, for example, doctors are flooded with enquiries after a particular health 'scare'. However, such responses are often very short-term. People are certainly not naive and unreflective media consumers, ready to absorb any message indiscriminately. If they were, then campaigns to encourage us to stop smoking or eat less fat would be more successful! On the other hand it is true that certain controversies, such as when questions were raised over the safety of the measles, mumps and rubella (MMR) vaccine, have had tangible effects. Even in this case, however, while vaccination declined by 10% the 'scare' did not have as big an impact as might have been expected. 'Most parents trusted health professionals, friends and family more than the media and continued to accept the MMR vaccine' (Boyce, 2007: 188).

Research into how people actually respond to the media tends to show that they act as sophisticated audiences, choosing how to engage with media facts, images, stories, characters and plots in relation to their own lives (Boyce, 2007; Henderson, 2007). In addition, each media 'message' competes with ideas and information from other media and broader cultural sources. How we respond also depends on social and economic context, the ease with which we can change our behaviour and the ways in which any particular media representation relates to our self-image, aspirations, group identity and networks. Sometimes the same media representations can even generate diametrically opposed responses from different social groups. For example, the British soap opera Brookside included a storyline about a businesswoman, Susannah, successfully standing up to a man who complained about her breast-feeding in a café-bar. This storyline was welcomed by middle-class breast-feeding women, who felt inspired by it. Reactions were strikingly different among a group of young working-class women. Susannah's strength of will did not fit with these women's self-perceptions: 'You need to be confident, which I'm not'. Clearly, if breast-feeding in a café-bar might cause a scene and necessitate a robust defence then trying to do it in the local burger joint would be likely to be even more controversial. For these women the Brookside episode seemed to reinforce the fact that breast-feeding in public was ill advised, rather than encourage them to think of it as an option (Henderson et al., 2000; see Case study).

It is thus important for all those working in health and medicine (whether, for example, as a medical researcher, a GP or a health promoter) not to assume they can easily predict how people will make sense of any information/representations. This is true whether the information is delivered via the mass media, personal communication or health promotion posters. It is also important to acknowledge the different levels at which influence may operate. Perhaps the mass media's most significant role may be in how they cultivate underlying common-sense understandings of the world. Newspapers, television, radio, magazines and, indeed, cinema, both reflect and promote ideas about what is normal – whether this relates to body weight, smoking or breastfeeding (see Case study). The media can also promote stereotypes by, for example, portraying people with mental illness as violent, thus encouraging fear and stigma (Philo, 1999). Fictional programmes may be particularly important in promoting emotional identification and can reach important new audiences. At the same time their power to provoke identification with particular characters and to convey forceful stories can mislead. The drama and human interest potential of stories about 'inherited' breast cancer, for example, generated many fictional TV representations and helped to raise its profile, but has also made many people overestimate the role of genetic risk factors (Henderson & Kitzinger, 1999).

On the other hand, it is easy to overexaggerate the power of fiction. Scientists and policy-makers sometimes blame science fiction for making the public worry about human cloning (for stem cell research purposes). Actually sci-fi may be used to *discredit* anxieties more often than to *underwrite* them. People are shame-faced about fears which 'sound like a sci-fi film'; they are more likely to back up their concerns about human cloning with reference to Nazi eugenics or news stories about rogue states misusing science or an international trade in organ transplants. It is profoundly unhelpful if scientists/policy-makers dismiss public concerns as simply a result of watching too many horror films (Haran et al., 2007).

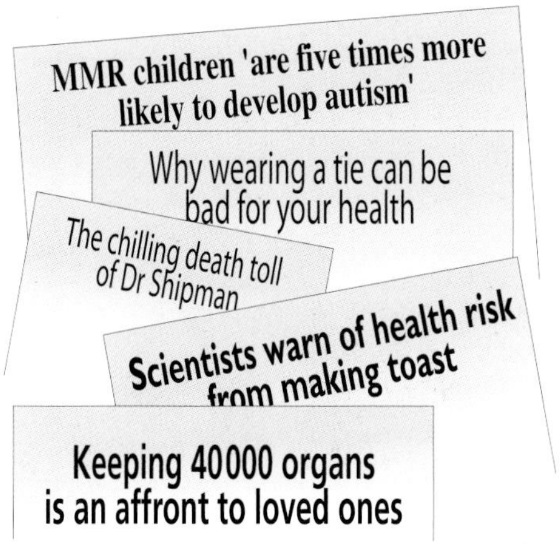

MMR children 'are five times more likely to develop autism'

Why wearing a tie can be bad for your health

The chilling death toll of Dr Shipman

Scientists warn of health risk from making toast

Keeping 40000 organs is an affront to loved ones

Fig. 1

Health and social issues

Newspaper reports and both factual and fictional television may also offer 'scripts' for thinking and talking about social and health issues. When the media started to acknowledge incestuous sexual abuse during the 1980s, this allowed some children and adult survivors to talk about such abuse for the first time (Kitzinger, 2001). The media breaching of taboos about bowel and testicular cancer have been similarly important. The media also played a vital role in putting AIDS and safer sex on the public agenda. However, the coverage has also been limited. One study of TV fiction found that, although young people were shown talking about sexual attraction and whether or not they wanted sex, condom use was never discussed, offering no 'scripts' and modelling of behaviour for young people (Batchelor & Kitzinger, 1999).

Another study revealed that the media's early voyeuristic fascination with the gaunt, sickly 'face of AIDS' encouraged people to think you could tell by looking who was infected (Kitzinger, 1995). Sometimes a message can also be confusing because the producers/scriptwriters or health educators attempt to avoid explicit language. The term 'body fluids' often adopted in AIDS discussions allowed some people to believe that saliva was dangerous. The advice to use a condom unless you are '100% sure of your partner' backfired – associating condom use with a lack of trust (Miller et al., 1998).

Medicine and the media

The medical profession is also acutely aware of how the profession as a whole is represented in factual and fictional media. Doctors may be heroes in fiction, but intense public attention has also been given to the villains: the Alder Hey hospital scandal about the use of children's organs, for example, or the doctor turned mass-murderer, Dr Harold Shipman. The mass media also have a crucial role to play in the development of scientific and medical research. In the field of human genetic research, for example, public acceptability is increasingly important. The ground was prepared for changing legislation on stem cell research, for example, by intense media lobbying. Interestingly, the resulting coverage, although arguably 'balanced' around the 'rights of the embryo' debate, excluded wider social and political questions and gave little opportunity for explorations of ambivalence (Williams et al., 2003).

Understanding how the media represent all aspects of health and illness is important for medical students. Indepth research about media representations and audience responses suggests that the relationship with public attitudes is more complex than might at first appear. It is important to go beyond personal impressions and anecdotes to take into account the diversity of the media and of audiences, and to consider the implications of the associated research.

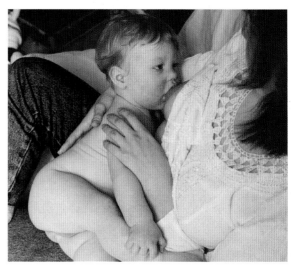

Fig. 2

 STOP THINK
- How do media representations influence how you think about your own health or how you respond to patients? Has the media influenced your images of the type of person liable to engage in particular risk behaviours?
- If you were going to design a campaign to promote a health behaviour, what media factors would you take into account?

The media and health

The mass media can:
- Put new health issues on the public/policy agenda or help raise their profile.
- Provoke debate about the ethics of scientific and medical developments.
- Invest public hopes in particular types of scientific research (e.g. stem cell research) as promising cures.
- Convey factual information and advice.
- Promote or challenge stereotypes (e.g. about people with schizophrenia or about who is likely to contract HIV).
- Cultivate common-sense understandings of health and illness and support ideas about what constitutes appropriate behaviours.
- Play a key part in short-term health 'scares' (whether that be about using the contraceptive pill or about a threat such as bird flu).

However, media influence is not straightforward or all-powerful:
- There is a large gap between what people know and what we do.
- Wider social issues are often more important than health messages on their own.
- The impact of media representations varies depending on format (e.g. fictional versus factual programmes) and the type of narrative, vocabulary, images and associations used.
- The impact will vary depending on how much the public trusts the sources of the story (e.g. government scientists).
- Different audiences may respond to the same programme or report quite differently depending on their identities and the context of their own lives.

Case study

Infant-feeding in the media

A systematic content analysis of 1 month's UK press and TV coverage showed that the overall pattern of coverage implies that breast-feeding is odd or problematic whereas bottle-feeding is largely normalized, associated with 'ordinary' families and problem-free feeding.
- Breast-feeding is rarely shown (Fig. 2). There was only one scene on TV of a baby on the breast and nine of a breast pump (not in use), but 170 scenes with babies' bottles.
- Babies' bottles have become a routine and iconic way of visually representing babyhood.
- Whereas a baby may be bottle-fed in a background scene on TV, breast-feeding, where it does feature, is foregrounded as a focus for debate.
- Breast-feeding is used to characterize particular types of women, e.g. middle-class 'earth mothers'.
- Bottle-feeding is used to symbolize positive male involvement in fatherhood.
- Problems with breast-feeding are highlighted, whereas difficulties with bottle-feeding are rarely mentioned. For example, there was only one reference to potential difficulties associated with bottle-feeding ('hassle' of bottle-washing) but 42 references to problems attributed to breast-feeding (sore nipples, saggy breasts, sleepless nights).
- Routine mass-media coverage rarely acknowledges the health implications of bottle-feeding. There was only one oblique reference within the entire sample to the potential disadvantages of formula milk (Henderson et al., 2000).

Housing, homelessness and health

Housing affects health directly and indirectly. Lack of adequate housing causes both mental and physical ill health. It can make existing illness and health problems worse, and delay recovery from illness (Fig. 1). Lack of adequate housing has detrimental social and economic consequences, which reduce people's opportunities to protect and promote their own health. Energy-inefficient housing contributes to fuel poverty and is detrimental to the environment and this has consequences for the health of the whole population.

Housing and health

In Victorian Britain, concerns about housing conditions causing ill health led to programmes of slum clearance. This commitment to improving public health by changing harmful social conditions contributed to the decline in infectious diseases and increases in life expectancy (see pp. 42–43).

The 1950s and 1960s saw growth in public-sector housing. The focus on quantity rather than quality brought problems such as dampness and lack of sound insulation and privacy, as well as social isolation. Research evidence emerged during the 1970s and 1980s showing the negative health impact of these 'new' housing problems, but health policy focused on individual behaviour as the cause of ill health rather than social conditions such as housing.

The late 1980s and 1990s saw a decline in the availability of affordable housing and a rise in the numbers of homeless people who were roofless or in temporary accommodation. In the early 21st century concerns about energy efficiency, the environment and fuel poverty have begun to reinforce the centrality of housing to public health.

Homelessness and health

The term 'homeless' is used to describe people who are 'roofless' and living on the streets and those living in temporary accommodation. People who are homeless are exposed to extreme environmental hazards such as damp, cold and noise as well as overcrowding, risk of violence, risk of accidental injury, poor hygiene and poor access to health services. Figure 1 shows the main illnesses associated with homelessness.

Housed but homeless

Social policy currently distinguishes between people who have permanent accommodation and the homeless. A definition of homelessness based on the 'lack of a right of access to own secure and minimally adequate housing space' (Bramley et al., 1987) would mean that people are seen as homeless if permanently housed in accommodation that is harmful to health or deprives them of resources that are necessary to maintain or protect health.

The health impact

How does lack of adequate housing affect health? The housing environment can affect health both directly and indirectly (Box 1).

The direct effects of lack of adequate housing can be explained using a medical model whereby specific aspects of the environment have physical effects that lead to specific symptoms or illness.

Another model of illness is the *general susceptibility model*, in which aspects of the environment act as stressors that make people more susceptible to illness. Specific features of the environment are not linked to specific illness as they are in the medical model. This model takes some account of the indirect effects of housing on health.

In both models researchers have to rule out the possibility that associations between housing and health occur as a result of other factors. The two most common artefact explanations that have to be ruled out are those of confounding factors and downward drift (Box 2). If researchers have data on other social conditions and past health and housing history, statistical techniques can be used to take account of these factors and assess the independent contribution of housing to health.

A third model that can be used to understand the health impact of housing is a socioeconomic model. This holistic model recognizes that it is important to understand the experience of living in inadequate housing, the impact on daily life and the compound effects of different aspects of inadequate housing and other conditions of social deprivation.

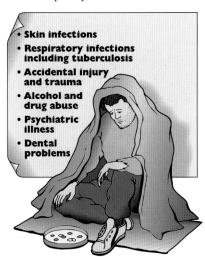

- **Skin infections**
- **Respiratory infections including tuberculosis**
- **Accidental injury and trauma**
- **Alcohol and drug abuse**
- **Psychiatric illness**
- **Dental problems**

Fig. 1 Illnesses associated with homelessness.

Box 1 **Lack of adequate housing: effects on health**

Direct effects
- Exposure to physiological effects of the environment or harmful agents fostered by environmental conditions

Indirect effects
- Exposure to poor living conditions in childhood may have consequences for health in later life
- Causes stress or discomfort, which increases general susceptibility to physical illness and emotional problems
- Exacerbates or delays recovery from existing health problems
- Undermines social relationships
- Makes it difficult or stressful to get on with the tasks of daily life
- Makes it difficult to access other resources which are necessary to sustain or promote health
- Can drain other household resources, including income, that protect and improve health
- Has an impact on energy efficiency and the environment, which in turn has an impact on public health

Box 2 **Key problems in establishing the links between lack of adequate housing and ill health**

Confounding factors
Lack of adequate housing is frequently associated with other factors which are known to cause ill health, such as unemployment or low income

Downward drift
People in poor health drift into poor housing or homelessness because of the consequences of ill health

Overcrowding
- Has a detrimental effect on relationships within dwellings
- Leads to loss of privacy which adversely affects mental health
- Increases the risk of infections particularly where there are shared amenities such as kitchens and toilets

Noise
- Unpredictable intermittent noise (e.g. from noisy neighbours or traffic) has psychological consequences including sleep disturbance, irritability and poor concentration

Dampness
- Causes poor respiratory health
- Acts as a stress which leads to depression, emotional distress and increased risk of physical illness

Cold
- Exposure to cold is a direct physiological stress and source of discomfort which increases general susceptibility to illness
- The elderly, people with an illness, young infants living in cold housing and people who are roofless are at risk of hypothermia

Poor architectural design
- Unsafe building design can increase the risk of accidental injury
- Lack of play space (both inside and outside) for children, dwellings which are easy targets for burglars and vandals, where the design restricts access (dark and threatening stairways or footpaths, high-rise accommodation, accommodation which has too many stairs for the residents) are stressful and affect mental health
- Lack of adequate insulation and ventilation makes dwellings difficult and expensive to heat, leading to problems of cold and dampness

Being roofless or living in temporary accommodation
- Can be a source of disruption and stigma which makes it difficult to get jobs and maintain or access health services

Living in a 'bad' area
- Makes it difficult to access resources which would maintain or promote health, including healthy food, leisure and entertainment facilities, health services and employment opportunities

Energy inefficiency
- Energy inefficiency causes fuel poverty. The compound effect of inadequate housing and low income is likely to impact on resources for healthy eating, socialising and other behaviours that can promote health or prevent illness
- Energy inefficiency impacts on the economy and the environment as a whole, with long-term health impact on the population

Fig. 2 Features of inadequate housing which are detrimental to health.

STOP THINK
- For a family with young children living in damp and overcrowded conditions, what are the possible consequences for the health service of housing-related illness?
- What are the possible costs to the health service of inadequate housing?

A range of factors associated with housing have been shown to cause physical illness and discomfort as well as depression and emotional distress (Fig. 2). *It's very noisy right by the motorway but we couldn't open the windows anyway because of all the break-ins. The walls are damp and there's mould on our walls, our clothes and shoes. It's freezing cold most of the time and in winter we all huddle into the one room. The kids are always sick and I'm at my wits' end (Hunt, 1997).*

Work on the energy efficiency of housing has drawn attention to the fact that people with low incomes are more likely to live in poorly constructed, least energy-efficient housing – they live in fuel poverty. A greater proportion of lower incomes is spent on energy and this may still not alleviate the problems of cold and dampness. Poor housing is seen to compound the problems of living on a low income rather than low income being seen as a potential confounding factor in the relationship between housing and health.

Case study

The direct effects of dampness on health

A study in the UK (Platt et al., 1989) looked at whether toxic fungal air spores which are present in damp and mouldy houses could explain the association between dampness and respiratory symptoms. The study involved the collection of health information from around 800 respondents. Measures of the internal housing environment were then taken by an independent team of surveyors who were 'blind' to the results of the health survey.

Reporting of respiratory symptoms was higher when the levels of damp and air spore counts were higher, indicating a dose–response relationship. The health survey asked about other factors which might influence respiratory health such as smoking, ownership of pets and the use of indoor appliances as well as other social factors known to be associated with poor health. The relationship between respiratory symptoms, dampness and air spore count remained after all other possible explanatory factors were statistically ruled out.

Indirect effects of dampness on health

Dampness can lead to overcrowding when occupants avoid using a damp room. Dampness and mould cause damage to property and add to the financial burden of those on low income. Keeping the house clean can be difficult, and visible mould and the smell of dampness may lead to embarrassment about inviting friends and family in. Concerns about the impact of dampness on the health of children can be an additional stress.

Working in the home

There are fitness standards for formal work environments such as offices (see pp. 56–57), but not for domestic housing. People who are not in formal employment may spend substantial amounts of time in housing environments which would not meet the minimum occupational health standards. Carrying out housework such as child care, cleaning and cooking is particularly stressful in poor conditions.

Housing and health services

Health professionals must consider the extent to which patients' illness or distress is the result of their living conditions. Health professionals are sometimes asked to comment formally on this in assessments of medical priority for rehousing or assessments for community care (see pp. 156–157). The moves to day-case interventions and early discharge from hospital make it even more important that health professionals know about patients' housing conditions and ensure that poor living conditions do not exacerbate illness or prejudice recovery.

Housing, homelessness and health

- The housing environment affects health directly and indirectly.
- Overcrowding, noise, dampness, cold, poor design and poor neighbourhood are detrimental to health.
- Being housed does not necessarily imply having a home.
- Housework is often carried out in conditions that would not satisfy Health and Safety at Work standards.
- Provision of adequate, affordable housing is an important component of a policy for health.

Work and health

The United Nations Declaration of Human Rights states that 'Everyone has the right to work'. Does this imply that work is 'good' for us and for our health? Is all work good for us? Table 1 summarizes some of the characteristics of work which have been identified as important for health. The other side of this picture is that the absence of these criteria can lead to ill health and injury. World Health Organization statistics tell us that 2 million people worldwide die each year from work-related accidents and disease. The 'right to work' is, therefore, complemented by the United Nations International Labour Organization's (ILO) commitment to 'adequate protection for the life and health of workers in all occupations'.

The world of work is changing in the 21st century. The health of working people will be affected by these changes, which include: increased use of information technology; increase in small businesses; falling trade union membership; more women and older people in the workforce; intensification of work; 24-hour society (e.g. call centres); increased demand for flexibility; more temporary/short-term contracts; growing inequality in skill levels; downsizing; privatization of state-owned industries. Globalization of industry is accelerating and can lead to the export of health and safety risks from the developed to the developing world. The ILO estimates that the fatal injury rate for established market economies is 5 per 100 000 workers whereas that for Asia reaches 23 per 100 000 workers.

Work-related ill health and injury

Discovering accurate information regarding the extent of work-related ill health and injury is difficult. In the UK there is systematic underreporting. The government accepts that less than half of non-fatal incidents reportable by law to the Health and Safety Executive are in fact reported (Health and Safety Executive, 2000a). As well as official reporting mechanisms, data come from a number of sources, including voluntary reporting schemes by occupational physicians and regular Labour Force surveys at both UK and continental European levels. The latter indicate that about 2 million people in the UK are suffering from work-related ill health and that 27% of European workers consider their health to be at risk from their work.

Accidents

At the turn of the new century, the UK government launched a strategy to address the continuing toll taken by workplace injury and ill health. One of the targets of the strategy *Revitalising Health and Safety* (Health and Safety Executive, 2000a) was to reduce fatal and major injuries by 10% by the year 2010. Sadly, progress toward that goal is low. Figures released for the year 2006–2007 show that 241 workers died in that year from work injuries, 11% higher than the previous year and the highest since 2001–2002. In 2006–2007, 274 000 reportable injuries occurred, according to the Labour Force Survey, a rate of 1000 per 100 000 workers (Health and Safety Executive, 2008). It is important to recognize that risk of accidents is not uniform, but is concentrated in certain industries, e.g. construction and agriculture, and among certain groups of workers, for example young workers, who are at 37% higher risk of injury.

Occupational ill health

A less visible but more extensive problem is that of work-related ill health and disease (Fig. 1). Common work-related conditions are back and other musculoskeletal problems, respiratory conditions such as asthma and bronchitis, work-related dermatitis and psychological conditions. With changes in the working environment, some conditions decline – for example, bladder cancer in the rubber industry – but others increase, for example, dermatitis and occupational asthma caused by exposure to a wide range of substances, including latex in disposable gloves, and stress-related conditions. Deaths related to work-related disease are over 20 times those of work accidents. The majority of these deaths are due to occupational cancers. Recent research indicates that 12% of all cancer deaths in the UK are caused by work. Of particular concern is the fact that this burden of death does not fall equally, but is concentrated in skilled and unskilled manual workers.

Responsibility for health at work

There is an apparent conflict for employers in the implementation of a healthy and safe environment. Creating such an environment can be costly in terms of both time and money. However, this must be balanced against the greater cost of not taking action, including sickness absence, increased turnover, compensation costs, damage to morale and industrial relations and, most importantly, the personal cost to the individual worker. Employees too may be caught in an economic conflict and may ignore health and safety in some situations, for example, where pay is related to speed or levels of production.

The law places the responsibility for workplace health firmly with the employer, although employees too have duties to take care of themselves and others and to follow health and safety rules. Most accidents are systems failures. Two independent studies have found that in only about 18% and 11% of cases respectively was the employee responsible for the accident and even in these cases part of the cause may be lack of training, low morale or pressure of work.

Prevention through risk assessment

Throughout mainland Europe, and increasingly internationally, the accepted place to start in addressing workplace health protection is risk assessment. In the UK this principle is now enshrined in the Health and Safety at Work Act 1974 through its many sets of regulations. It entails:

Table 1 **Characteristics of 'healthy' jobs**	
Pay and conditions	Good wages/benefits
	Security
Physical environment	Protection from physical, chemical and biological hazards
Demands	Neither too much nor too little work. Not excessive hours
	Clarity of role and no conflicting demands
	Minimal unsocial hours or shiftwork
	Minimum conflict between demands of home and work
Skills	Ability to use skills and be creative
	Opportunity to develop new skills
Control	Ability to control how you work
	Participation in decision-making
	Ability to organize independently
Support	Collaboration and collective effort. Good communication
	Good relationships with colleagues and supervisors
	Being valued and respected. Equality of treatment

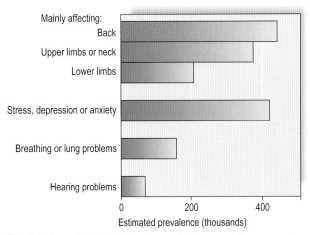

Fig. 1 Estimated 2005–2006 prevalence of self-reported illness caused or made worse by work, by type of illness, for people ever employed (from www.hse.gov.uk/statistics).

- Proactive, detailed consideration of the work environment and all work tasks; identification of hazards (something with the potential to do harm).
- Assessment of levels of risk (the likelihood of harm occurring) and severity (how serious the harm would be).
- Planning and implementation of action to eliminate hazards or reduce risk.
- Monitoring to ensure the effectiveness of that action.

By definition, risk assessment is a management responsibility, must be carried out by a competent person and should involve consultation with the workforce.

One of the key groups in effective prevention are occupational health physicians, nurses and other occupational health professionals. However, Health and Safety Executive figures indicate that two-thirds of working people in the UK have no access to occupational health expertise and support. The UK situation compares badly with continental Europe, where in some Nordic countries coverage nears 100%. Another key group is the trade unions. Research shows that workplaces with active unions show a 50% reduction in workplace injuries.

Stress at work

Stress is now the second largest cause of work-related ill health and sickness absence in Europe, next only to back and other musculoskeletal conditions. Research has shown that failure to provide the elements listed in Table 1 can result in work-related stress (Cox et al., 2000). Evidence of the link between stress and ill health is growing. Research shows that job insecurity leads to increased self-reported ill health and clinical symptoms, with those at the lowest levels of the company being worst affected. The introduction of new technology can lead to psychological distress, particularly among lower-paid, less-skilled and older workers. There is clear evidence of links between stress and coronary heart disease but conflicting evidence about which stress factors are most implicated. Overtime work is associated with high blood pressure. It is known that stress can suppress the immune system (Platt et al., 1999).

It is now accepted that organizational solutions (primary prevention) aimed at addressing the causes of stress are more effective than interventions targeted at individual coping skills (secondary prevention) or counselling (tertiary prevention), although the best employers will provide all three. Factors that potentially lead to stress are now included in those which employers must risk-assess.

Work–life balance

A problem reported by workers throughout Europe is the difficulty in achieving a healthy balance between work and life outside work. This is exacerbated in the UK by the longest working hours in Europe. Women bear the brunt of this. Even when working full-time, women still carry much higher levels of responsibility for the home, including care of children and other dependants. On the other hand, there is now clear evidence that financial and physical well-being are strongly linked to paid employment. Domestic labour can be routine, boring, unpaid and undervalued. However, when women choose to enter paid employment they are consistently paid less than men, which means that childcare costs take a proportionately higher percentage of their income. There is now pressure on employers to consider the introduction of family-friendly policies to address this issue, for example, flexible working hours, home working, term-time working, job shares and subsidized childcare. In the case of parents and carers, employers are under a legal obligation to consider employee flexible-working requests.

 STOP THINK When making diagnoses and considering causes of ill health, it is important for doctors to think and ask about work as well as biological and social factors. Did you know that approximately 8% of patient visits to GPs are about work-related conditions? Higher numbers will be suffering from some form of condition caused or made worse by work.

Case study

Clare, a young textile worker, went to her GP complaining of episodes of dizziness and fainting. Her symptoms were worse during the working week and improved when away from work. This pattern suggested that her ill health might be the result of chemical exposure at work. She was referred to an occupational physician, who confirmed that this was the likely cause. The chemical was probably formaldehyde, a chemical used to pretreat permanent-press garments. It was recommended that exposure levels be limited as far as possible. After communication between her GP, the occupational physician and Clare's employer, her employer agreed to improvements in ventilation and in the chemical process involved, and Clare's symptoms subsequently disappeared.

Work and health

- Official figures for occupational death, injury and disease underestimate the total amount of occupational ill health.
- It is crucial in occupational health as well as any other health field to prioritize prevention.
- Worldwide trends in employment have important implications for occupational health and safety.
- High-demand and low-control jobs create stress, which can cause ill health.
- One major issue facing all workers but particularly women is finding a balance between demands at work and at home.

Unemployment and health

As we move into the era of what has been called 'liquid' capitalism, we are witnessing increased part-time employment, more flexible work patterns and more self-employment. At the same time unemployment over the life course will become a more common experience for a sizeable section of the population. Unemployment will be especially high for young men (Luck et al., 2000). There will be more chronic unemployment and more workless households. Medical professionals will increasingly be faced with having to deal with the health effects of unemployment (Wadsworth et al., 1999).

The evidence and mechanisms

It is now accepted that unemployment is a stressful life event that can cause ill health and even mortality (Table 1). Research has also been able to capitalize on the volume of work carried out since the 1990s which gives more attention to the mechanisms that cause ill health. One way to summarize the research evidence is by considering causality and the possible links between unemployment and ill health and mortality (Fig. 1). We can consider each pathway in turn.

The stress pathway – psychological morbidity and mortality

Stress is strongly associated with lowered mental well-being and becoming unemployed is a serious stressful life event. A study by Weich & Lewis (1998) on 7726 adults drawn from the British household panel study found that unemployment was associated with the maintenance of episodes of most common mental disorders. An important series of studies on psychological well-being was carried out by Warr (1978) and colleagues on different subgroups of the unemployed. An index of present life satisfaction was found to be strongly negatively associated with unemployment for both redundant steelworkers and men attending unemployment benefit offices. On the other hand, a measure of constant self-esteem yielded no differences between managers with or without a job.

A similar pattern emerged for measures of positive well-being, where a person was asked if he/she had experienced positive events in the past few weeks. Positive effect in recent weeks among redundant steelworkers was clearly associated with their employment status at the time of interview. Indicators of negative well-being, where the interviewees were asked if they had experienced negative events – for example, feelings of loneliness – in the past few weeks, showed the clearest overall relationship, with significant differences between employed and unemployed respondents in every case.

Importantly these studies also threw light on some of the factors that moderated the negative impact of unemployment:

■ People who were committed to their work and who became redundant were found to be particularly disadvantaged.

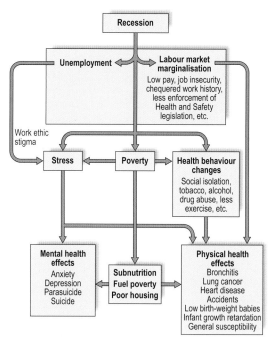

Fig. 1 How might unemployment lead to poor health?

■ Age and length of unemployment were likely to be inter-correlated, and so older people were less likely to become re-employed and were more likely to be sick. The middle-aged unemployed, in fact, were found to have the lowest well-being scores.

■ Although they found differences between the sexes, with men having higher rates of psychological morbidity than women, this was thought to be related to personal commitment to their work. When the variable of personal work involvement was held constant, the sexes were equally affected.

Death rates have also been found to rise in times of economic depression; unemployed people have higher death rates than the employed; and death rates rise with the increasing duration of unemployment. A British study (Moser et al., 1984) looked at 5861 men aged 15–64 years who were waiting to take up a job or were seeking work in the week before the 1971 census. The standardized mortality ratio for 1971–1981 for men aged 15–64 years at death who were seeking work in 1971 was 136. It was particularly high among those under 54 years, reaching over 200 in those aged 35–44 years. The causes of death that predominated among the unemployed were malignant neoplasms (particularly lung cancer), accidents, poisonings and violence (particularly suicide). The stress pathway is partly implicated in some of these causes of death.

Association or cause?

Any cross-sectional analysis comparing groups of employed workers with unemployed men and women shows that employed people are healthier despite occupational hazards. These studies also give us some interesting pointers towards the health condition of the long-term unemployed (for more than 1 year), among whom there are likely to be far more health problems than among the short-term unemployed. Such studies cannot, however, tell us whether these effects are specifically caused by unemployment. Selection processes operate; individuals may have become unemployed because they had health problems to begin with. It is also difficult to separate out the direct effect of

Table 1 **Trends in death rates/100 000 persons by employment status and social class among men aged 36–64, 1971 cohort, England and Wales**

Social class		Follow-up period			
		1976–81c*	1981c*–1985	1986–1991c*	1991c*–95
Employed	Non-manual	3361	2518	2178	1642
	Manual	4105	3281	3281	2455
Unemployed	Non-manual	4689	3980	2500	2889
	Manual	5917	4505	6059	4113

*1981/91 refers to day before census day in the first time period and census day onwards in the following time period. Adapted from Harding et al. (1999).

unemployment from any indirect effect of poverty, bad housing conditions, geographical location and social class. Although most research produces correlations between unemployment and health, the establishment of causality requires studies over time, looking at workers before termination of their employment and following them through and after redundancy.

An important American longitudinal study looked at 100 men who lost their job and 74 controls who did not as a result of two factories closing. The study followed the cohort from preclosure to 2 years postclosure. The controls were found to be healthier than the terminees. Myocardial infarction was at the expected level, but the risk of coronary heart disease had increased among the terminees. Research by Beale & Nethercott (1985) on a factory closure in south-west England found increased consultation rates with GPs and increased referral rates to hospital among redundant workers and members of their families compared with controls.

Ferrie et al. (2001) considered the health effects of privatization after one department of the civil service was sold to the private sector. Eighteen months after privatization they analysed the results for two groups: (1) the insecure re-employed and unemployed; and (2) those permanently exited from paid employment. Within group 1, they found significant increases in minor psychiatric morbidity and consultations with a GP. Within group 2 levels of long-standing illness were significantly different, but not the rest of the measures. This demonstrates that both insecure re-employment and unemployment were associated with increased minor psychiatric morbidity and that being permanently out of paid work was associated with long-standing illness.

As mentioned above, death rates are elevated among the unemployed. For example, the British Regional Heart Study (Morris et al., 1994), after controlling for social class and health at time of entry into the study, found that unemployed men aged 40–59 years were 1.7 times more likely to have died after 5-year follow-up than men who were not unemployed during that time. The study by Harding et al. (1999), analysing data from the Office for National Statistics longitudinal study, found that from 1976 to 1995 mortality among the unemployed was higher, within each class grouping, than among the employed (Table 1). As Drever & Whitehead (1997) state: 'Losing his job doubles the chances of a middle-aged man dying within the next five years.'

Relative poverty of health related behaviour

The work of Wadsworth et al. (1999) and Weich & Lewis (1998) stress the interplay between unemployment itself and linked financial elements, and we can see the central position of this element in Figure 1. Psychological health is seen to be affected by financial problems that increase the frequency of stressful life events. Mental health is also affected by decreasing social activity and participation, and diminishing social support. Although alternative social networks may eventually be formed, these may involve groups who have withdrawn from the norms and values of mainstream society. They may, thus, be more likely to indulge in health-damaging behaviours: tobacco and alcohol use, drug-taking and bad diet. In terms of physical health the 'stress pathway', involving physiological changes (for example, raised cholesterol and lowered immunity), is believed to be the main mechanism. The importance of relative rather than just absolute disadvantage has also been highlighted in the recent literature (see pp. 44–45, 48–49). Work by Wadsworth et al. (1999) looked at a longer timeframe, focused on younger age groups and considered the effects

of today's increasingly fluid labour market. They concluded that: 'prolonged unemployment early in the working life of this population of young men was likely to have a persisting effect' on their future health. This has obvious implications for the importance of targeting our efforts towards reducing unemployment among the young.

Conclusion: policy implications

So how can we mitigate the worst effects of unemployment upon health? In Figure 1 we can see the centrality of poverty within the unemployment and health nexus. Government policies directed at alleviating economic disadvantage will therefore cushion the worst health-related effects of unemployment. Research carried out by Wilkinson (1998) (see pp. 44–45) on different European countries has already demonstrated the moderating health effects within those countries with the best social security provision. But of course GPs and hospital doctors have their own part to play in giving advice to patients to reduce secondary health effects related to stress and disadvantageous behavioural change, and to ensure that they also claim the benefits to which they are entitled (see pp. 44–45).

STOP THINK Social scientists are now predicting rapidly increasing trends towards flexibility in the world's labour markets (Westergaard et al., 1989). They also believe that detrimental health effects will be particularly bad for young people (Lewis & Sloggett 1998).
■ What do you think?

Case study

The personal effect of unemployment

CM is an unemployed 28-year-old and lives with his partner in obvious conditions of hardship. I could do better. I could pack up the fags with an effort of will. I think I could stop drinking. But there is a kind of need there as well. When I go for a drink, I don't really feel like it's enjoyment. I feel it's a need to get pissed, a need to get stoned… because you kind of feel shit that you have got no money so you try to look for a release or escape from that and then because it costs you money to do that so you end up on this downward spiral… There is also a big tension because I know quite a bit about health and diet. It was always an interest of mine. The impact of the way you lived on your health and stuff. So I do feel a total idiot sometimes that I smoke, because I know all the stuff and I never wanted to see myself as a 'smoker'. I wanted to be healthier than that… People say you drink and smoke and take drugs and it is seen that you do that because you like to have fun, but it is not about that at all. They are missing the point totally. It is a form of escapism if you like… You do sort of push things aside. Like you numb your brain with certain chemicals and things and that is the escapist aspect of it. (from A. Dolan, PhD thesis, University of Warwick, 2003).

Unemployment and health

■ All cross-sectional studies show the employed to be in better health than the unemployed. Longitudinal studies strongly suggest that the contrast is caused by unemployment rather than by selection within the labour market.

■ The main causes of mortality among the unemployed are malignant neoplasms (particularly lung cancer), accidents, poisonings and violence (particularly suicide).

■ Relative poverty, social isolation and lack of self-esteem, and damaging health-related behaviours are the major factors associated with the production of ill effects among the unemployed.

Labelling and stigma

We all use labels to name and describe things. Such labelling can have both positive and negative associations, for example the 'good doctor', the 'caring nurse' or the 'lazy medical student'! Labelling and its associated idea of stigma are useful in understanding the importance of the *social* consequences of medical diagnosis. We are particularly interested here in the way neutral medical labels acquire negative and stigmatizing connotations. Labelling and stigma are important for medical practitioners for two reasons. Firstly, negative labels are often applied by the public at large to people with particular diseases such as epilepsy, schizophrenia or psoriasis which are thought to signify some moral failing, social disgrace or separation from normal society. Such beliefs may be rooted in superstition, fear and ignorance but they are quite common. Secondly, medical practitioners act as important arbiters of the labels that get applied in much of what they do.

Doctors and labelling

A medical diagnosis is also a social label with potentially powerful negative consequences. For example, a psychiatrist in diagnosing mental illness is doing more than prescribing a course of treatment. Such a diagnosis may result in significant restraints on liberty if institutional care is involved. General practitioners sign sick notes and declare people unfit to work and eligible to receive financial benefit from the state. A chest physician may be called upon to assess the degree of loss of lung function in a man with asbestos-related illness who is making a claim against his former employer. In each of these three examples the medical diagnosis is also an important social label with social consequences and moral and financial implications.

The medical diagnosis is a biological or medical explanation of some underlying pathology in the body or mind. However, that diagnosis has social effects that go well beyond biology and may have significant social and psychological consequences for the person and perhaps his or her family and employer.

Social reaction

The behaviour of the public is strongly influenced by medical labels. Think of the types of reaction that are often made to diagnoses of cancer. But it is not only life-threatening illnesses that produce strong reactions. For example, knowing that someone has epilepsy, or has been a patient in a psychiatric hospital, can strongly affect the way others respond to them. People react not just to the biological pathology, but to what they regard as its social significance. When the social significance of the label carries a strongly negative connotation, this is an example of what sociologists and psychologists call *stigma*. The two terms – labelling and stigma – are not interchangeable because some labels are highly positive. However, in the context of medical work, it is the negative attributions by self or others that are of particular significance.

The case study shows that an important distinction needs to be made between the presence of some deviation from normality – in this case the presence of unrecognized coronary heart disease – and the social reaction to the subsequent diagnosis – the change in the man's behaviour

and the response of his wife and the insurance company. Sociologists have called this distinction primary and secondary deviation (Lemert, 1951). *Primary deviation* is some kind of physical or social difference of an individual or a group. *Secondary deviation* is the response of self and others to the public recognition – the label – of that difference.

This idea of primary and secondary deviation was originally developed in a classic text about crime by Edwin Lemert (1951). Lemert observed that many people commit crimes. He also noted that for the vast majority of people this is only a brief excursion into things like petty shoplifting, under-age drinking, pilfering in the office, fiddling their expenses or speeding in their car. The point was that these activities did not lead to a life of crime. Indeed, the vast majority of people who have at one time or another transgressed the law actually regard themselves as morally upright citizens. For most people, in other words, their law-breaking has no long-term effects because it is not detected and it is not punished and very few others know about it. Their law-breaking is the primary deviation since a deviant act has been committed. Secondary deviation occurs if and when the general public, the courts and the police respond to an individual as a criminal and that person's whole life gets caught up in that social role. Career criminals are classically involved in the reinforcement of their own secondary deviation.

Stigma

The term 'stigma' is most usually associated with the work of Erving Goffman (1968a) in another classic text. He was particularly interested in the public humiliations and social disgrace that may happen to people where highly negative labels are applied. He made the distinction between *discreditable* and *discrediting* stigma. A discreditable stigma is one that is not known about by the many people with whom the person with the stigma comes into contact everyday. Only the person with the stigmatizing condition and a few close intimates will know about it. A discrediting stigma, on the other hand, is one that cannot be hidden from other people because it is obvious and visible. People respond to the condition rather than to the person (Fig. 1).

A good example of a discreditable stigma is a patient who has had a mastectomy or an ileostomy (see pp. 116–117). To people in the street such patients look quite normal when they are fully clothed. Apart from their closest friends and relatives, their doctor and the few other people they might wish to inform, their's is a hidden stigma. Other people do not react to it because it is not obvious and they therefore do not know about it. Individuals with a mastectomy or an ileostomy may go to great lengths to conceal their physical difference – say by not going to a swimming pool and never getting undressed in front of strangers. The existence of mastectomy or ileostomy will be very important to them, and will have an effect in their own thoughts, feelings and behaviour. To other people, because it can't be seen and is therefore not known about, it is irrelevant (Kelly, 1991).

In contrast, someone with an amputation, or who is in a wheelchair, or who has lost an eye, does not have the option of concealing these things from others very easily and people respond on the basis of the visible difference

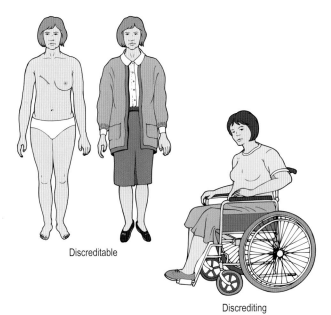

Discreditable

Discrediting

Fig. 1 Discreditable and discrediting stigma.

rather than the person (Fig. 1). What this means is that, for some disabilities and diseases, individuals have little control over the publicly available information about them. As that information may be the basis of judgements, both positive and negative, and these judgements can have profound social and psychological effects, they are important medical issues.

Felt stigma and enacted stigma

A distinction that is sometimes made is between *enacted* stigma and *felt* stigma. Enacted stigma is the real experience of prejudice, discrimination and disadvantage as the consequence

STOP THINK

- What are likely to be the primary and secondary deviations as a consequence of screening for disease? Note: no screening test is 100% accurate.

- What are some examples of screening tests which might produce stigma?

- Not all medical conditions carry negative labels. Patients with the common cold, chickenpox, measles and influenza, or who fracture their leg playing soccer, do not generally attract stigmatizing labels, and the social response of the general public is usually unremarkable. Indeed, such illnesses may attract sympathy. Why do these illnesses attract sympathy?

- Problems such as alcoholism, schizophrenia, syphilis, HIV/AIDS and epilepsy, however, frequently do attract highly negative labels. What is the reason for these conditions attracting negative labels?

- Are smoking-related diseases and obesity stigmatized conditions?

- What are the implications of the existence of groups of illnesses that are stigmatized for the provision of care?

- Do you think that treatment decisions and decisions to fund certain drugs are linked to issues of stigma?

Case study

Negative labels applied to self: the case of coronary heart disease

A middle-aged man has begun to experience the early symptoms of angina. He does not know what the pains are and he merely assumes they are typical for a man of his age and are caused by his playing vigorous games of cricket with his grandson. So long as he believes his pains are the harmless consequences of ageing, he will do nothing to alter his behaviour; indeed he continues to smoke and to drink alcohol as he has done for the last 40 years. A biological abnormality is present that could be medically detected but has not been yet and the disease has not yet reached a point where it is significantly debilitating. Therefore, it has had no social consequence for the man or his family.

However, let us assume this man goes for a routine insurance medical because he wants to alter his pension plan. He describes his symptoms and the doctor suspects heart disease. Following investigation, coronary heart disease is diagnosed. The medical label is applied and treatment can begin. But let us also imagine how the man feels. He is now a patient who thinks of himself as a cardiac case. He is very frightened. He immediately stops smoking. He also gives up drinking and goes on to a low-fat diet. He becomes extremely concerned about overexertion and gives up playing cricket with his grandson. His wife also becomes anxious and discourages him from digging the garden and insists that he sit in an armchair at home. Finally, he is unable to get additional insurance and alter his pension. We can see that this man's life has been transformed, even though biologically speaking his angina is no worse now than it was before he had his medical check-up. However, his own behaviour, that of his wife and, indeed, that of his insurance company have all changed as a consequence of the medical label.

of a particular condition, say epilepsy. However, the research shows, at least in the case of epilepsy, that such frank negative stigmatization and labelling is thankfully relatively rare (Scambler & Hopkins, 1986). However, it is the fear that such discrimination might occur – which is defined as felt stigma – that can be so worrying. This is why the degree to which people feel able to be in control of information about themselves is so important. In epilepsy, for example, the worry may stem from the fact that the disease is not well controlled, and the concern is about having a seizure in public.

Labelling and stigma

- In the social and behavioural sciences labelling refers to the social response of individuals and groups to physical, psychological or social characteristics and particularly differences in others.

- Medical diagnoses are an extremely important example of labels in this sense, and doctors are key people in some labelling processes through the act of diagnosis.

- Not all labels are negative, but some medical ones certainly are.

- Primary deviation refers to the fact of biological, physical or social difference.

- Secondary deviation refers to the social response of the individual and others to the difference.

- Stigma is a particularly negative form of labelling.

- The fear of stigmatization is a very powerful force affecting people's behaviour.

- Stigma and labelling may play a part in some medical decision-making.

Perceptions of risk and risk-taking behaviours

The identification of risk factors for disease is important for prevention. We know that social as well as biological factors are implicated in the patterning of ill health. However, there is also increasing emphasis on the importance of lifestyle and the role of health-related behaviours in both preventing and causing disease and ill health. Those behaviours that are deleterious to health can be termed risk-taking behaviours, because of the known risk they pose for an individual's health. In recent years there has been a growing emphasis on individuals' responsibility for their own health and the promotion of behaviour change to reduce an individual's risk of disease and ill health (pp. 74–75).

This has brought with it an emphasis on self-control, on moderation in behaviour and on the provision of information to inform people of the risks to health associated with certain lifestyles and behaviours. However, it is important to recognize that individuals' potential for control over their lifestyles, behaviours and health is limited by the social circumstances in which they live and which shape their lives (pp. 44–45). Understanding people's own perceptions of risk and the contexts within which their risk-taking behaviours occur is important for doctors and others who may be assessing a patient's risk of disease and encouraging a healthier lifestyle.

Perceptions of risk

Ignorance is often considered to be a major barrier to following lifestyle advice, although there is much evidence to suggest that the lay public are well aware of the publicized risks to health, such as the relationship between smoking and lung cancer or the range of risk factors associated with heart disease. In fact, research suggests that knowledge itself is not a powerful predictor of behaviour.

People may view a range of risks very differently. For example, salmonella infection from egg consumption was viewed as very risky when this was highlighted in the media, although the chances of infection were small. However, the longer-term risks of cholesterol and heart disease were not viewed in the same way. These different perceptions of risk may influence behaviour in different ways, with reactive lifestyle changes around egg consumption occurring quickly, but modification of diet to prevent heart disease being much harder to achieve.

People have a tendency to believe that their chances of experiencing a negative event, including illness, are less than average, but that their chances are higher than average for a positive event. This is called 'unrealistic optimism' or 'optimistic bias' (Weinstein, 1982). Factors regarded by individuals as decreasing their risk include both personal actions (for example, engaging in preventive health behaviours or seeking appropriate help) and psychological attributes such as personality, values held, likes and dislikes (for example, being the type of person who does not let things get you down, or being 'health-conscious'). These are both associated with perceived controllability of the event. Environmental or hereditary factors are not perceived in the same way. The predominant characteristics affecting optimistic bias are: the belief that if the problem has not yet appeared, there will be an exemption from future risk; that

the problem is perceived as preventable through individual action; that the hazard is perceived as infrequent; and that there is a lack of experience with the hazard (Weinstein, 1987). Some research has suggested that people nonetheless overestimate their absolute risk of a disease, such as breast cancer, and also overestimate the chances of surviving 5 years after diagnosis, of the cancer being curable and the chances of cancer being detected by mammogram (Clarke et al., 2000). However, in relation to perceived risk of disease, although people overestimate their own risk, they do this to a lesser extent than they do for others. In other words, they still retain an optimistic bias about themselves relative to similar others.

Optimistic bias may result in weakened intentions to prevent future ill health. However, in some cases, optimistic bias (in relation to control) may strengthen intentions to take preventive action because optimistic bias enhances self-efficacy (see pp. 142–143) and belief in the controllability of negative events (Weinstein & Lyon, 1999). For example, a man might overestimate his ability to make lifestyle changes (such as giving up smoking or taking up exercise) but also overestimate the extent to which changes will reduce their risk of disease (e.g. eating less high-fat food will not remove the risk of heart disease). There is also some evidence that unrealistic optimism is associated with positive well-being. The relative importance of the positive or negative aspects of optimistic bias will depend very much on the nature of the health problem – compare a patient recovering from a heart attack, for example, with an intravenous drug user. It is important to understand risk perception as individuals are unlikely to engage in health-protective behaviours unless they perceive themselves to be susceptible (Weinstein, 1984; Petrie et al., 1996).

Differences between lay and expert perceptions of risk in relation to health can be better understood when lay knowledge is viewed in the context of people's lives and experience. It is important that lay perceptions of risk are not just seen as wrong or based on ignorance, but rather as embedded in particular social and cultural circumstances, as examined in the following example.

Example 1: lay understanding of heart disease

A large, indepth study of people living in south Wales investigated lay explanations of heart disease. This research took place during a large campaign to prevent heart disease (Davison et al., 1991). The results showed that people had their own explanations for the causes of heart disease, which drew on, yet differed from, the publicized lifestyle risks. In this 'lay epidemiology', people drew on a range of knowledge and experience to explain who was a candidate for heart disease (Box 1). This included lifestyle factors, heredity, social environment such as work, physical environment such as climate, and a degree of randomness attributed to luck and chance.

This demonstrates that people understand the range of risks associated with heart disease, not just those associated with lifestyle. However, people are also well aware, from their personal observations, that those at high risk of getting heart disease do not always suffer from it, and that sometimes those at low risk do. People know that predicting who will actually get ill is difficult for those conditions that are multifactorial

Box 1 **People who may be identified as coronary candidates**
- Fat people; people who don't take exercise and are unfit
- Red-faced people; people with a grey pallor
- Smokers
- People with a heart problem in the family
- Heavy drinkers
- People who eat excessive amounts of rich, fatty foods
- Worriers (by nature); bad-tempered, pessimistic or negative people
- People who are under stress from:
  - Work
  - Family life
  - Financial difficulty
  - Unemployment/retirement
  - Bereavement
  - Gambling
- People who suffer strain through:
  - Hard manual labour
  - Conditions of work/home
  - Excessive leisure exercise
  - Overindulgence (sex, dancing, drugs, lack of sleep, etc.)

(From Davison et al., 1991, with permission.)

(i.e. caused by several different factors). Any attempt to oversimplify this with an emphasis on behaviour such as eating is likely to be sceptically received, as lay people's own experience and knowledge tell them that the process is more complicated and less certain than that.

Risk-taking behaviour

Just as it is important to understand lay perceptions of risk, risk-taking behaviour must also be examined in the context of individuals' lives. Risk-taking behaviours often do not take place in isolation, but in interaction with others. This can explain why some people indulge in behaviours that are considered to be, even by themselves, detrimental to health. The following example will help to demonstrate the importance of social context in understanding risk-taking behaviour: it considers the practice of unsafe commercial sex between men. The case study focuses on young people and smoking.

Example 2: unsafe commercial sex between men
A study by Bloor et al. (1992) of the risk-taking behaviours of male prostitutes in Glasgow, Scotland, demonstrated the importance of social interaction and social relations in determining behaviour. All but one of the 10 male prostitutes they contacted were practising unsafe commercial sex. However, these same prostitutes knew that this behaviour was risky, especially in terms of HIV transmission, and also knew that they were vulnerable to infection. It was the social

STOP THINK
- Why might knowledge of risk factors for ill health not influence an individual's behaviour?
- In what ways are individuals constrained in their actions?
- Think of some 'unhealthy behaviours' that you engage in. Now think about some others that your friends engage in. What explanations can you think of for both your own and your friends' behaviours?

circumstances surrounding male prostitution that led to the practice of unsafe sex. Unlike much female prostitution, where negotiation of fee and terms is established by the prostitute at the start of the encounter, the male prostitutes studied were subjected to client control – they themselves had little say over what should happen. This situation can partly be explained by the covert and stigmatized nature of the activity: it is neither legal nor socially sanctioned.

Practical applications

Recognition of the social context of risk, in terms of both perceptions of risk and risk-taking behaviours, is important for doctors as they become involved in public health and health promotion as well as in dealing with individual patients. Doctors should try to elicit people's own explanations and treat these as reasonable and based on experience. This should lead to greater understanding and empathy between doctor and patient (pp. 94–95). Similarly, account must be taken of the circumstances within which people live and how this may influence their behaviour. Doctors should not promote 'victim-blaming', where those who engage in behaviours considered damaging to their health are deemed to be irresponsible. Often such behaviour can be considered a rational response to poor social conditions, or the only choice in a situation where the individual has little control.

Case study

Young people and smoking
In a qualitative study of young people's perceptions of smoking, Allbutt et al. (1995) found that those studied were well aware of the risks associated with smoking: indeed, some had direct experience of its effects within their own families. However, both smokers and non-smokers discussed the positive aspects of smoking, such as the image, weight loss or relaxation. These are some of the things they said: 'It felt good, I felt big.' 'It relaxes you, that's why I like it.' 'If you've got a drink or a cigarette it's easier to talk to somebody because you can do something with your hands if you're not talking to them.' 'It helps me when I'm stressed.'

Smoking itself was experienced as an activity that took place within a group, where friendship is important. These positive aspects encourage risk-taking behaviour. Attempts to prevent young people smoking should go beyond the provision of relevant information, and acknowledge the meaning that the behaviour has for them, in the context of their own lives.

Perceptions of risk and risk-taking behaviours
- The concept of a risk factor for disease is important for both professionals and the lay public.
- Risk perceptions and risk-taking behaviours are part of a wider social context, including both social conditions and social interactions.
- These may constrain the choices that individuals can make; risk-taking behaviours should be seen, at least in part, as socially determined.
- Promoting healthy behaviours means more than encouraging individuals to change. People's own risk perceptions must be understood.

What is prevention?

The goals of prevention are to preserve and promote good health in society by preventing disease and minimizing its consequences. It is useful to distinguish between three types of prevention, usually referred to as primary, secondary and tertiary prevention. The distinction between these three types of prevention is that each has a different goal. Have a look at Table 1 before you read on.

Primary prevention: disease incidence

The incidence of disease is measured in terms of the number of new cases of disease occurring in society, usually during a specified time period, such as 1 year. Primary prevention can be undertaken whenever the cause of disease has been identified.

Perhaps the best-known form of medical intervention in primary prevention is mass immunization. Over the years, immunization has been introduced against poliomyelitis, tuberculosis, measles and many other diseases. However, since it usually takes several years of medical research before a virus is identified and a vaccine developed, the impact of immunization on disease incidence is sometimes very small. Poliomyelitis immunization is probably one of the few medical interventions to have had a demonstrable primary prevention effect in the last century (Fig. 1).

Health education (e.g. advice to use condoms during sex) and public health measures that help people avoid contact with viruses and bacteria may be particularly valuable early interventions.

The major causes of death in developed countries today are

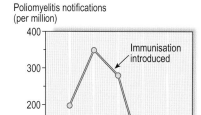

Fig. 1 Poliomyelitis notifications before and after introduction of immunization: England and Wales (adapted from McKeown, 1979, with permission).

diseases of the circulatory system and neoplasms (see pp. 42–43). These diseases have been linked to particular behaviours, such as smoking cigarettes. Figure 2 shows that smokers' life expectancy during the last century has increased only half as much as that of non-smokers, a remarkable finding given the improvements in nutrition and sanitation that have occurred during the same period. In developed

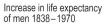
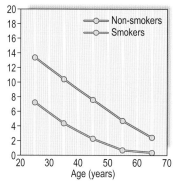

Fig. 2 Increase in expectation of life of men 1838–1970 (adapted from McKeown, 1979, with permission).

countries primary prevention efforts have been particularly concerned with health education regarding personal behaviours (see pp. 74–75).

Secondary prevention: disease prevalence

Prevalence is defined as the number of people who have a particular disease at any one time. Clearly, if diseases are left untreated and new cases are occurring all the time, the prevalence of a disease will increase. Although doctors are continually involved in secondary prevention, from time to time campaigns are mounted to increase the likelihood of doctors detecting particular diseases. For example, skin cancer may go unrecognized by patients and doctors unless specific efforts are made to identify it during consultations. Some forms of secondary prevention, such as screening for relatively rare diseases such as cervical cancer, require the participation of practically all women in society if those with the disease are to be detected and the screening programme is to prove cost-effective. Efforts to persuade people to take part may, therefore, be seen by some as efforts to compel people to participate in secondary prevention programmes, and doctors delivering these services need to be aware of the anxieties people have about screening tests (see pp. 68–69).

Tertiary prevention: adverse consequences of disease

As a result of increased life expectancy there is increasing concern for the care of people who survive treatment of, for example, heart disease, cancer or stroke. This means ensuring that patients experience the best possible health for the longest possible period of time following diagnosis. Tertiary prevention is concerned with a wider range of health indices than either primary or secondary prevention. For instance, tertiary preventive interventions might have as their goals the reduction of disability and promotion of psychological well-being. Exercise and rehabilitation programmes may be

Type of prevention	Distal goal	Proximal goal	Behavioural goal
Primary prevention	Prevent new cases of disease Prevent new cases of AIDS	Prevent infection with HIV	Use of condoms during sexual intercourse
Secondary prevention	Reduce number of people with disease at a given time Reduce cases of cervical cancer	Identify cervical cancer early and detect pre-cancerous cell abnormalities and treat effectively	Uptake of test to detect cancer and pre-cancer Uptake of treatment
Tertiary prevention	Minimize consequences of disease or impairment Minimize disability in children with cerebral palsy	Identify disability	Uptake and maintenance of skills training

Table 1 **Goals of prevention**

Table 2 **Levels of intervention to achieve behavioural change: fat in the diet**		
Level of intervention	**Example of intervention**	**Behavioural changes**
Governmental/societal	Legislation requiring manufacturers to specify the fat content of products on packaging	Agricultural policies to restrict animal fattening Research investment to develop low-fat food products Department of Health incentives to doctors to undertake prevention
Social/environmental	Mass-media health education	Provision of low-fat choices in schools/worksite canteens
Individual	Screening by doctors to assess risk and provide motivation and healthy-eating advice	Rehabilitation programmes by nurses and doctors to promote diet change, e.g. following heart attacks Food and cookery demonstrations and workshops in community centres School health education to provide motivation and skills

provided in medical settings and during follow-up care to enable stroke survivors to walk and acquire control over a range of movements (see pp. 118–119).

Chronic conditions that are genetically acquired or acquired during childhood or early adulthood are also a focus of tertiary prevention. These conditions cannot be cured, but much can be done to minimize the extent to which they result in disability or distress. A person with asthma can exercise control over his or her condition by using medication effectively and practising behavioural strategies to avoid attacks.

Levels of intervention

The success of prevention depends to a great extent upon the ability of the health care system and health care professionals to deliver preventive interventions to people who believe themselves to be in good health, and on the extent to which people take up interventions and are motivated and able to comply with behavioural recommendations. In order to bring about behavioural change, it is important to acknowledge the cultural and social influences that govern behaviour (see pp. 72–73).

Strategies to change behaviour occur at many different levels (Table 2). Action by governments is important in facilitating health-related behavioural change among both doctors and patients. For instance, in 1990 the British government changed the GP contract in order to encourage greater participation in preventive health care. One target for change was in primary and secondary prevention of heart disease. GPs were offered financial inducements to encourage them to screen patients with respect to their diet, smoking habits, exercise and blood cholesterol levels, and to offer appropriate treatments or behavioural change clinics to help people to modify their lifestyle. Governments may also seek to prevent heart disease by imposing taxes on cigarettes to limit their consumption or passing legislation that ensures that the fat content of food is clearly marked on labels so that people are able to make informed choices about their diet.

A second level of change concerns attempts to modify the social environment or commonly held views about health and health-related behaviours. People will be unable to change their diet if they have limited access to fruit and

vegetables in local shops or works canteens. Community- and organizational-level interventions can do a great deal to assist individual behavioural change. People are very much influenced in their behaviour by what they see or believe others do, and by what they think will be approved or disapproved of by others (see pp. 52–53).

At an individual level, health care professionals are directly involved in communicating to patients what preventive strategies they might use and advising them on how to implement these strategies. Doctors' advice to patients can be very effective in motivating people to change. Many preventive behaviours require people to acquire new skills and confidence in their ability to control or promote their own health. It is on the development and delivery of effective behaviour change strategies that much of primary and tertiary prevention depends (see pp. 74–75).

Dilemmas and problems in prevention

For many years, prevention has been seen to be the province of a specialty known as public health medicine. A shift towards prevention requires that all health professionals acquire new skills in the effective communication of health education messages and behaviour change strategies.

Some forms of prevention rely upon the participation of everyone in society in order to make them cost-effective. For example, infectious disease control depends, to a large extent, on what is known in epidemiology as herd immunity. These considerations may have led some to question how we distinguish between education, persuasion and compulsion. Other forms of prevention that are now becoming available rely on the detection of fetal abnormalities. The introduction of genetic screening has raised concerns about the ethics of parental choice and society's view of those with genetic disorders (see pp. 68–69).

STOP THINK

- How might you go about making a case for spending money on prevention?
- What ethical issues are associated with preventive programmes to: (1) immunize all children; (2) screen all women for cervical cancer; (3) ban smoking in public places; and (4) conduct genetic tests for fetal abnormalities?
- What skills do doctors require in order to practise preventive medicine effectively?

What is prevention?

- Primary prevention refers to the prevention of disease incidence.
- Secondary prevention refers to the prevention of disease prevalence.
- Tertiary prevention refers to the prevention of disease impact.
- Preventive efforts occur at many levels: the governmental or societal policy level, the social or environmental level and the individual level.

What are the objectives of health promotion?

The objectives of health promotion are: (1) to prevent disease; and (2) to promote health and well-being. The two are related. For example, the management of chronic pain involves supporting patients in maintaining as full and positive a life as possible, that is, maximizing well-being, which, in turn may reduce pain experience.

Health promotion is relevant to almost all areas of medicine but most attention is focused on diseases that have a substantial lifestyle component (Box 1).

Tones & Tilford (1994) have suggested three philosophies of health promotion: (1) social engineering; (2) individual prevention; and (3) individual empowerment.

> **Box 1 Main areas for health promotion**
>
> ■ Smoking
> ■ Diet and weight
> ■ Contraception and HIV prevention
> ■ Blood pressure monitoring
> ■ Screening for cancers
> ■ Alcohol and substance abuse
> ■ Responsible medication use
> ■ Child care
> ■ Exercise

Social engineering

Social engineering assumes that ill health is caused by social phenomena such as poverty, poor living conditions, lack of education, inappropriate cultural norms and inadequate health care. Consequently, health promotion objectives should be to improve living standards, change norms and improve health care access. Social engineering can be effective: for example, in southern India for cultural reasons birth control was often not used, but increasing women's literacy there also increased the adoption of birth control. Unfortunately, mass social engineering is often expensive and it can also be criticized for imposing change against some people's will or without consultation. For example, some people are opposed to the fluoridation of water, despite the dental benefits.

Individual prevention

This school of thought believes that health is strongly influenced by the behaviour and conditions of individuals and can, therefore, be improved by changing the individuals' health behaviours by education, advertising, technological interventions, such as seat belts, or making the holes in salt cellars smaller, as well as special medical treatment and screening. This approach fits with much medical thinking, which tends to be oriented towards treating individual patients. The most common form is probably the provision of leaflets informing patients about lifestyle factors (Fig. 1). Unfortunately, individualistic prevention involving education alone is rarely effective (see pp. 76–77). Also, there can be an element of patient-blaming in individual health promotion. This may be inappropriate because in most diseases addressed by health promotion, such as cardiovascular disease, the patient's behaviour is only one causal factor among many.

Individual empowerment

Individual empowerment involves giving people the means to take responsibility for their health and to change their social conditions. Empowerment can be effective, but people may choose not to make health their priority. It requires patients to become educated about health, disease and treatment so that they can make informed decisions (have a look at the NHS Choices website at http://www.nhs.uk/Pages/homepage.aspx). When patients are not fully informed, there are ethical issues involved in medical professionals deciding which health-related decisions the patient has a right to make. Most would agree that patients are free to choose their own diet, but few would allow patients to decide which anaesthetic they would prefer. The difference is in the level of knowledge and expertise involved in making the decision and in the risks involved. Another difficulty is that much health promotion claims to be empowering, while strongly encouraging people to make the 'correct' health decision. There are also contradictions, for example society is currently concerned about both a rapid rise in obesity and an increase in the prevalence of excessive thinness and eating disorders (see pp. 86–87).

The practice of health promotion

Health care practitioners can provide patients with information via leaflets (Fig. 1), other written sources, such as self-help books (Heather & Robinson 1996), computer systems and other media such as posters or multimedia displays in waiting areas. Health care practitioners can also facilitate social change, for example, by pressing for improved housing conditions. However, practitioners probably do most health promotion via personal contact. A doctor's attitude and approach to patients can also promote health. A paternalistic pill-pusher is liable to develop patients who believe in quick medical repairs for their ailments, rather than prevention. A doctor with better communication skills may listen to patients and discuss how they should deal with their health problems. This may help inform and empower patients on health issues (see pp. 96–97).

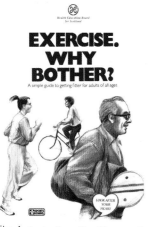
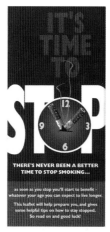
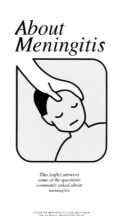

Fig. 1 A selection of health promotion leaflets found in a GP's surgery.

STOP THINK

- What is the difference between health education and health promotion?
- When might giving patients leaflets about their condition not affect their behaviour?
- What steps might a doctor take to ensure that leaflets were effective?
- Health information is sometimes seen by patients as patronizing and unrealistic. Why might this be so?

Many consultations provide scope for opportunistic health promotion, where the doctor promotes health in a consultation concerning something else. Two examples would be the following: a patient with a head injury from falling may also have an alcohol problem and the doctor should take the opportunity to enquire about this; and patients over 40 years of age attending their GP these days are likely to have their blood pressure monitored, whatever the presenting problem.

A related way of promoting health is to take detailed histories of health behaviours and social circumstances. Until recently health behaviours were rarely recorded. Accurate histories allow patient behaviours to be followed up on subsequent visits.

Primary care also provides specific facilities, programmes and clinics for different health behaviours. It is often appropriate to offer patients available aids for behaviour change. These range from simply monitoring change, for example by weighing the patient on each visit, to prescriptions, for instance for nicotine gum or patches for heavily dependent smokers, to advisory leaflets (Glanz et al., 2002). Many health centres now also have access to dieticians, specialist nurses and psychologists to help with a range of health behaviours.

Brief interventions

If doctors systematically ask all patients about their smoking or drinking and simply suggest to the smokers that they stop, or the drinkers that they cut down, without providing further intervention, then this has a small but significant impact on behaviour. About 5% more smokers quit than a control group who did not receive advice (Pieterse et al., 2001) and over 15% more drinkers reduce their alcohol intake to safer levels (Raistrick et al., 1999: 168). Although effects are modest, brief interventions are quick, cheap and not subject to the problems of successfully recruiting and retaining patients in more intensive interventions. They are suitable for all who have less serious problems (Dunn et al., 2001). See the following website for further expert advice information on smoking cessation interventions: http://www.cochrane.org/cochrane/revabstr/ab001292.htm.

Avoid fear messages

It is commonly believed that the best way to change people's behaviour is to frighten them. Fear can be a powerful motive for changing behaviour, but fear messages can easily misfire because their impact depends upon a number of complex factors (Ruiter et al., 2001). Greater objective risk of harm (or greater fear) does not necessarily lead to greater behaviour change or compliance with medical advice.

Case study

Andrea is a married woman aged 48 years. She is severely obese, with high normal blood pressure (140/95 mmHg). She is moderately active, given her obesity. Andrea attended because she wanted help to lose weight. In what follows the GP expresses concern about her smoking, but does not risk alienating the patient by pushing the issue.

GP:	*'So you take about five or six drinks a week. That's well within the safe limits and I don't think it will be having much effect on your weight. Do you smoke?'*
Andrea (laughs):	*'Yeah, I've always got something in my mouth.'*
GP:	*'How many a day?'*
Andrea:	*About 40.'*
GP:	*'That's quite a lot. Have you ever thought of quitting?'*
Andrea:	*'One thing at a time, doctor. I don't need to put on more weight.'*
GP:	*'Actually, your smoking is worse for your health than your weight problem. I would like to see you try and stop.'*
Andrea:	*'I'd rather get this fat off first.'*
GP:	*'OK. Would you like to make an appointment with our dietician? I'll talk to you about smoking again in a few months.'*

Arousing fear can inhibit appropriate behaviour change, rather than facilitating it. Fear can lead patients, particularly those who perceive themselves at risk, to fail to attend properly to the relevant information. Patients may try to reduce fear by avoiding thinking about it, or may minimize the dangers, to reduce cognitive dissonance (see pp. 72–73). This may result in their rejecting the doctor as a credible source of information on the topic, or avoiding the entire issue. It is important also to emphasize the positive aspects of behaviour change, to increase patients' motivation to protect themselves from risk and develop a workable plan of action (see pp. 76–77).

Mass-media fear campaigns remain popular. Shocking approaches to topics such as child abuse, drunk driving, drug overdose or lung cancer attract publicity and debate, but generally, the people most impressed by such campaigns are those least at risk. Such campaigns may raise awareness of issues, but they are unlikely to change behaviour by themselves.

What are the objectives of health promotion?

- The objectives of health promotion are to prevent disease and promote health.
- Objectives can be achieved by: (1) social engineering; (2) individual prevention; and (3) empowerment.
- Health care professionals can promote health through:
  - Information provision
  - Facilitating social change
  - Setting an example
  - Communicating effectively with patients
  - Including health behaviours in history-taking
  - Recommending healthy behaviours
  - Providing support for behaviour change.

Health screening

Health screening plays a valuable role in the prevention of illness and the promotion of health. For those who screen positively there is the possibility of early diagnosis or early identification of risk with the resulting benefits of early medical intervention. Those who screen negatively are likely to benefit from reassurance. However, the usefulness of health screening may be limited if the uptake rate is low or if no benefits are obtained by patients found to be positive. In addition, there may be disadvantages to patients if the techniques simply serve to increase their anxiety.

Patients can be screened for the presence of existing disease (e.g. phenylketonuria, breast cancer), for precursors of disease (e.g. cervical cytology, HIV test and tests for chromosome abnormality) or for risk factors for disease, which may take the form of negative health behaviours (e.g. smoking, poor diet) or biological or genetic factors (e.g. hypertension, Huntington's disease, *BRCA* gene mutations in breast cancer).

Screening: process and results

Usually those found to be positive will go on to have further tests which will determine whether the first result was a true or false positive. Since no screening test is perfect, there will always be a number of false positives and false negatives and the number will depend on the sensitivity and specificity of the test. The four possible outcomes of screening are shown in Figure 1.

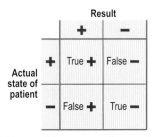

Fig. 1 Four possible outcomes of a screening test.

Uptake of screening

No test achieves 100% uptake by the relevant population. Doctors may fail to offer the test and patients may not accept it if offered. While the reasons for patients declining a test have been investigated in some detail, research suggests that doctors may not offer a test even when it would be appropriate, perhaps when the doctor thinks the test is ineffective or believes the patient would not take the appropriate actions (e.g. change diet, adopt safer sex procedures), or simply forgets to offer the test. If a test is not offered, the patient will be unable to make an informed decision.

Those offered a test may refuse to take it because it is incompatible with their health beliefs (see pp. 72–73); for instance, they may not think they are susceptible to the condition being tested. For example, women were more likely to have amniocentesis if they thought they were likely to have a Down's baby; and uptake was related to perceived risk, but not to actual risk as indicated by the maternal age. Patients may also decide not to have a test, e.g. declining a faecal occult blood test for colorectal cancer because the test is unpleasant.

Adverse effects for those tested

Patients show high levels of anxiety when being screened and awaiting results. Informing the patient that the test is negative lowers anxiety more effectively than telling them to assume the result is normal if they hear nothing more. However, even communicating a negative result can have adverse effects. A false-negative result can be harmful if it prevents the patient from receiving appropriate treatment or advice on lifestyle; a false-negative HIV test might result in the patient putting his/her partner at risk by sexual transmission and remove his/her motivation to adopt safer sexual practices. Similarly, a true-negative result can also be harmful, e.g. a patient with a familial risk of type 2 diabetes may be reassured by a negative diabetes test and may fail to make the necessary preventive changes to diet and exercise, thereby increasing the risk of developing the disease in the future.

Patients testing positive

Following a positive screening test result, there are further stages of tests, results and medical management. Each of these involves further social and behavioural processes, as shown in Figure 2.

When the initial test result is positive or ambiguous but is followed by a clear negative result, i.e. the patient has received an initial false-positive or invalid result, patients may continue to be anxious long after being told the negative result.

If the result is a true positive, patients' reactions will tend to vary with the implications of the results, depending on the seriousness of the condition and the available preventive or curative medical treatment. Nevertheless, there may be unexpected reactions. For example, individuals found to be positive for genetic diseases such as Huntington's chorea or polyposis have reported feeling relieved, perhaps because their uncertainty was reduced.

When screening identifies people at risk of disease, there may be adverse effects of labelling the individual and it has been found that they may respond as if they are ill rather than just at risk (see pp. 60–61). Studies of people shown on screening to have hypertension have found that they subsequently show higher levels of distress, report more symptoms, take more time off work and participate less in social activities. The level of distress is affected by the way in which the diagnosis is communicated. For example, those informed that they were hypertensive and given leaflets describing hypertension as 'the silent killer' were more anxious months later than those fully informed that it was a risk factor and reassured about management (Rudd et al., 1986).

Implications of a positive result

For some test results, such as Huntington's chorea, the result carries no specific implications for action in a clinical context, although the recipient may choose to make relevant plans for the future. For other tests, such as genetic tests with a probabilistic rather than certain result, there may be continued uncertainty and further clinical monitoring will be required. For yet others, such as hypertension,

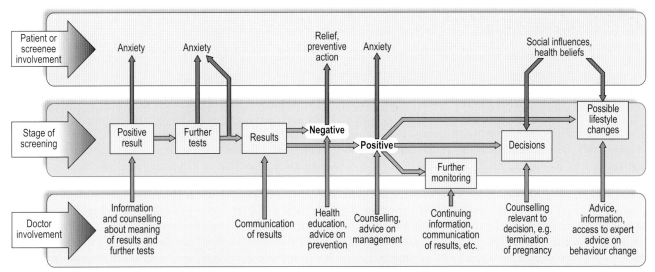

Fig. 2 Schematic outline of health screening and the social and behavioural factors involved – the process following a positive result.

appropriate medical management may reduce the likelihood or severity of the condition.

Other positive results may require the recipient to make critical decisions (such as whether to terminate a pregnancy) or to consider changes in behaviour and lifestyle (such as reducing fat intake or practising safer sex). While there is ample evidence that many people will make these changes successfully, a substantial number of people will attempt to change and fail. The overall success of the screening programme may be limited by failures to change behaviours in those screening positive.

The role of doctors in screening

Doctors may play key roles at every stage (see Fig. 2 and list below). The results of screening, both in terms of successful detection and management of clinical conditions and in terms of the potential adverse effects for those tested, depend on the doctors' behaviours. The role of doctors in screening includes:

- Offering screening: inviting the individual to attend without raising unnecessary fears.
- Counselling about screening: giving information about procedures, potential benefits and limitations, and checking comprehension, thereby enabling the individual to reach an informed decision.
- Providing health education: before screening, e.g. for serum cholesterol or HIV; after positive screening, e.g. for risk factors for cardiovascular disease.
- Communicating results that may be complex: providing enough information to enable patients to understand; achieving a balance between raising unnecessary anxiety and giving inappropriate reassurance.

STOP THINK Think of one area of health screening, such as in pregnancy, for genetic disease, or for cardiovascular risk factors. Follow the flow charts in Figure 2 and consider what adverse effects might arise at each stage. How might doctors minimize these adverse effects?

- Advising on decisions following positive results: giving information to enable informed choice and consent.
- Clinical management: varies depending on the type of screening.
- Assisting individuals to make necessary lifestyle changes, e.g. quitting smoking, improving diet, increasing exercise, taking medication, safer sex, repeated screening or monitoring.

Case study

Mrs Green had been alarmed to be recalled for further tests after blood tests suggested something might be wrong with her baby. She had taken a long time to conceive and this was a much-wanted child. Although she thought the pregnancy might already show, she felt she could not tell her friends at work until she got the result of the amniocentesis and could be sure the baby was all right. After the amniocentesis, the obstetrician said there was nothing to worry about as the test result was normal. However, Mrs Green continued to be concerned: why had the original test been positive? Surely that indicated something was wrong; after all, 'there's no smoke without fire'. If one test was positive and one was normal, how could the doctors be sure which one was right? Her continuing anxiety led her to be on the lookout for signs that things were going wrong even after the birth of her normal healthy baby.

Health screening

- For any screening test, a substantial number of those offered the test do not accept – a result of poor information, social influences or, in some cases, good decisions.
- Screening may have adverse effects, especially raised anxiety, which may persist even when the result is normal.
- The way in which results are communicated can affect the impact of the results on the individual.
- Those being screened require information and counselling before and after screening.
- For some tests, those being screened may need health education and advice on behaviour and lifestyle change.
- People do not always succeed in making lifestyle changes without further professional assistance.

The social implications of the new genetics

Developments in molecular genetics have major implications for society and individuals, doctors and patients. The knowledge and techniques which have arisen from the development of recombinant DNA are likely to affect profoundly how we think about and deal with health, risks to health, disease and illness (Cunningham-Burley & Boulton, 2000; Pilnick, 2002). The search for genetic components to a range of diseases, behaviours and traits is well under way.

These developments influence the social, cultural, ethical and personal realms as well as the biological, and have implications for some of the fundamental principles that guide research and clinical practice – confidentiality, autonomy, informed consent and individual choice. Scientific developments in genetics promise great improvements in health, understanding and treating disease and increased control and choice for individuals, especially in relation to reproduction. Many scientists, clinicians and others take the social and ethical implications seriously and contribute to the important debates about how this knowledge may be used (Nuffield Council on Bioethics, 1993; www.hgc.gov.uk).

Genetic testing

The genes for many single-gene disorders have been identified, and genetic components in common multifactorial conditions are now being researched. Testing for a range of genetic diseases (e.g. for late-onset dominant conditions or for carrier status for single-gene recessive disorders) is now available in many industrialized countries. Experience gained in the introduction of existing genetic-testing programmes provides a good illustration of the social, cultural and ethical issues involved, and may help shape the application of scientific development in the future.

Predictive testing: Huntington's disease

Huntington's disease is an autosomal-dominant condition. All those who inherit the gene will develop the disorder; it is of late adult onset, fatal and untreatable. Definitive testing is now available that can identify those who will develop the disease. At first glance, the provision of predictive testing within families known to be at risk of Huntington's disease may seem to be desirable, not least because individuals who have been identified as inheriting the gene may wish to make particular reproductive choices or plan for their own future. However, the possibility raised by genetic testing brings with it specific concerns about the rights of individuals to know or not know their genetic status, the rights of other family members to information and the psychological impact of a positive result. Moreover, the experience of introducing predictive testing for Huntington's disease has thrown up other pertinent issues, and few individuals have actually come forward for testing (Richards, 1993). Those who have fall into three different groups:
1. Those who want to be tested in order to plan their lives or avoid passing the gene on to children.
2. Those who want to obtain an early diagnosis (they are already suspecting symptoms).
3. Those who want to establish that they are free from the disease (they are past the age when they would be likely to develop symptoms).

Several reasons have been identified to explain why people have not come forward for testing. Firstly, a positive test result would have implications for their existing children, some of whom may have inherited the disorder. Secondly, there is no effective treatment for the disease, so testing may not bring any medical benefits. Thirdly, some people were worried about the loss of health insurance (where applicable). Lastly, some felt that the completion of their own child-bearing removed any reason to have the test. It has also been found that both positive and negative results can cause distress to individuals and their families. Those found to be free of the disease may experience survivor guilt. The certainty provided through testing is not always welcomed. Families have lived with uncertainty in terms of the risk status of its members, and this uncertainty forms a crucial part of identity and experience (Richards, 1993). The experience of introducing testing for Huntington's disease suggests that the information is not always desired by those at risk, and that an individual's right to refuse to be tested must be preserved. The situation is even more uncertain in relation to genetic susceptibility for disease (see Case study).

Carrier testing for recessive disorders: beta-thalassaemia

Beta-thalassaemia is an inherited blood disorder. If both parents are carriers of the trait, there is a one in four chance of passing the disease on to their child, while carriers themselves remain free from the disease. The disease can be fatal without proper treatment, and the treatment is complex. Knowledge of carrier status makes possible greater reproductive choice, particularly the use of prenatal diagnosis and the abortion of affected fetuses where this is personally and culturally acceptable. In Cyprus, where the trait is common, the orthodox church insists that people are aware of their carrier status for beta-thalassaemia when they marry. Where both partners are carriers, the couple then use prenatal diagnosis and abortion to avoid the birth of an affected child. Abortion is accepted on these grounds, but not on others. This programme has virtually eliminated the births of children with beta-thalassaemia in Cyprus.

Screening for carrier status can raise a range of other issues too. For example, screening for sickle-cell trait in the

Case study

Susan is 32 years old and has two young daughters. Her mother died from breast cancer at the age of 56 years. She thinks that other female relatives may have had breast cancer. Susan had not really given her risk of breast cancer much thought and certainly viewed herself as a healthy person. However, when her older sister was diagnosed, she began to think it might be 'in the family'. She had read that susceptibility genes had been identified (BRCA1 and 2) for some familial breast cancers and that a test was available to those at risk. She wondered whether this could explain her family history and what the consequences of that would mean. Would she want to be tested? How would she discuss this with her sister? What might happen to her – would she have to have both her breasts removed or would she just have regular check-ups? After worrying about all these things for several weeks, she decided to see her GP. On the basis of her family history, the GP referred her to a clinical geneticist.

USA demonstrated that stigma can be attached to carrier status, leading to further discrimination of black people (see pp. 48–49). Where people do not perceive themselves to be at risk, because they have little direct knowledge of the disease being detected, uptake has been low, for example, with testing for cystic fibrosis carrier status in parts of the UK (Marteau & Anionwu, 1996).

Understanding susceptibility to common diseases

Most diseases are multifactorial in aetiology, involving the interaction of genes with each other and with the environment. Research may lead to tests to identify genetic susceptibility to a range of common diseases in individuals. One major research investment in the UK is the UK Biobank (www.ukbiobank.ac.uk), where 500 000 healthy volunteers aged between 40 and 69 years will contribute genetic, lifestyle and medical histories so that researchers can study why some people develop certain diseases and others do not. The sample will be followed up through their medical records. The study aims to improve the prevention, diagnosis and treatment of common diseases such as cancer and heart disease.

Population screening

Population screening for susceptibility to disease could be beneficial where treatment or lifestyle modification improves health outcome. With the development of pharmacogenetics, treatments may become better suited to an individual's genotype. However, population screening raises ethical and other concerns (Clarke, 1995; Willis, 2002). Firstly, screening whole populations in order to identify individuals with genetic susceptibility to common diseases is commercially attractive to those corporations developing tests and treatments. Secondly, like other forms of screening, those not considered at high risk may view themselves as invulnerable to disease, while those at high risk may not necessarily be helped, especially if lifestyle modification is difficult or treatment options limited. Thirdly, population screening may lead to a view that genes determine health. The geneticization of disease may result in neglect of other solutions to the problem of ill health, such as social and environmental interventions. Specific screening programmes may be very useful where early intervention in those identified as at risk will improve outcomes.

Limits to the use of genetic technology and genetic explanations for disease

Two general issues are relevant to the application of knowledge gained from research into the genetic components of diseases and behaviours: eugenics and individual choice.

Eugenics

Concerns about eugenic control of populations are sometimes raised. The identification of genes implicated in disease can quickly lead to the availability of tests, such as those for Huntington's disease and beta-thalassaemia, outlined above. Where such testing aims to provide people with the information to make informed decisions (e.g. greater choice in relation to reproduction in order not

STOP THINK
- Will research into the genetic basis of disease lead to geneticization, where other causes are ignored?
- How can we avoid the stigma and discrimination that those with genetic disease may face?
- What sort of information will help informed decision-making for patients?

to pass on the disease to their children), this can mean aborting affected fetuses. The elimination of disease in this way may add to the stigma and discrimination currently experienced by disabled people in our society, and may affect the resources available for their care. Concerns also relate to the potential increase in the number of tests available and, therefore, the range of diseases that may be deemed serious enough for interventions of this kind.

Individual choice

Many of the concerns expressed about eugenics are muted by individual choice in democratic societies. The rights of individuals to choose whether to be tested and whether to abort affected fetuses are considered paramount: there should be no coercion to make a particular decision. While the preservation of individual choice is important, it is also crucial to recognize that decisions are not made in a social vacuum. There are many constraints on individuals that can make one choice more favoured than another. There may be subtle rather than overt pressures to conform to what is expected to be the obvious or right decision, or people may not have sufficient information with which to make informed decisions. Where there are inequalities, discrimination and concerns about the costs of care, the extent of choice available to individuals is culturally and socially constrained.

Practical application

Those involved in health care should be aware of the developments in genetics and their effects on individual patients and on society more generally. Within consultations, it will be important to discuss social and ethical issues with patients, and consider the context within which decisions are made, in particular about genetic testing. It is also important for doctors to work towards ensuring that the possible negative outcomes of genetics (e.g. increased discrimination, stigma and inequality) are minimized. This can be achieved through self-regulation, through engaging in open and public discussion and through actively promoting regulation and control of those institutions whose functioning is likely to be directly influenced by genetic research and its application – insurance, employment and health care provision.

The social implications of the new genetics

- Research into the genetic basis for disease can lead to applications in clinical practice, but we need to be sure of the ethical and social consequences.
- Genetic testing raises important social and ethical issues for individuals, doctors and society, and these need to be discussed and debated openly.
- Decisions taken by patients and doctors should be understood within their social, cultural and economic context; these may vary across cultures and social groups.

Health beliefs, motivation and behaviour

Health can be promoted through adoption of health-promoting behaviours and avoidance of health risk behaviours (see pp. 64–69) and the impact of illness can be minimized by seeking medical help and complying with treatment (see pp. 88–89 and pp. 94–95). So how can people be encouraged to adopt behaviours which promote health and minimize the impact of illness?

If we can identify beliefs, attitudes and intentions (collectively termed 'cognitions') that distinguish between people who do and do not undertake health-related actions then we may be able to change these cognitions and so promote health behaviours amongst the general population. Research in this area focuses on individual differences in what people think but these differences often reflect social and cultural differences.

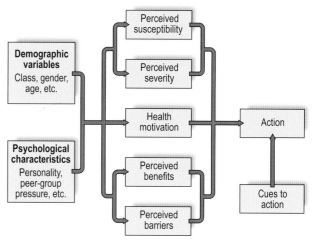

Fig. 1 The Health Belief Model (based on Becker et al., 1977).

The Health Belief Model (HBM)

In the 1950s US public health researchers began to investigate which beliefs were associated with health behaviour. The resulting model focused on people's beliefs about the threat of ill health and the costs and benefits of health behaviour (Fig. 1). Threat perception involved perceived susceptibility to illness or health breakdown (e.g. 'How likely am I to suffer from breathing difficulties or contract lung cancer if I smoke?') and the anticipated severity of the consequences of illness (e.g. 'How bad would it be if I suffered from breathing difficulties or contracted lung cancer?'). The model also included beliefs concerning the benefits or effectiveness of a recommended health behaviour (e.g. 'If I give up smoking, what will I gain?') and the costs or barriers associated with the behaviour (e.g. 'How difficult will it be to give up smoking and what will I lose?'). Two other factors were included: cues to action which trigger health behaviour when people are aware of a health threat and convinced of the effectiveness of action (e.g. advice from a doctor) and general health motivation (i.e. how highly a person values good health).

How useful is the Health Belief Model?

Reviews of research into the HBM (Janz & Becker, 1984; Harrison et al., 1992; Abraham & Sheeran, 2005) confirm that measures of the beliefs highlighted by the model provide useful predictors of a range of preventive behaviours (e.g. breast self-examination) and sick role behaviours (e.g. taking medication). However, these reviews also suggest that the beliefs included in the model are not strong predictors of behaviour. This implies that other cognition differences may help distinguish between those who do and do not take health-related action.

Reviews have also shown that perceived costs or barriers are especially important, suggesting that minimizing the degree to which health behaviours are thought to be painful, time-consuming, expensive or embarrassing will help promote them. Perceived severity has been shown to be less important in relation to prevention than responses to symptoms or medical advice. Thus stressing susceptibility to future health problems is likely to be more effective in promoting preventive health behaviour than emphasizing severity (see pp. 94–95).

Health-related intentions: the theory of planned behaviour

King (1982) extended the HBM in a study of hypertension screening. She designed a HBM-based questionnaire which included measures of intentions. Her model correctly predicted whether people did or did not attend later screening in 82% of cases. Measures of intention were found to be the most powerful predictors. A number of cognitive models have proposed that intentions are important indicators of whether or not people will take action. The most popular of these models is the 'theory of planned behaviour' (Ajzen, 1991; Fig. 2). Ajzen (1991) notes that 'intentions are assumed to capture the motivational factors that influence a behaviour; they are indications of how hard people are willing to try, of how much of an effort they are planning to exert, in order to perform a behavior' (p. 181).

The theory of planned behaviour has sucessfully predicted a range of behaviours (Ajzen, 1991; Armitage & Conner, 2001). It proposes that *perceived control* is an important determinant of intention. Perceived control refers to individuals' assessment of their ability to undertake an action or sequence of actions and includes awareness of barriers to performing actions. Perceived control affects our intentions because we do not usually intend to undertake the impossible. However, perceived control, which is closely related to self-efficacy, can also affect performance because those who believe in their ability are more persistent and devote more effort to trying to succeed (Bandura, 1997).

The theory of planned behaviour proposes that intentions are also determined by attitudes towards the action and by

> **STOP THINK** Mr Davidson is a 48-year-old lorry-driver who has seen his doctor about a series of illnesses over the past 6 months. He always complains of stress and overwork and his doctor thinks he needs to take more rest and exercise and reduce his working hours. List some helpful remarks his doctor could make to change Mr Davidson's view of his health.

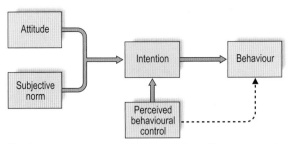

Fig. 2 The theory of planned behaviour (adapted from Ajzen, 1991, with permission).

subjective norms. Attitudes refer to our overall evaluation of an action and encompass many of the health beliefs included in the HBM. For example, if a smoker believes that giving up smoking will reduce her chances of contracting a serious illness then she will evaluate this action positively. However, if she also believes that she is more likely to feel more positive and relaxed when smoking and highly values such mood control, she may accept the increased chances of lung cancer, while acknowledging that this outcome would be disastrous. Subjective norms refer to individuals' beliefs about others' approval of the action in question. When we value others' approval and know that have strong views about what we do (e.g. 'Do my friends think I should not smoke?' or 'Does my partner think we should use a condom during sexual inter-course?'), this can have an important impact on our decisions.

The theory of planned behaviour has two advantages over the HBM. First, the research-supported proposal that beliefs have their effects on behaviour through intentions provides an explanation of how many (frequently contradictory) beliefs culminate in a decision to act. Secondly, the focus on action-specific cognitive measures shifts attention away from general representations of illness to representations of particular actions and enhances behavioural prediction. Thirdly, the theory acknowledges the impact of social influence on individual behaviour.

Implications of cognitive models for health promotion

Davis (1968) found that 44% of patients who had not followed their doctor's advice had not in fact intended to do so and only 8% of those who had not intended to follow the advice actually did so. These findings strongly suggest that people's intentions provide an important indication of whether or not they will perform preventive and sick-role behaviours. Doctors might enhance the effectiveness of their advice by finding out what their patients' intentions are and promoting health-related intentions.

Individuals are more likely to intend to take action and actually act when they believe:
- Their health is important.
- They are susceptible to a health threat which could have serious consequences.
- The proposed action will be effective and does not have too many costs.
- Others who are important to the person approve of the action.
- They can successfully carry out the action.
Perceived control can be increased by:
1. Teaching someone how to do something (e.g. explaining how to take the progestogen-only oral contraceptive so as to maximize its reliability).
2. Encouraging people to believe in their own abilities (e.g. by discussing how they gave up cigarettes successfully in the past).

3. Modelling a behaviour so that the person can watch a successful performance (e.g. seeing someone use an inhaler correctly on video).
4. Encouraging practice of preparatory behaviours (e.g. encouraging buying and carrying condoms in order to prepare for condom use).

Motivation can also be increased by encouraging people to make a commitment to act, for example, by discussing their intention with them and getting them to sign a behavioural contract specifying the behaviour to be carried out in a specified context over a specified period of time (e.g. 'I will run to work every day this week').

Case study

Health beliefs and condom use

John and Mary are heterosexual teenagers. They are motivated to protect their health. They acknowledge the potential seriousness of sexually transmitted diseases and know that condoms offer good protection. However, John believes that only gay men and drug injectors are at any appreciable risk of HIV infection and that other sexually transmitted diseases are not very serious. He has never used a condom and believes that they may reduce intimacy and sensation during intercourse. Consequently, he does not buy or carry condoms.

Mary takes oral contraceptives. She is concerned about her susceptibility to HIV and *Chlamydia* infection and has consistently used condoms with her last two partners. She does not find them off-putting and thinks they provide good protection against infection. Mary no longer has a regular sexual partner and does not carry condoms because she is worried that her girlfriends and boyfriends will think she is regularly seeking casual sex and question her morals if they see her carrying condoms.

John and Mary become attracted to each other in a night club and go back to John's home because his parents are away. When Mary mentions condoms, John rejects the implication he is infected and declares that he 'never' uses condoms. In fact, he does not have any and is unsure about using them. Mary is very attracted to him and decides to take a risk rather than lose John's affection. The next day Mary has a hangover and is worried about the risk of infection. John also has a hangover but he is not worried and intends to go clubbing again that night.

Health beliefs, motivation and behaviour

- Identifying beliefs associated with health-related behaviour and seeking to change those beliefs is an important part of promoting health-related behaviour.
- The Health Belief Model highlights the importance of perceived susceptibility and severity, perceived costs and benefits of health behaviours, general health motivation and cues to action.
- The theory of planned behaviour highlights the importance of intentions as predictors of future behaviour and the impact that others' approval may have on intention formation.
- In addition to attitudes and subjective norms, high perceived control or self-efficacy promotes intention formation and makes successful performance more likely.
- Health beliefs can be targeted in individual consultations and mass-media campaigns to increase patient adherence.

Changing cognitions and behaviour

Often we can change people's behaviour by changing their environment. For example, making condoms, dental care or medication easy to access and inexpensive is crucial to health promotion. Similarly, banning smoking in public places is likely to be more effective in reducing smoking and its health impact than individual smoking cessation programmes (Sargent et al., 2004).

The Health Belief Model (HBM), for example, has been used to design behaviour change interventions which have successfully changed behaviour (Abraham & Sheeran, 2005). For example, Champion (1994) evaluated an intervention designed to increase mammography attendance amongst women over 35 years old. A randomized controlled trial was used to compare four conditions: (1) a no-intervention control group; (2) an information-giving intervention; (3) an individual counselling intervention designed to change HBM-specified beliefs; and (4) a combination intervention designed to provide information and change health beliefs. Controlling for attendance levels prior to intervention, the results indicated that only the combination intervention had a significantly greater postintervention adherence rate than the control group. This group was almost four times more likely to be adherent to attendance guidelines. This indicates that both information provision and belief change are required to maximize mammography adherence, as would be suggested by the Information–Motivation–Behavioural (IMB) skills model (Fisher & Fisher, 1992). In this case the belief change interventions resulted in greater perceived seriousness, greater benefits and reduced barriers but not increased susceptibility.

Contradictions and change

Festinger (1957) and others have observed that people tend to seek consistency in their beliefs. Festinger's cognitive dissonance theory proposes that being aware of two inconsistent cognitions (e.g. beliefs or attitudes) causes an aversive psychological state, which we are motivated to eliminate through cognitive change. For example, being aware that smoking makes one susceptible to serious illnesses and that one is a smoker may facilitate cognitive change.

An experiment by Stone et al. (1994) shows the relevance of cognitive dissonance theory to health promotion. In this study participants were randomly allocated to four conditions: (1) receiving information about condom use (information only); (2) receiving information and giving a talk promoting condom use that might be used in health education in schools (commitment); (3) being made aware of past failures to use condoms by recalling these failures (awareness), and (4) a combination of the commitment and awareness conditions. All participants were then given an opportunity to buy condoms. Figure 1 shows that generating commitment and making participants aware of their own past failures led to greater condom purchase than the other three strategies. Participants in the combined condition (4) would have found it difficult to change the belief that condom use was worthwhile, because they had been persuaded to promote the importance of condom use. Yet they could not change their awareness of their own past failures to use condoms. In these circumstances,

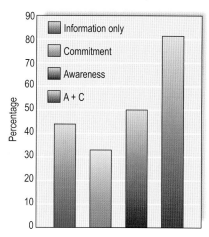

Fig. 1 Cognitive dissonance and health promotion. Percentage buying condoms. A, awareness; C, commitment (from Stone et al., 1994, with permission).

cognitive dissonance theory predicts that they would seek to reduce their cognitive dissonance by distancing themselves from their past failures. Affirming the intention to use condoms in the future, and regarding themselves as different from the person who failed to use condoms in the past, resolves the cognitive contradiction created by the 'awareness' condition. Hence many more people in this commitment and awareness group (82% versus 50% in the awareness condition) took the opportunity to buy condoms. This study also emphasizes that providing people with information alone may not be enough to motivate them to take action (only 44% bought condoms in the information-only condition).

In the experiment described above the researchers made it easy for participants to buy condoms. However, perceived control over action is not always high. For example, a smoker may not find it easy to distance herself from her smoking past and so may not resolve to give up. Instead, she may resolve her dissonance by changing her beliefs about susceptibility to future illness. She may, for example, convince herself that her genetic make-up will protect her from the risks of smoking or, alternatively, that other risks mean that she will die prematurely whether or not she smokes (see pp. 62–63). Thus it is critical to take account of perceived barriers and perceived control when attempting to make people change their behaviour (see pp. 72–73). In some cases, this may mean that people have to learn new skills before they can change their behaviour. For example, how to cook tasty meals with vegetables, how to relax without smoking or drinking alcohol, or how to discuss condom use with a partner.

How people process persuasive messages

The way in which people are persuaded by a message designed to change their beliefs or attitudes can also affect the extent to which they remain persuaded and the impact that such persuasion has on their behaviour. Petty & Cacioppo (1986) argued that people put more or less cognitive effort into the way in which they process persuasive messages. They called this *cognitive elaboration* and their model is known as the *elaboration likelihood model* (ELM). When people think about the content of a message, and consider and evaluate the arguments put forward in terms of what they already know, this is known as *central route* processing (involving cognitive elaboration). Persuasion by this route is most likely to lead to longer-term changes in attitudes and to influence action. However, people may not always be willing or able to devote the cognitive resources necessary for central route processing. In this case, they may make decisions about persuasive messages without properly understanding and evaluating the arguments. For instance, when people are under time pressure, or do not understand what's being communicated, or think that the issue is not especially relevant to them, they may be persuaded without central route processing. They may decide on the basis of what they feel about the message or use simple rules such as 'expertise = accuracy', i.e. she's an expert so that must be right, or 'consensus = correctness', i.e. if so many people agree, they must be right (Chaiken, 1980). This kind of cognitive processing is called *peripheral route* processing. When people are persuaded in this way, the apparent belief changes may not be sustained because underlying knowledge and beliefs have not been related to the new information.

If we want to persuade people of health-promotion messages (see pp. 66–67), we need to ensure that they have the opportunity and motivation to engage in central route processing. One barrier to understanding messages is a lack of knowledge. If we cannot understand a message we cannot engage in central route processing (see pp. 94–95). Peripheral route processing also makes it more likely that people will be persuaded by weak arguments because they are not evaluating the arguments, whereas those who use central route processing will be able to dismiss weak arguments. We can see this effect in data from an experiment by Wood et al. (1985). They compared the impact of messages containing weak and strong arguments on people who had either good or poor prior knowledge. Figure 2 shows that those with good knowledge changed their attitudes in response to the strong arguments, but were not persuaded by weak arguments. By contrast, those with poor knowledge, who we can assume were engaged in peripheral route processing, showed almost as much attitude change in response to weak as strong arguments. This illustrates why the information component of the IMB model is important.

Encouraging people to take greater responsibility for their health is an important aim for health services. This will be facilitated when people develop good knowledge; for example, knowledge of how their body works, what symptoms mean and how medication has its effect. Presenting well-informed people with well-argued messages that appear relevant to them, in a manner that allows them to concentrate on and revisit presented information, will enhance cognitive processing and persuasion. Persuading people of a new position and then contrasting this with their current behaviour can generate cognitive dissonance and thereby motivate change. However, behaviour change is only likely to follow from attitudinal and motivational change when people have confidence in their ability to change and can do so in a supported and graded manner. Where this is not possible people may reject health promotion messages and reaffirm attitudes associated with health risk behaviours (see pp. 26–27, pp. 62–63 and pp.76–77).

STOP THINK Imagine you want to persuade an over-weight patient to take more exercise. What would you say to her? Why might giving this person free membership of a gym fail to increase the amount she exercised?

Case study

Henry has been intending to stop smoking for a number of years and had stopped for a day or two on a few occasions. He now feels he cannot stop because it makes him feel so bad. Henry is reluctantly persuaded to go to a smoking cessation clinic. They offer him nicotine patches and teach him simple relaxation procedures. They point out that this will help him give up without feeling as bad as he did on previous occasions. They also demonstrate to him that, although he thinks that smoking makes him feel better and more relaxed, the continual nicotine withdrawal actually has a negative effect on his mood for which he is continually trying to compensate. Explaining how nicotine affects him helps Henry understand why he has found it so difficult to give up, and the patches and relaxation techniques bolster his confidence that he can quit. The clinic staff emphasize the consequences for him and his friends and family if he does contract lung cancer and help him acknowledge that he is worried about becoming ever more unfit. They talk through what he sees as the main barriers to giving up and plan what he might do in the first couple of weeks to overcome these various difficulties. In Henry's case this includes going to the non-smoking coffee room during breaks at work and not going to the pub for 2 weeks. They pair Henry up with another person who is trying to quit and talk to him about what he will say to his partner about quitting. They also provide Henry with a contract that asks him to specify his reasons for (or the advantages of) quitting and the day on which he will start his quit attempt. Henry begins his quit attempt the next day.

Changing cognitions and behaviour

- Cognitive dissonance theory proposes that being aware of two inconsistent cognitions causes an aversive psychological state, which we are motivated to eliminate.

- Attitude change may be prompted by cognitive dissonance but if behaviour change is thought to be difficult, people may reject health promotion messages rather than change their intentions.

- People may process persuasive messages using the central or peripheral route. Central route processing is more likely to lead to enduring attitude change and action.

- Providing information alone is unlikely to change behaviour, but knowledge is important to central route processing of health-relevant messages. Hence information, motivation and behavioural skills are all crucial to successful behaviour change.

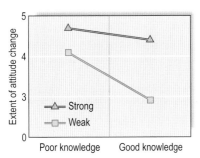

Fig. 2 Prior knowledge and the effect of argument strength on persuasion (from Wood et al., 1985, with permission).

Helping people to act on their intentions

The theory of planned behaviour (see pp. 72–73) highlights intention as an important cognitive antecedent of action. Strength of intention is a good indicator of how motivated individuals are to act and how much effort they will put into trying to enact that intention. If people do not intend to change their behaviour, they are unlikely to do so. For example, across a series of studies of health-related behaviours, Sheeran (2002) found that only 7% of those who did not intend to act subsequently did so. Thus, if a patient leaves a consultation without intending to pick up a prescription and then take prescribed medication as directed, she is very unlikely to do so. Consequently, a crucial first step in health promotion (whether encouraging exercise, smoking cessation or adherence to medication regimens) is persuading people to decide to change, that is, motivating them to act.

Even when people intend to change they do not always succeed. Sometimes this is because they have diminished control. For example, approximately half of all smokers intend to quit over the next year but only about 30% of them try and only about 2% succeed. In this case both pharmaceutical (e.g. nicotine patches) and behavioural interventions (e.g. support groups) can help translate quitting intentions into action (Fiore et al., 1996). Even when there are no issues of dependence, people often fail to act on their intentions. Across studies of screening attendance, exercise and condom use, Sheeran (2002) found that 47% of intenders failed to act on their intentions. This has been called the *intention–behaviour gap* and has prompted psychologists to investigate cognitive processes that make it more likely that people will act on their intentions. Increased self-efficacy, anticipated regret and task analysis have been found to increase the likelihood that people act on their intentions (Fig. 1).

If we lack prerequisite behavioural skills then we may fail in our attempt and abandon our intention. However, even when we just lack confidence, this low perceived self-efficacy may result in reduced effort or poorer performance (see pp. 72–73). Consequently, it is helpful to focus on past successes, the ease with which others like oneself accomplish tasks and small steps towards a goal when learning a new skill or trying to change an established behaviour. For example, Fisher & Johnston (1996) manipulated self-efficacy by inviting chronic pain patients to reflect on past experiences of high or low control and found that this manipulation altered levels of self-efficacy which, in turn, accounted for different performances on a lifting task. Those who had focused on past success were more successful at the task.

Anticipated regret can also prompt people to act on their intentions rather than remaining inactive. Regret is a powerful negative emotion that people want to avoid. Consequently, making future regret salient can help people maintain and enact intentions. In a series of studies, Abraham & Sheeran (2003) found that people with higher anticipated regret were more likely to sustain their intentions to exercise over time and to take more exercise as a result. Even amongst those with strong intentions to exercise, people with high levels of anticipated regret exercised more often than those with low levels of anticipated regret. Thus prompting people to think about the regret they will feel if they do not seize opportunities to act can help them bridge the intention–behaviour gap.

Health-related intentions may also require planning and preparatory actions. For example, one may need to acquire condoms before using them or obtain sportswear before exercising. Thus planning a sequence of actions focusing on achievable steps that lead towards an intended outcome can facilitate the enactment of intentions. Studies have found that such task analysis can enhance perceived control. Stock & Cervone (1990) report that dividing a complex task into a series of subgoals led to higher self-efficacy at task outset and heightened self-efficacy and satisfaction at the point of subtask completion. This also resulted in greater overall task persistence. Consequently, helping people plan out a sequence of steps involved in what they intend to do can help promote the enactment of intentions.

People often explain why they did not do the things they intended by saying that they forgot, were too busy or did not get round to them. This usually means that they had more important or more pressing intentions which took priority over the intention that was not enacted. Thus, the intention–behaviour gap is partially created by competing intentions or goals. We intend to do many things but only act on a proportion of our intentions. Consequently, if we can prioritize any particular intention we increase the likelihood of acting on it. Linking intentions to particular environmental contexts and to one's representation of oneself can boost their priority.

Gollwitzer (1999) has shown that turning an intention into an *implementation intention*, which specifies a condition under which an action will be performed using an 'if–then plan', facilitates the translation of intentions into action. For example, resolving to take one's medication in the bathroom, immediately after a morning shower, or to go swimming at the local pool at 2.00 p.m. on Friday afternoons makes it more likely that one will act in these specified contexts than the intention alone.

Implementation intentions can be used to help people prioritize action in the face of distractions (e.g. 'if I have lots of work to do at 2.00 p.m. on Friday, I will just ignore it'). This can be important to shielding an intention (e.g. to go swimming) from other goals. Similarly, implementation intentions then may be used to suppress unwanted responses

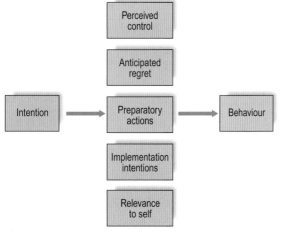

Fig. 1 Bridging the intention–behaviour gap.

('If I begin to feel angry I will stay calm and not react aggressively').

Of course, the success of implementation intentions plans depends upon identifying key barriers to action and making corresponding if–then plans (Gollwitzer & Sheeran, 2006). If the problem is remembering when to act when one has the opportunity, then specifying where and when to act can enable aspects of the environment to prompt intended actions, so giving them priority in that context at that particular time. So once an implementation intention is made to take medication in the bathroom after a morning shower, stepping out of the shower can be enough to prompt taking the medication. Implementation intention formation has been shown to have this effect for a variety of health-related behaviours such as breast self-examination (Orbell et al., 1997; see Case study), taking vitamins, attending screening and rehabilitation after surgery (Sheeran, 2002).

Whether we translate intentions into action also depends on the relevance of intentions to our self-representation. If a person sees herself as the type of person to whom exercise is important then she is more likely to act on an intention to begin running or swim regularly than someone who sees exercise as less relevant to who she is. If an intended action seems peripheral to our sense of self then that intention may be more likely to change over time as it is overridden by intentions more relevant to the self. Thus if someone decides to take exercise to please his partner he is less likely to take action than someone who decides he will exercise because he wants to feel fit. Similarly, someone who decides to take medication to please her doctor may be less likely to succeed than someone who decides to do so because she believes the medication is important to her health. Feeling 'I want to do that' (as opposed to 'I should do that') can help prioritize an intention. Therefore, if an intention can be anchored in a person's self-image or seen to serve another important personal goal (Fig. 2), it is more likely to maintain priority in competition with other intentions. Thus achieving concordance with a patient (see pp. 94–95) is likely to involve linking new health-related intentions to the patient's view of himself and his important goals.

When encouraging people to change their behaviour it is crucial to focus on realistic intentions. When people intend to do things for which they lack the skills or things that are difficult within their environment, they are not likely to succeed. Behaviour change must begin with things we can achieve. Hence walking from home may be a more realistic approach to initiating exercise than joining a gym or resolving to travel to a public pool. Once a small change is established, further change may be easier to initiate. Even when people's intentions are realistic there are a variety of ways in which we can facilitate the translation of intentions into action: enhancing confidence or self-efficacy; highlighting anticipated regret; realistic task analysis and planning; implementation intention formation; and linking intentions to important goals.

 STOP THINK Imagine a patient who tells you that she always intends to take her preventive medication but never seems to manage it. What would you ask her? What might you say to help her take her medication?

Case study

Orbell et al. (1997) promoted implementation intention formation in relation to breast self-examination (BSE) in a survey of women on a university campus. Women were asked about past BSE and their intentions to perform BSE in the next month. Intervention questionnaires were randomly distributed to half the sample. These questionnaires informed women that:

You are more likely to carry out your intention to perform BSE if you make a decision about when and where you will do so. Many women find it most convenient to perform BSE at the start of the morning or last thing at night, in the bath or shower, or while they are getting dressed in their bedroom or bathroom. Others like to do it in bed before they go to sleep or before getting up. Decide now where and when you will perform BSE in the next month and make a commitment to do so.

This text was absent from the control questionnaires. Women in the control and intervention groups did not differ in intention to perform BSE or experience of BSE. However, a follow-up questionnaire 1 month later found that 64% of women in the intervention had performed BSE whereas only 14% in the control group had done so. All of the intervention group women who had intended to perform BSE (in the first questionnaire) did so but only 53% of control-group women who had intended to perform BSE did so over the month.

This study demonstrates how forming if–then plans, in this case specifying when and where you will perform an intended action, makes it more likely that you will act on your intention.

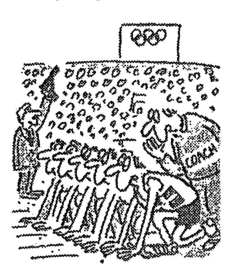

'Psst, there's someone at the finishing line who's interested in buying your house'

Fig. 2 Linking intentions to pre-existing self-relevant goals can increase the likelihood of action. Copyright the *Daily Telegraph* 2001. Reproduced with permission.

Helping people to act on their intentions

- The intention–behaviour gap may be partially bridged by enhancing perceived control and by making anticipated regret salient.
- Planning a series of preparatory actions leading to a health goal may also make it more likely that people act on their intentions.
- Specifying when and where one will undertake a particular action makes it less likely that it will be forgotten or postponed in the specified context.
- Forming other if–then plans can also help shape behaviour.
- Linking a new intention to individuals' sense of themselves or to their important goals increases the likelihood they will act on that intention.

The social context of behavioural change

Few would dispute that good health is a worthy goal for individuals and states or governments to pursue. In most industrialized countries, health education bodies promote healthy, and discourage unhealthy, behaviour. The emphasis on the individual's responsibility to make good health choices is literally evident in the message from the Scottish Health Education Board: 'Choose to be different'. However, individuals operate within a social context and we need to appreciate this when considering the notion of choice in behaviour change.

This spread looks at two ways in which behaviour change can be seen in a social context: firstly, the social context in which individuals come to alter their behaviour; and secondly, the role society plays in influencing citizens' health behaviour.

The social context of individual behaviour change

There is clear evidence that behaviour such as smoking, eating large quantities of salt or certain fats and failing to exercise is detrimental to health. Lay people are not necessarily unaware of this (health warnings are printed on the sides of cigarette cartons, for instance) and it seems only common sense that people will make sensible decisions to change their behaviour on the basis of such information. So why do people often fail to do so?

You will see that behaviour prediction models like the Health Belief Model endorse the assumption that the individual will indeed think rationally about costs and benefits before engaging in particular behaviour. This model has demonstrated fairly good predictive power in certain health domains. However, to the extent that it forefronts the role of a person's cognitions (e.g. perceived susceptibility to disease) in influencing specific behavioural intentions, it is heir to early research in persuasion which assumed that influencing behaviour was simply a matter of targeting people's thoughts (attitudes/beliefs), on the basis that attitudes *cause* behaviour in a fairly unproblematic way. Pioneer health promoters therefore believed that *information*, once disseminated, would be sufficient to alter beliefs and hence behaviour: they were wrong!

Interestingly, advertising companies had long recognized that the most successful of campaigns will usually only be effective in altering the consumption habits of a small percentage of the targeted audience. Early health education initiatives probably had too high expectations of behaviour change and, importantly (unlike advertising campaigns designed to, say, switch the consumer's allegiance to another brand of soap powder), they were often aimed at altering behaviour that was *pleasurable*, such as smoking. Further, in some cultural contexts, hazardous behaviour may be valued and engaged in precisely because of the associated risk, e.g. a type of cigarette marketed under the brand name Death Cigarettes has sold successfully (Bunton & Burrows, 1995).

Note that someone's established behaviour may also become habitual (automatic; independent of conscious thought). As there is evidence that such a person is less likely to attend to information relating to his/her habit, persuasion is even more problematic as a behaviour change strategy. If a habit is addictive as well, persuasion becomes only one element in a battery of potential interventions and supports for behaviour change.

Investigating 'unhealthy' behaviour

Specific behaviours such as smoking occur in a social context – a web of interdependent causes and cultural meanings. A classic study that illustrated the importance of investigating the context and complexity of the role played by smoking was that by Hilary Graham (1984). She argued that caring for children and managing the financial and organizational burdens of domestic life may be so stressful that smoking can be conceptualized as a coping strategy. One of her respondents said:

> After lunch, I'll clear away and wash up and put the telly on for Stevie (her son). I'll have a sit down on the sofa, with a cigarette… It's lovely, it's the one time in the day I really enjoy and I know Stevie won't disturb me. I couldn't stop, I just couldn't. It keeps me calm. It's me (sic) one relaxation, is smoking (Graham, 1984, p. 172.).

Smoking actually enabled this carer to be a more effective mother. Graham termed this phenomenon 'the responsibility of irresponsible behaviour'. Note that nicotine does, indeed, act neuropharmacologically to reduce stress (File et al., 2001).

Studies like Graham's (and see Copeland, 2003, for similar, more recent work) give us some indication of how behavioural change is constrained by social circumstances and hint at some of the reasons behind social class differences in health behaviour (and outcomes), e.g. why working-class mothers (with fewer material resources) may find it harder to give up smoking than middle-class mothers. It would be difficult, indeed, to get an idea of the

---

Case study

Mrs Berry, a 34-year-old mother, visited her GP, Dr Hall, concerned about the weight of her 14-year-old son. While she had tried to improve meals at home and encourage him to eat more healthily, he refused to do so and she knew that outside the house he was buying a lot of junk food. He also spent most of his time in sedentary pursuits – watching TV or playing computer games. Dr Hall recalled a study in New Zealand in which young people's love of technology – specifically of their personal cell phones – had been used to help them quit smoking. Researchers had texted messages to them such as: 'Write down 4 people who will get a kick outta u kicking butt' every day for 6 weeks (Rodgers et al., 2005). This stratagem had proved really successful in changing behaviour and in engaging the target audience's interest. Dr Hall wondered whether a similar project could be set up in relation to resisting junk food and to taking up exercise. It might also have the benefit of getting children together and widening their circle of friends and activities. Dr Hall's imagination began to take off: she had a vision of a group of fit, enthusiastic young people relentlessly texting their MPs and local councillors to lobby for improved local sports and leisure amenities…

sheer complexity of the role played by smoking in Graham's respondent's life by looking solely at isolated psychological factors, such as her attitude towards, or knowledge about, quitting the habit.

If smoking (and therefore how to eliminate it) appears much more complicated once we begin to examine it in context, consider obesity. Obesity is not a specific behaviour; rather, it is a state which is implicated in many health problems and whose incidence is increasing, such that it has been suggested that, for the first time in centuries, life expectancy in the UK may start to downturn. Despite the fact that obesity does not directly lead to poor health outcomes (fit fat men outlive slim unfit men, for example) and despite evidence that the causes of obesity are many and varied, ranging from the biological through psychosocial to sociological, societal concern has overwhelmingly focused on the role of lifestyle.

Social context of mass behaviour change

Mass education campaigns directed at people's attitudes may have limited success in changing behaviour. Sometimes the state targets the actual behaviour by introducing sanctions: just as we might privately decide to deny ourselves a chocolate bar if we fail to complete an assignment on time, the state might implement external incentives – perhaps legal penalties – if we do not conform to a particular behaviour.

In Scotland, the government banned smoking in public places in 2006. Research has already been published showing improvements in the health of bar staff as a consequence (Menzies et al., 2006). Many people would probably agree however that it would be unacceptable for the state to legislate to forbid practices like smoking or drinking in the private sphere (though taxation may be used to discourage them). In these cases, persuasive health promotion campaigns aimed at our views and beliefs are the alternative.

But can you choose to be healthy?

The UK government's current approach to health education represents us as having responsibility for our health and the freedom to choose a healthy lifestyle.

There are some problems with these ideas. Dentistry, for example, is becoming increasingly privatized, so the poor may be unable to afford oral health no matter how strongly they value it. The classic Alameda County study in California (Berkman & Breslow, 1983) demonstrated that, even after taking into account the influence of all known behavioural risk factors, there were still substantial differences in morbidity and mortality between high- and low-income families. Material and environmental conditions thus play significant roles in generating health inequalities (Acheson, 1998; Graham, 2000).

Clearly governments have conflicting interests: while wishing to promote their citizens' health, they must also generate wealth by supporting industrial development but in so doing produce the pollution and dangerous work conditions that make some of us ill (as indeed does the prosperity – witness the stark rise in obesity in China). So, while 'choose to be healthy' is a liberal sentiment in that it allows individuals control over their lives, it also serves to deflect attention from the role material and environmental factors play in illness causation, and can therefore be seen as a politically expedient message. Prior (1995) has likened the use of individualistic explanations of ill health to explaining

variations in the homicide rate in Northern Ireland during 'the troubles' in terms of personal shortcomings, such as failing to belt one's flak jacket. It is as absurd to ignore cultural/political factors in explaining illness.

In addition, most governments receive vast revenues from the sale of tobacco and alcohol, and it is perhaps not surprising that they allow companies producing such products to advertise themselves, e.g. by sponsoring sports events. The 'look after your own health' philosophy has also spawned a burgeoning health industry; we are enjoined to purchase every conceivable 'health' product from yoghurt to gym membership! The tensions governments experience in trying to offer citizens the kind of information they need to 'choose' healthy options, and, on the other hand, attempting to control the choices which are available, is well illustrated in relation to obesity. Food manufacturers are now required to provide information about fat, salt and sugar levels, yet the advertising on TV of 'junk' food is to be banned around programmes aimed at young children. The overall context in which we play out our behaviour is thus ultimately determined by political and economic considerations and, therefore, can only be influenced by collective action.

The role of health professionals

Health professionals are high-status repositories of knowledge about the lives of lay people and can operate as powerful influences on individuals (e.g. by advising patients to alter their behaviour), on local government (e.g. by supporting community self-help groups) and on national government (e.g. by recommending a reduction in the amount of alcohol that drivers may legally consume).

STOP THINK
- The needs of non-smoking patients requiring high-cost cardiac surgery might in future be prioritized over those of heavy smokers. Would you support such a strategy?
- Which would you support: the addition of a health warning about saturated fats to packets of butter and cheese, or increased tax on those products?

The social context of behavioural change

- The social context of behavioural change can refer to the background to an individual's efforts to stop a deleterious (or start a beneficial) behaviour or to the overall societal influences upon how we behave and think.

- Attempts to effect mass behaviour change may be more successful if behaviour itself (rather than attitudes) is targeted.

- The idea that individuals can exercise choice over their health status can deflect attention from environmental/material explanations of health inequalities.

- Health professionals have the power to help individuals and groups to change their behaviour.

- Trying to influence behaviour always has ethical implications.

Illegal drug use

Illegal drug use has become common, particularly amongst younger people, and this has created extensive concern. The UK has one of the highest drug-use prevalence rates in the world, with perhaps 300 000 problematic drug users and more than 11 million people who have ever used an illegal drug. Figure 1 shows the most widely used types of drug in the UK in 2006. Some forms of drug use, such as cannabis smoking, which is as common as tobacco smoking amongst younger people, are ceasing to be unusual or deviant in the UK, and many illegal drug users, particularly the more moderate ones, probably suffer few problems, just like many alcohol drinkers. This is no reason for complacency, for as prevalence has increased, drug-related problems have increased and diversified. Whereas 20 years ago drug services mostly saw heroin or cocaine users, these days people who seek help for drug-related problems commonly include people whose primary problems are one (or more) of the following:

- Cannabis abuse or dependence (Box 1), usually with alcohol and occasional use of other drugs. Because cannabis is the most prevalent illegal substance, there are more people dependent on cannabis than on all other drugs combined (Dennis et al., 2002).
- Heroin or opiate abuse or dependence, sometimes combined with benzodiazepines and other drugs, and typically involving drug injection (Neale, 2002).
- Cocaine or crack cocaine abuse or dependence. The likelihood and severity of cocaine dependence have sometimes been overstated (Ditton & Hammersley, 1996). Yet cocaine is becoming even more prevalent, which will lead to more widespread problems.
- Amphetamine abuse or dependence (Klee & Morris, 1997).
- Psychotic or delusional symptoms related to drug use. This is more likely for people with pre-existing mental disorders and is most commonly found with amphetamines or cocaine (Farrell et al., 2002), although it can also occur with cannabis or hallucinogens such as LSD (Abraham & Aldridge, 1993). People already vulnerable to schizophrenia may have symptoms triggered or worsened by illicit drugs, most commonly cannabis (Moore et al., 2007).
- Overdose, most commonly on opiates, alcohol or benzodiazepines, or mixtures of such drugs.

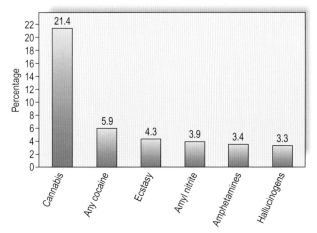

Fig. 1 Percentage of 16–24-year-olds reporting use of the most prevalent drugs in the previous year, 2005–2006 (adapted from Home Office 2005/06, with permission).

Box 1 Diagnosing drug problems

The DSM-IV (American Psychiatric Association, 2000) recognizes two forms of drug problems:
- Drug abuse: involves use over at least 12 months, with repeated problems interpersonally, or in social roles such as education or work, or legal problems, or dangerous behaviour linked to use and significant concern about those problems, but without dependence
- Drug dependence: can additionally involve unsuccessful attempts to quit, classic signs of addiction, such as increased tolerance (taking higher doses over time) and withdrawal symptoms, spending excessive time seeking and taking drugs, and having difficulty controlling intake

- Ecstasy-related deaths are not overdoses but have a different aetiology, which is not yet entirely clear, though it includes hyperthermia (overheating) (Burgess et al., 2000).

People who seek help for drug problems often have other psychological, social and physical health problems (Table 1), which may also need attention (Klee & Morris 1997; Orford 2000; Dennis et al., 2002; Farrell et al., 2002; Neale, 2002).

Table 1 Situations where drug users may require special treatment

Situation	Special problems
Obstetrics	Maintenance or reduction of prescribing and counselling may be required to minimize harm to mother and fetus
Surgery	May show high tolerance to anaesthetics and sedatives May be HIV-positive
General practice	Can be disruptive and deceptive May require specialized support services
Internal medicine	May fake pain to obtain painkillers May continue to use drugs that interact with their prescribed medicines
Infectious diseases	HIV, hepatitis
Casualty	Overdose, injuries through accidents while intoxicated, violence related to the drugs trade

Treatment

Drug users seeking help include some who are doing so mainly because of the concern of other people. Many drug users have mixed feelings about use, which they enjoy and find beneficial in some way, and can sometimes fail to recognize the development of a problem as quickly as others do. Techniques for motivational enhancement (Miller & Rollnick, 1991) can be particularly important to get users to consider frankly the costs and benefits of use; this is particularly useful in the form of brief interventions for people who are not dependent, which can be appropriate in primary care (Dunn et al., 2001).

Treating drug dependence is difficult. It can take a decade before drug-dependent individuals stop, during which time they typically have repeated involvement with health and other services. They will usually have tried to stop or moderate their use several times. Relapse management is an important component of any competent antidrug treatment. Users should also be provided with the information and means to minimize the harm their drug use causes. Information also benefits users who are not dependent (Box 2). For opiate users, methadone or buprenorphine maintenance can allow users to stabilize their lifestyle and reduce the problems related to a criminal, drug-injecting lifestyle. Ideally, prescribing should occur in a way that makes it difficult for people to abuse their prescribed drugs or sell them on the black market and it should occur with regular, competent counselling, for example from the community pharmacist doing the dispensing.

Box 2 Harm minimization strategies for drug injectors

Education
- Hazards of injecting (especially equipment-sharing)
- Safer sex
- Getting sterile equipment and   condoms
- Cleaning equipment
- Avoiding overdose
- First aid

Direct action
- Hepatitis B and C immunization
- Provision of sterile injecting equipment and condoms
- HIV testing (with counselling)
- Substitution of oral methadone

(adapted from Department of Health, 1991)

Case study

Mike is a 23-year-old drug injector with a history of criminal convictions and drug misuse going back to age 14 years. Two years previously he had been discharged from a residential detoxification programme for using drugs. He told the GP that he was now highly motivated by having a steady partner and a newborn daughter, but cannot give up heroin. The GP prescribed methadone and established a good relationship with Mike. With the prescription his general health improved and his previously hostile approach to NHS staff decreased. He was also referred for dental treatment because of numerous caries due to neglect and a sugary diet; the pain of these had previously been concealed by high doses of drugs. Unfortunately, 6 months later Mike was arrested for burglary. He denied involvement and the GP testified in writing on his behalf, but as a persistent offender he was nonetheless convicted and sentenced to 2 years. In prison his maintenance regime was replaced by a rapid reduction of methadone dose. Mike was unable to manage and began to inject again occasionally, sharing a syringe. As a result he contracted hepatitis C. On release he was determined to stop injecting. However, his GP was now reluctant to prescribe methadone as Mike had not used opiates regularly in prison. This, and a serious quarrel with his partner, led Mike to resume heavy drug use and crime for some months. He returned to the GP requiring treatment for a large abscess (Fig. 2). He is now back on methadone, requires regular monitoring for liver damage from hepatitis C and has re-established a relationship with his family, although he no longer lives with his daughter's mother.

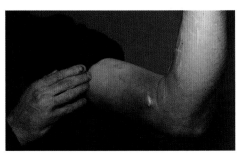

Fig. 2 Damage to arm by use of injectable drugs.

No single treatment works best. A good relationship between the therapist and the patient is very important and it is best to see treatment as enabling clients to change themselves (see pp. 132–135). Cognitive-behavioural approaches (see pp. 138–139) can help, particularly in changing negative drug-related behaviours, such as harmful injecting practices (see Platt et al., 1991, for review). Motivational interviewing is also widely used to help clients ready themselves to make change and prepare for the difficulties and possible relapses that will follow (Miller & Rollnick, 1991). Involving the client's relatives in family or systemic therapy can also be helpful, particularly for younger drug users. The Minnesota model of treatment using a '12-steps' approach and focusing on abstinence can also work. When treatment is evaluated, only 20–30% will quit or reduce drug use and stay that way for 6 months or more. Treatment needs to be extended over weeks or months, rather than necessarily being intensive or residential. Alleged higher success rates tend to be due to biased selection of patients or weak measures of outcome (Miller & Sanchez-Craig, 1996). Treatment is more difficult when the client has little social support, a chaotic lifestyle and also has other major psychological, health or social problems. Most substance users modify or quit drug use without treatment, leaving a residue of people with severe problems who require extensive help; however, encouragingly, recovery rates from substance-use disorders are higher than from most other mental health disorders (Orford, 2000).

For people under 18, abuse or dependence may not be clearly diagnosed and it may be better simply to describe them as having drug problems (Newcomb, 1995).

 STOP THINK
- Should illegal drugs be regulated, or should they remain illegal? Many of the harms of illegal drugs are caused by the fact that they are illegal, hence sold by a dangerous industry – one of the largest in the world – in unsafe ways and unsafe forms with no controls over who uses when and how (RSA, 2007). Attempts to stifle use have not been effective.
- In the UK cannabis was reclassified from a class B to a class C drug in 2004, which decreased the possible prison sentence for possession from 5 to 2 years (see the Home Office website for details: http://www.homeoffice.gov.uk/drugs/drugs-law/Class-a-b-c/?view=Standard). This may have increased recognition that it can be dangerous but there is no evidence that such measures increase use (see www.drugpolicy.org).

Illegal drug use

- Illegal drug use is quite common.
- Much illegal drug use is not a medical problem, but most drugs do cause occasional acute problems, even deaths.
- There are a number of different common patterns of drug problem.
- The dependent drug user may take a long time and repeated attempts to stop. Before stopping he or she may benefit from help with:
  - Harm reduction, including substitute prescribing, such as methadone for heroin, or advice on safe injecting.
  - General medical care.
  - Life problems as well as drug dependence.

Alcohol use

Alcohol is the most widely used recreational drug in the western world (Anderson & Baumberg, 2006). Although many users come to no harm, its use can cause medical, psychological and social problems. The management of alcohol should be a major public health and public policy issue, but historically people have resisted alcohol regulation (Anderson & Baumberg, 2006; Measham, 2006).

The medicalization of alcohol problems

Between about 1850 and the late 1950s alcoholism came to be considered a disease caused by some biological reaction to alcohol. This reaction was supposed to be permanent, so the only palliative treatment for alcoholism was permanent abstinence. Still widely believed, this idea is faulty:

- Many problem drinkers come to harm from drinking but are not alcoholics. The most notorious contemporary example is the rise in binge drinking, mirrored in the UK by a rapid rise in liver cirrhosis (Leon & McCambridge, 2006). Average personal intake in Europe, excluding abstainers, is in excess of recommended safe limits (Anderson & Baumberg, 2006); we all drink unhealthily and it is counterfactual to stigmatize alcoholics.
- Even dependent drinkers have some control over their drinking and some people with severe alcohol problems can moderate their drinking to problem-free levels, often without help (Heather & Robinson, 1983).
- Some very heavy drinkers survive unchanged for 30 years or more (Valliant, 2003).

Alcoholics Anonymous (AA) emphasizes abstinence, as do some professional treatments. Other treatments include monitored detoxification for severely dependent drinkers, counselling (see pp. 132–135) to enable the patient find methods of coping other than drinking, or therapeutic communities where patients stay off alcohol and undertake group therapy. Given a choice, some patients opt for abstinence and some for moderating their drinking. Occasional relapses to heavy drinking are common, even amongst those trying to abstain, and patients are taught to expect and cope with this. Controlled follow-up studies suggest that approximately 80% of people treated for alcohol dependence by any method have relapsed within 2 years. Alleged better rates tend to be due to bias (for example, treatment programmes that only admit people who have virtually stopped drinking already) or poorly controlled research (Miller & Sanchez-Craig, 1996).

The 12-steps approach

AA (http://www.alcoholics-anonymous.org) consists of groups of recovering alcoholics who provide one another with mutual support to achieve complete abstinence. Their philosophy is the famous 12-steps approach, which requires that alcoholics surrender to a higher power (or God), admit their wrongs and try to rectify them (see pp. 142–143). People who were heavily dependent, have religious or spiritual feelings and accept abstinence as a goal are likely to benefit most from this approach. AA has less to offer people who are not dependent. Doctors often suggest AA as a supplement to treatment.

Drinking problems and government advice

Even quite moderate drinking increases morbidity (Table 1) and mortality. Consequently, the UK government advises that women should not regularly drink more than 2–3 units of alcohol a day, men should not regularly drink more than 3–4 units of alcohol a day and pregnant women or women trying to conceive should avoid drinking alcohol (National Alcohol Strategy, 2007). A unit or standard drink is usually defined as a half-pint of beer, a small glass of wine or a standard measure of spirits. However, many people, especially young men, drink above these limits (Fig. 1), often due to going out a few nights each week (Hammersley and Dittan 2005).

At the legal limit for driving (UK: 80 mg alcohol in 100 ml blood), reactions are slowed by about 20% and thought is impaired. People who are drunk may generally behave in risky, antisocial or foolish ways without adequately considering their actions. This causes some of alcohol's pleasurable effects – people are more likely to dance, flirt or converse. Unfortunately, drunkenness also contributes to quarrels, violence, disorder, suicide, fires, road-traffic accidents, other accidents, child abuse and other problems (see Raistrick et al. (1999), Chapter 4 for a useful summary). It is also quite easy to overdose on alcohol, which can kill through respiratory depression.

There is currently great social concern over links between alcohol, violence and disorder and there are initiatives to manage this such as banning the consumption of alcohol outside, and the use of plastic glasses to reduce injuries. However, increasingly liberal licensing laws in the UK have probably led to increased alcohol consumption (Measham, 2006; Anderson, 2007), worsening a major public health problem.

Controlling the nation's consumption

Increasing the price of alcohol by taxation can reduce national consumption, which in turn reduces alcohol-related problems (Anderson, 2007). Alcohol advertising in the mass media may influence children, but it has little effect on consumption levels (see Raistrick et al. (1999), Chapter 8). However, the portrayal of alcohol in TV programming and writing is predominantly positive (or melodramatically negative) and there is scope for using mass media more skilfully to promote safer drinking. Other approaches try to change the way people drink by:

Table 1 **Alcohol, disease and possible benefits**

Disease	Beneficial effects
Liver disease – fatty degeneration, fibrosis, acute alcoholic inflammation, cirrhosis	1–2 units per day may reduce the risks of coronary heart disease
Cardiovascular disease – hypertension. Heavy drinking increases stroke risk and coronary heart disease	Red wine lowers cholesterol levels
Cancer – oesophageal cancer, possibly stomach cancer	Small occasional dose of alcohol may serve as a sedative or tranquillizer
Neurological disease – Korsakoff's syndrome, alcoholism	

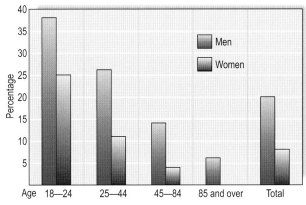

Fig. 1 Percentage drinking above safe limits – note that some of all age groups drink heavily (from Lader & Meltzer, 2001, with permission).

- Education about safe levels and risks. This may have helped change society's attitude to drunk-driving. A simple message to drink less may offset people's tendency to treat safe limits as 'allowances'.
- Continued control over where, when and by whom alcohol may be consumed, with licensing laws. For example, decreasing under-age drinking may require a reduction in tolerance of violations of existing law.
- Manipulation of th̶ ̶ ̶ ̶l and social settings where drinking problems̶ ̶ ̶ ̶ ̶ ̶ ̶mple, the banning of alcohol on foot̶ ̶ ̶ ̶ ̶ ̶ ̶s to prevent disorder.

A major barrier t̶ ̶ ̶ ̶
to and minimizatio̶ ̶
The health professional's ̶ ̶ ̶
related problems, by routinely taking al̶ ̶ ̶ ̶ ̶
treating alcohol use as a priority health care issue.

The role of medicine

Alcohol consumption has a direct impact on patient care. At peak times, up to 70% of all admissions to accident and emergency units are related to alcohol consumption and the total cost of alcohol misuse to the health service is estimated to be in the region of £1.7 billion a year. The medical profession can:

- Be aware of the contribution that alcohol can make to illness and injury in general practice and hospital specialities (Table 1 and Box 1).
- Counter the drinks industry's promotion of its products.
- Press for better controls on the sale, marketing and pricing of alcohol.
- Routinely ask patients about their drinking and relate this to illness and disease.
- Advise patients of safe drinking levels and suggest that they adopt these levels.
- Monitor patients' drinking, and praise and encourage reduced drinking.

Box 1 **Alcohol in medical practice**
Alcohol abuse can play a role in:
- Depression
- Anxiety and other psychiatric problems
- Problems of the digestive system
- Cardiovascular problems
- Neurological problems, apparent dementia and headaches
- Abuse of other drugs and medicines
- Family problems
- Falls and accidents
- Obesity
- Insensitivity to anaesthetics and pain relief

- Serve as a role model by drinking moderately, within safe limits.
- Be aware of and refer to local specialized alcohol treatment services.

For more detail, see the British Medical Association's policy positions (http://www.bma.org.uk/ap.nsf/Content/Alcomisuse#background).

Alcohol use
- Alcohol is often involved in many health, psychological and social problems.
- Alcohol use should be a routine part of history-taking.
- Some people require treatment for dependence.
- Others require advice to moderate their drinking.
- Drinking beyond 2–3 drinks per day, 14 a week (women) or 21 a week (men) is not unusual, but it endangers long-term health.
- Society tends to be complacent about the health risks of alcohol.

STOP THINK

- Some medical students and doctors drink excessively. Could you, or your colleagues, benefit from cutting down? How might you go about this? Doctors often drink as part of medical school culture, to cope with stress and to relax, although drinking can end up worsening the stress and work can be affected by drinking or hangovers. What other methods of coping might be more constructive?

̶ ̶se study

̶ ̶ ief intervention with a heavy drinker
Ralph is 35 years old and a travelling salesman. He presented with frequent abdominal pains, which he attributed to stress. From examination and tests there was no evidence of physical abnormality and non-specific gastritis was diagnosed. When Ralph attended the GP again to discuss the test results, the GP asked him to go through the previous 7 days and list all the alcohol he had consumed (a retrospective drinking diary). Ralph was drinking over 50 units of alcohol a week – about 2 pints (4 units) or equivalent at lunchtime and a further 2 pints in the evening to relax.

GP: *You don't drink that much a day, but it's steady. Now the recommended safe limit for men is 21 units a week – that's about 10½ pints of beer a week.*

Ralph: *Is that all? How much did I get through last week then?*

GP: *A bit too much, 58 units. I think that your stomach pains are made worse by your drinking. I'd like you to stop for a week or so and see what happens to your pain.*

Ralph: *I can't give up drinking! It goes with the job. A lot of my clients wouldn't stand for it if I didn't have a couple with them.*

GP: *I'm not suggesting you give up for ever, just for a week to see what happens, then maybe try and cut down a bit. Try not to drink every day, or have some soft drinks sometimes, or low-alcohol beer.*

Ralph: *That's going to be hard, but I guess I have to, don't I, doctor, if it's affecting my stomach and that?*

GP: *Yes. Come back and see me after you've stopped for your week. If you want to know more about cutting down then there's a good book, Let's Drink to your Health! (Heather & Robinson, 1996).*

Ralph now has the advice of the doctor as a motive for cutting down and as an excuse when he feels social pressure to drink.

Smoking, tobacco control and doctors

The global picture

Smoking is the largest preventable cause of premature death and disability in the UK and the world, and the largest cause of social inequality in health in most industrialized countries. Cigarettes kill half of lifetime users. Half of these deaths are under 70 years. Those dying before 70 lose on average 21 years of life. In 2000, tobacco killed over 4.8 million people. Half of these deaths were in developing countries. By 2020 deaths will double to 10 million, 7 million of these in developing countries (Mackay et al., 2006; Davies et al., 2007). Death rates are higher in men than women as men have a longer history of smoking. In countries such as the UK, where women have smoked for several decades, the gap is closing rapidly.

The costs of smoking in the UK

Smoking affects health throughout the life course. Each year 112 000 people in the UK are killed by smoking – one-fifth of all deaths (ASH, 2006a). Most die from lung cancer, chronic obstructive lung disease (bronchitis and emphysema) or coronary heart disease. Smoking is also a risk factor for other cancers (e.g. mouth, larynx, liver,

bladder, cervix), strokes, miscarriage, cot death, infertility, impotence, osteoporosis and many other diseases. Breathing in other people's smoke, second-hand smoke (SHS), causes around 12 000 deaths in the UK each year (ASH, 2006b). Children are particularly vulnerable. SHS increases their risk for diseases such as pneumonia, bronchitis, glue ear and worsens asthma (Muller, 2007).

The NHS spends £1.5 billion a year treating diseases caused by smoking (ASH, 2006c). This includes 364 000 hospital admissions, 8 million GP consultations and over 7 million prescriptions. Other costs to the state include sickness/invalidity benefits, widows' pensions and social security benefits for dependants. Industry loses 34 million working days each year from smoking-related sick leave.

Smoking and inequalities

In the UK smoking has declined since the 1970s. In 2005, 25% of men and 23% of women smoked cigarettes. This decline has been faster in affluent than poorer groups. Smoking is a major cause of inequalities in health, accounting for over half of the excess deaths due to

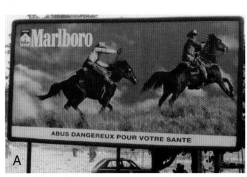
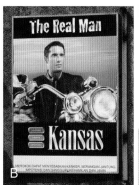
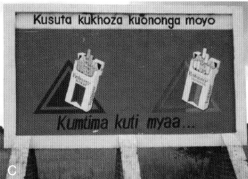

Fig. 1 Cigarette promotions in developing countries. (a) Marlboro – the most successful international cigarette brand, in the Ivory Coast; (b) Bali; (c) Malawi (caption: 'Smoking is good for your heart'). (courtesy of Campaign for Tobacco-Free Kids)

Case study

The Massachusetts tobacco control programme

In 1992 voters in Massachusetts agreed that 25 cents be added to the cost of a pack of cigarettes, with the extra revenue to be used to reduce smoking. Subsequently Massachusetts spent about $39 million a year on its tobacco control programme – $6.50 for each person in the state. This was the highest per capita expenditure on tobacco control in the world. The programme was designed to increase quitting, reduce uptake and reduce exposure to SHS. It included:

- Mass-media campaigns: to inform the public about the dangers of smoking and SHS.
- Services: local cessation services, youth leadership programmes, telephone counselling and educational materials.
- Promotion of local policies: funding local tobacco control policies, e.g. smoke-free public places, illegal sales to children.

The data in Figure 2 show a significant reduction in smoking in Massachusetts compared to little change in the rest of the USA (with the exception of California, which had a similar programme). The Massachusetts experience shows that a strongly implemented, well-funded, comprehensive programme can reduce smoking.

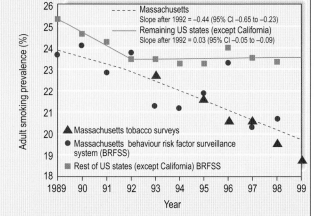

Fig. 2 From Biener et al. (2000), with permission.

inequalities in health in Scotland. The more disadvantaged you are, the more likely you are to start smoking and the less likely you are to quit. In 2005, people in routine and manual occupations (31%) had nearly twice the smoking rate of those in professional and managerial occupations (17%) (ASH, 2007).

The tobacco industry

Tobacco companies are in business to make profits. They need to recruit young smokers to replace the 50% of their adult customers who die from using their product. They need to keep their customers smoking as long as possible, by reducing motivation to quit and maintaining nicotine addiction. They achieve this through manipulating the marketing mix to appeal to different smokers and expanding their markets in developing countries.

The FCTC – a global tobacco control strategy

The WHO Framework Convention on Tobacco Control (FCTC) came into effect in February 2005 and has been ratified by over 140 countries. This is the first international treaty on public health and is based on evidence from around the world. It commits governments to take action to protect citizens from the harm caused by tobacco, including:

- Increase taxation of tobacco products and combat smuggling: the level of smoking is highly related to price. The cheaper the price the higher the level of consumption. For every 1% increase in the real price of cigarettes there is a 0.5% decline in adult consumption. The decline is even greater in young people. Tobacco tax can be used (hypothecated) to pay for other elements of the tobacco control strategy and to address factors (e.g. poverty) that make it difficult for smokers to quit.
- Ban tobacco advertising, promotion and sponsorship: tobacco companies argue that they do not target young people. Research studies and the companies' own confidential documents show that this is not the case. Banning tobacco promotion reduces smoking. Many countries have introduced bans. Bans must include: direct advertising and sponsorship, indirect promotion such as putting cigarette brand names on other products, e.g. clothes (brand-stretching), paying for cigarette brands to appear in films (product placement) and all types of media (Fig. 1), including the internet.
- Protect people from tobacco smoke in workplaces, public transport and indoor public places: people have the right to breathe smoke-free air. As well as reducing exposure to SHS, smoke-free policies increase smokers' motivations to quit and reduce uptake rates.
- Promote and strengthen public awareness of tobacco control: both prevention and cessation. For example, young people need to be aware of the health effects, how quickly addiction occurs and have the motivation and skills not to start.
- Regulate the content, packaging and labelling of tobacco products: this includes requiring large rotating health warnings on packaging and prohibiting misleading descriptors such as 'light' or 'mild'. This is important in developing countries where there is little awareness of the health effects. Warnings should include visual images, which can be powerful, particularly where literacy levels are low.

- Promote cessation and adequate treatment for tobacco dependence: two-thirds of smokers want to quit. Cessation support greatly increases success rates. This could include mass-media campaigns, quitlines, group or one-to-one support, and providing pharmacotherapy, such as nicotine replacement therapy (NRT).
- Prohibit sales to children: even in countries such as the UK, where it is illegal to sell cigarettes to under-18s, surveys show that young smokers can buy cigarettes. Laws need to be enforced.
- Research and evaluation, to develop more effective approaches: in particular, in relation to disadvantage, gender and ethnicity.

Doctors and smoking cessation

Helping smokers to quit is one of the most cost-effective interventions that doctors can take. For example, the cost of smoking cessation support ranges from £212 to £873 per life-year gained compared to prescribing statins (cholesterol-lowering drugs), which costs between £5400 and £13 300 per life-year gained (www.treatobacco.net). National evidence-based guidelines have been produced for doctors and other health professionals on how they can help patients quit (Health Scotland/ASH Scotland, 2004; Aveyard & West, 2007). Combining pharmacotherapy with behavioural support increases long-term quit rates to 15–20% – four times the unaided success rate. The UK is the first country to provide local specialist cessation services nationwide. These services were used by more than 600 000 smokers in 2005–2006.

Helpful websites include ASH (www.ash.org.uk); ASH Scotland (www.ashscotland.org.uk); Global Youth Advocacy Training Network (www.gyatnetwork.org); International Union Against Cancer (UICC) (www.treatobacco.net).

STOP THINK
- Around two-thirds of teenagers will try at least one cigarette, but fewer than half of these will become regular smokers. Thinking about yourself, what were the factors that influenced you whether or not (1) to take your first cigarette and (2) to continue to smoke?

Smoking, tobacco control and doctors

- Global deaths from tobacco are increasing rapidly and young people continue to take up smoking.
- Smoking in the UK is highly associated with disadvantage and is a major cause of inequalities in health.
- The tobacco industry needs to keep recruiting young people to replace smokers who quit or are killed by tobacco.
- Reducing the harm caused by tobacco requires comprehensive action to ban tobacco promotion, increase prices, reduce access to young people, increase health education, provide cessation support and reduce SHS exposure.
- Doctors have an important role to play in supporting both patients to quit smoking and wider action by the government and other agencies.

Eating, body shape and health

Although a large proportion of the world's population suffers from malnutrition, a growing proportion suffers from overeating and eating conditions are associated with a growing number of health problems. Problems with eating are the product of overabundance of palatable food and reduced exercise on the one hand, and unrealistic ideals about body shape on the other. The system responsible for appetite regulation is unable to cope adequately with these pressures. Most urgent is the increase in obesity in western society. Obesity has well-documented health risks, including heart disease (see pp 106–107), diabetes (see pp. 124–125), high blood pressure and stroke. Of particular concern is the increase in childhood obesity, resulting in a range of health-related complications (Malecka-Tendera & Mazur, 2006). Obesity also has psychological effects, with increased depression, feelings of ugliness and low self-esteem. Consequently, many overweight individuals diet to lose weight. However, disorders of eating associated with attempts to diet are also increasing, and the modern clinician is faced with the conundrum of how to promote healthy eating amongst people who are underweight through excessive dieting and how to help overweight individuals lose weight (see Case study).

Assessing weight status

The body mass index (BMI: Table 1) assesses weight status, and helps identify people who are outside the normal weight range. BMI figures are not definitive measures of health. The BMI of many elite athletes is above the 'normal' range, but their excess is muscle rather than fat. In general, however, BMI remains a good approximation of weight status.

Table 1 **Body mass index (BMI) calculation and classification***

BMI	Classification
<18.5	Underweight
18.5–24.9	Normal
25.0–29.9	Overweight
30.0–34.9	Mildly obese
35.0–39.9	Moderately obese
40.0 +	Severely obese

*BMI = weight (kg)/(height (m))^2.

The perfect body

The ideal body shape portrayed in magazines has changed markedly over time, and anyone looking at pictures of women used as models in art across the ages will see remarkable changes in physique. Today the figure portrayed as ideal, that is, excessively thin and athletic but often with enhanced breast size, is unattainable for the vast majority of women. This is most extreme in the use of 'size zero' fashion models in advertisements aimed at women. Even the dolls idolized by young girls have BMIs in the anorexic range (Fig. 1), coupled with a bust size that could only be obtained through surgery. While the ideal has got thinner, the average body size has increased, so the disparity between ideal and actual body shapes has grown. The result is widespread dissatisfaction with body shape, and it is perhaps no coincidence that levels of depression in women have risen in parallel with these concerns (Sawdon et al., 2007). Men, too, are increasingly concerned with body shape, although eating disorders for men are concentrated in professions where weight is an issue (e.g. ballet dancing, jockeys and some athletes) and in homosexual men, who appear more sensitive to societal pressures (Hospers & Jansen, 2005; see pp. 52–53).

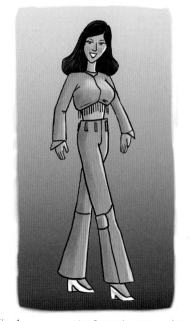

Fig. 1 A woman with a figure the same as that of a popular doll would have a body mass index of 16.6.

Dangers of undereating

The idea that healthy, often academically gifted and likeable girls should refuse to consume sufficient food to maintain a normal body weight has baffled clinicians since anorexia nervosa was formally defined in 1873. Descriptions of the disorder predate that time, challenging the common view that anorexia nervosa is the modern dieting disease. Anorexia is associated with excessive dieting and a morbid preoccupation with body shape, to the point where the sufferer refuses to consume adequate food to sustain a normal body size (Mehler, 2001). It remains a rare disorder, affecting 1/1000 even in the most at-risk groups (high-achieving middle-class girls aged 12–16). Claims that anorexia has become more frequent are hard to verify because of changes to diagnostic criteria, but many psychologists see the full disorder as the tip of an iceberg of women (and increasingly men) whose lives are controlled by attempts to diet. Although traditionally interpreted as a sociocultural disorder, there is increasing evidence for a genetic component which predisposes some individuals to develop anorexia (Kaye et al., 2000), and for a strong comorbidity with obsessive-compulsive disorder (Serpell et al., 2006). Mortality is high, and the disorder is very hard to treat.

Dangers of dieting

Guides to dieting feature heavily in the media and few people in western society have not at some time tried to restrict their eating. The increased prevalence of obesity indicates that these attempts rarely work, even though many diets result in initial rapid weight loss. One consequence of frequent failed attempts to diet is the phenomenon of weight cycling, where a *positive energy balance*, defined as energy intake in excess of expenditure, results in weight gain, which leads to short-term dieting and consequent weight loss, only for weight to be regained and the cycle continued. Research suggests that this pattern itself has adverse effects on health: weight cycling increases blood pressure more than sustained overweight and other illnesses (Foster et al., 1997). Health professionals recommend people who are not obese to maintain a stable weight to minimize these risks.

Binge eating: cause or consequence of dieting?

The defining feature of binge eating is the consumption of a much larger amount of food in a given time than is normal. Binge eating can be associated with obesity and a subtype of anorexia nervosa, but is best known in the specific disorder bulimia nervosa (Table 2). Here, the sufferer has a regular behaviour pattern of dieting followed by periods of excessive eating. Bingeing is followed by attempts to counteract the anticipated consequences of the binge on body weight by self-induced vomiting, use of purgatives or excessive exercise and dieting. The classic psychological model of binge eating was to see it as a secondary consequence of dieting. Accordingly, binge eating was characterized as compensation for the lack of food intake during dieting by overeating when the ability to maintain dieting broke down. The corollary of this is that binge eating should be seen only in people who are currently attempting to restrict their intake. However, sufferers from binge-eating disorder present the behavioural manifestations of binge eating but score low on measures of dieting (Dingemans et al., 2002). This suggests that the tendency to binge eat may be a characteristic of certain individuals, but since unrestricted binge eating will lead to weight gain, binge eating itself may lead to attempts to diet. Dieting may then exacerbate the tendency to binge, and so lead progressively to bulimic behaviour. Thus binging and dieting are interrelated, but one may not inevitably lead to the other (Polivy & Herman, 2002).

Promoting a healthy lifestyle

The increase in obesity and eating disorders in western society has occurred during a period when other aspects of eating have altered. Most notable has been the increase in use of 'fast foods' and pre-prepared meals at the expense of fresh produce. These types of food often have high energy density, and high fat and salt content. Increased energy density does not lead to equivalent increases in satiety, and so promotes passive overconsumption (Westerterp, 2006). Likewise, both variety and palatability promote overeating (Yeomans, 2007). With obesity and eating disorders both increasing in incidence, and dieting itself having potential harmful effects on health, how should society tackle these issues? Some see dieting as a necessary evil, since lack of dietary restraint in the face of plentiful high-energy food and low levels of exercise leads to obesity. Most health care professionals concur that promotion of a healthy lifestyle, including healthy eating together with increased energy expenditure, is preferable. Indeed, many clinicians now routinely prescribe exercise as a component of their treatment for obesity but poor adherence (see pp. 94–95) can render such interventions ineffective. Nonetheless, a lifelong commitment to exercise programmes is recognized as the most effective alternative to drug-based therapy for obesity (McKinnis, 2000). However, excessive exercise and dieting together are also features of anorexia (Bergh & Soderston, 1996), so it is important to monitor effects of prescribed dieting with exercise to ensure that this does not lead to a secondary eating disorder.

Many obese individuals falsely attribute their problems to genetic influences associated with disturbed metabolism and/or appetite, whereas less than 4% of morbid obesity can be traced to a specific genetic disorder. Obesity is commonly related to our sedentary lifestyle, including convenience shopping and the replacement of walking and cycling by the use of the car. Only major changes in society, such as promotion of healthy eating, reduced portion sizes, reduced availability of energy-dense foods, designing amenities in ways to promote exercise, and increasing the opportunity for safe walking and cycling will ultimately solve the dual problems of obesity and disordered eating.

Useful websites include those of the National Institute of Diabetes and Digestive and Kidney Diseases' (NIDDK) site on weight loss and control (http://www.niddk.nih.gov/health/nutrit/nutrit.htm); the Eating Disorders Association: http://www.edauk.com/); and the American Obesity Association (http://www.obesity.org/).

 STOP THINK What are the consequences for health and psychological well-being of:

- being constantly overweight?
- cycling between overweight and normal weight?
- being underweight?
- alternately binge eating and dieting?

Case study

The following description was provided by a GP during a discussion on eating disorders.

A family (parents in their early 30s, daughter aged 14) were seen during a routine 'well-family' surgery. The daughter was in perfect health, but both parents were overweight and so were advised to increase their levels of exercise and reduce their fat intake. One year later, both parents were still overweight but the daughter has lost considerable weight as a consequence of excessive dieting and is now diagnosed as having anorexia nervosa.

The GP had no intention of drawing the girl's attention to her weight. However, adolescent girls have a heightened awareness of issues relating to body shape, and awareness of this sensitivity is crucial when communicating health advice.

Table 2 **Clinical diagnoses associated with binge eating**	
Characteristics	**Clinical diagnosis**
Binge eating with no dieting	Binge-eating disorder, often leading to obesity
Binge eating with dieting, excessive exercise, self-induced vomiting or use of purgatives, but no excessive loss of weight	Bulimia nervosa

Eating, body shape and health

- Being obese has serious consequences for physical and mental health.
- Anorexia nervosa has a high mortality rate.
- Repeatedly gaining and losing weight (weight cycling) has more health risks than remaining mildly overweight.
- The ideal body shape depicted by society is unattainable for most people.
- Binge eating can be found in obesity, anorexia nervosa and bulimia nervosa.

Deciding to consult

Understanding why people with symptoms do or do not consult a doctor is important because some doctors feel frustrated and angry about 'inappropriate or trivial' consultations, and some patients feel frustrated and angry about doctors whom they perceive as uninterested in their problems. Both sets of feelings influence subsequent consulting behaviour, medical treatment, adherence and health. Delay may seriously affect a patient's risk of disease progression and the development of complications.

Understanding why people consult or delay consulting is also important because changes in access to doctors and other health professionals (particularly nurses and pharmacists) may significantly affect GP workload and quality of patient care.

The symptom iceberg

Estimates of the proportion of people who experience symptoms of ill health vary from survey to survey, though the 2003 Scottish and English health surveys generally reveal similar prevalence rates. Box 1 summarizes some of the results of the Scottish Health Survey.

Figure 1 is easier to remember and, although the proportions are not strictly accurate, the general picture is valid. Over a 2-week period, about 75% of the population will experience one or more symptoms of ill health. About one-third of these people will do nothing about their symptoms. About one-third will self-medicate or seek the advice of an alternative practitioner (see pp. 146–147), and about one-third will consult their GP. How high/low the iceberg sits in the water will reflect access to doctors and other health care professionals (including complementary and alternative medicine) and patients' confidence in their self-care abilities. In some areas, patients are now being offered alternative ways of accessing doctors using telephone or e-mail consultations. NHS Direct (NHS-24 in Scotland) provides a 24-hour information service (by phone and on the web) and a nurse-led advice service uses nurses to triage the nature and urgency of the caller's problem, and directs the caller to the most appropriate health care professional.

Hannay (1979) has shown that the proportion of people with significant medical symptoms who do not consult a doctor is higher than the proportion of people with minor medical symptoms who do consult a doctor (26% and 11% respectively). More recently, a Department of Health publication has suggested that as many as 40% of GP consultations are for minor ailments that people could take care of themselves (Department of Health, 2005), but this ignores patients' confidence in their diagnosis and self-care abilities. Morris et al. (2003) have found that 40% of 240

patients they interviewed indicated that they were consulting about a minor ailment but that, in approximately half these cases, their GPs thought that the patient was right to consult. Women, preschool children and adults aged 65+ are the people most likely to consult a GP over a year.

Differences in symptom perception

Three features of symptoms are important for people's perceptions of their seriousness: (1) the intensity or severity of the symptom; (2) the familiarity of the symptom; and (3) the duration and frequency of the symptom. For example, a severe headache may cause a person who has rarely had a headache to go to the doctor, whereas a person who has experienced migraine for some years is unlikely to consult. This person may consult, however, if the symptoms are unusual in some way or if the headache persists for longer than usual or recurs more frequently than usual.

Differential explanation

At the same time as they perceive their symptoms, people try to make sense of them and to explain them within the context of their lives. They do this using their own lay knowledge and experience and the knowledge and experience of their family and friends (pp. 100–101). Lydeard & Jones (1989) investigated the health concerns of a sample of consulters with symptoms of dyspepsia and a sample of non-consulters with similar symptoms, and found that consulters were significantly more likely to be worried that their symptoms indicated a serious or fatal condition, particularly heart disease or cancer. People with a family history of stomach cancer were also more likely to consult, seeing themselves as 'more vulnerable'.

Differential evaluation

People weigh up for themselves what the relative costs and benefits will be of going (and of not going) to the doctor or other health practitioner (see pp. 38–39). People often decide that other things in their lives are more important than dealing with symptoms of ill health; indeed, doctors themselves are classic examples of people who battle on at work because they perceive themselves as indispensable. Many patients temporalize: they wait, possibly take some medication that they already have with them, and see if the symptoms go away over time and only decide to consult if they do not.

People also weigh up what they think the doctor will think of them, and what the doctor or other health worker can

---

Box 1 **Prevalence of ill health in the Scottish Health Survey 2003 (8148 adults, 3324 children)**

- 75% of adults reported their health as good or very good
- 25% reported disability which limited them (50% of adults 75+ years)
- 16% reported acute sickness in previous 2 weeks
- 17% of females and 13% males had raised GHQ (mental ill health) scores
- 36% attended hospital outpatient departments in the past year
- 11% were admitted to hospital in the previous year

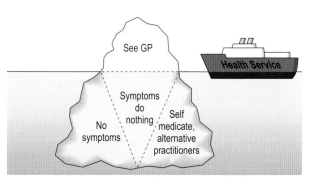

Fig. 1 The symptom iceberg.

actually do for them and their symptoms. Research with people with breathing difficulties has shown that people who perceive their symptoms to be serious may delay going to see their doctor if they believe that they will not be able to communicate the seriousness to the doctor.

It is also common for people to consult their doctor with symptoms that appear minor to the doctor but the decision to consult reflects anxiety that things might be serious, and they are consulting in order to confirm that they've reached the right explanation and to reassure themselves that there is nothing seriously wrong. In a qualitative study of parents' concerns when their preschool children became acutely ill, Kai (1996) found that parents felt particularly anxious when their self-care management failed to control their child's symptoms and the threat that these symptoms could imply.

Mothers of children are also very aware of the moral dilemma they face every time they perceive their child not to be well: do they consult with what might be trivia and risk being seen as 'bad' consulters, or do they delay and risk being labelled as 'bad' parents

STOP THINK   Two studies of patient information leaflets written with the intention of reducing GP consultations by patients with symptoms of minor illness have found no change in consultation rates (Fitzmaurice, 2001).
- Does this surprise you?
- Why do you think they had no effect?

Access

People experiencing symptoms are less likely to visit their doctor if they live further away from the clinic/surgery.

Access to child-care arrangements or the provision of a sitting service for a dependent relative, the availability of a telephone to make an appointment, the availability of a suitable appointment slot, and the approachability and friendliness of the doctor and the practice staff are also important factors affecting accessibility.

In some countries, but less so in the UK where most medical care is free at the point of use, the financial cost of payment may act as a deterrent to consulting a doctor.

Influence of family and friends

According to some studies, up to 50% of symptoms are taken to a doctor on the advice of family or friends. It appears that family are more likely than friends to recommend a visit to the doctor, possibly because they have the responsibility for caring for the individual.

Research with pregnant women has found that social class IV and V women with extensive and strong lay support and advice, sometimes referred to as people's lay referral network, are less likely to attend hospital antenatal classes compared with women from social classes I and II with less lay support. It has been suggested that both the relative number of lay advisers and the degree of congruence in culture between the woman and the doctor will affect the woman's decision whether or not to consult.

People who move to a new area away from their friends and family have been found to make more visits to a doctor in their first year after moving. This raised consultation rate may reflect

not only the absence of social support, but also the increased risk of ill health arising from the stress of moving house.

Triggers

Several studies have shown that it is not always the experience of symptoms that brings a person to see the doctor. A symptom or an anxiety may have been present for some time, but something else in the person's life triggers the person to consult. A relative may become concerned about a continuing problem and suggest a visit to the doctor; a change at work or in one's personal life may make the symptom more noticeable or incapacitating than before, precipitating a consultation.

Delaying

A good example of the problems associated with patients who delay when they experience symptoms relates to the symptoms of having a heart attack. There is good evidence that delay in receiving medical care is associated with higher mortality, which might have been avoided had treatment (defibrillation and/or thrombolytic therapy) been instituted earlier.

Ruston et al. (1998) found that people who did not delay seeking medical care had a better knowledge than 'delayers' of a wider range of symptoms of a heart attack, and were more likely to consider themselves at risk. Delayers were more likely to be taking medicines for other conditions, like dyspepsia, and would take these medicines and temporalize. Similarly, Horne et al. (2000) identified a mismatch between symptoms expected of a heart attack and symptoms actually experienced, leading to delay.

> ### Case study
>
> In a study of people experiencing angina (chest pain on exertion), Richards et al. (2002) found that, compared to residents living in an affluent area of Glasgow, residents from a deprived area reported greater vulnerability to heart disease but that this was not associated with higher reported use of a GP. Instead, they interpreted their symptoms as 'normal' and did not present to their doctor for fear that they would be reprimanded by the GP for bothering them with trivia.

Deciding to consult

- The decision to consult a doctor is a complex interplay of physical, psychological and social factors.

- Many people go with relatively minor symptoms because they are anxious that something serious may be indicated.

- People may delay with serious symptoms because of anxiety, lack of knowledge, mismatch of knowledge, use of substitute medication and the relative greater importance of other things in their lives.

- There is often a mismatch between what doctors and patients perceive as appropriate reasons for consulting.

- The perception of what the doctor can do for them and how they will treat them is a significant factor in individuals' decision to consult.

- A change in a person's social setting or relationships may trigger a consultation even when there has been no change in the symptoms.

Seeing the doctor

Every weekday in the UK, almost 1 million people consult their GP. The consultation between patient and doctor is at the core of all medical practice, be it with a GP or hospital doctor, be it in the UK or elsewhere. Although an intensely personal and private meeting, usually conducted behind closed doors or curtains, there are rituals and social norms (expected ways of behaving) that provide structure and coherence to what happens in a particular culture.

Doctor–patient relationship

Four models of the doctor–patient relationship have been described: (1) paternalistic; (2) mutual; (3) consumerist; and (4) default.

Paternalistic

The paternalistic relationship or *disease-centred* approach has, until recently, been the most commonly observed type of relationship. The doctor, a medical expert, makes a systematic enquiry with the patient answering relatively specific and closed questions, carries out appropriate tests and reaches a diagnosis or a range of possible diagnoses. The doctor then decides on the appropriate treatment, which the patient is expected to follow without question. The process is relatively technical and specific to the symptoms/problem that the patient presents.

In the 1980s, studies of doctor–patient relationships demonstrated that patients, particularly those with chronic illnesses, were also 'experts' in what the symptoms/problem meant to them and their families (Tuckett et al., 1985). This and other research suggested that patients sometimes held different ideas from their doctors about their illnesses, why they were ill or what they wanted to do about it.

Mutual

The mutual relationship is now becoming more common, partly as a result of greater patient knowledge, particularly about chronic disease, and partly because of a general cultural shift for individuals not to be passive followers of authority but autonomous agents in their own right. It is characterized by the doctor recognizing both this patient autonomy and the importance of the patient's own beliefs and knowledge of health and illness, and the social context in which the illness is dealt with. This model involves the doctor working with a *patient-centred* approach and is discussed in more detail below.

Consumerist

The consumerist relationship is becoming more common in the UK as a result of the extension of private health insurance, the introduction of patient charters, the increasing emphasis on extending patient choice and initiatives to provide quicker access to a doctor. It is characterized by patients 'shopping around' for their preferred care and is accompanied (as exemplified in the USA) by relatively high levels of investigation and treatment, and litigation.

Default

The fourth model, sometimes labelled default, is characterized by low levels of engagement between doctor and patient. It can be observed in situations where the doctor can find nothing organically wrong to explain the patient's symptoms, and where the patient is labelled as *somatizing*. There are very particular problems associated with the way patients and doctors respond to such situations, and there is a considerable risk that patients will become trapped in a cycle of overinvestigation and treatment.

The patient-centred approach

In its recommendations for undergraduate education in the UK, the General Medical Council (2002) emphasized the importance for all students of learning the patient-centred approach. Box 1 highlights five key features of the approach.

Stewart (2001) contrasts the patient-centred approach with 'what it is not – technology-centred, doctor-centred, hospital-centred, disease-centred'. This is unfortunate as there are good reasons for hospital doctors to use the patient-centred approach, particularly as many inpatients and outpatients are in hospital with acute episodes of illness often associated with, or complicated by, chronic illness. They have important information needs and have their own perspectives on what is happening to them (p. 102–103).

Box 1 **Patient-centred care**

- Explores the patient's main reason for the visit, concerns and need for information
- Seeks an integrated understanding of the patient's world – that is, the patient as a whole person, his or her emotional needs and life issues
- Finds common ground on what the problem is and mutually agrees on management
- Enhances prevention and health promotion
- Enhances the continuing relationship between the patient and the doctor

(Adapted from Stewart, 2001.)

The skilled doctor, whether in hospital or in the community, should be able to move easily between dealing quickly and effectively with acute, life-threatening symptoms using a disease-centred approach to taking a more patient-centred approach as soon as the threat to life has diminished (see pp. 96–97). Furthermore, the acute, disease-centred approach does not have to be at the expense of treating the patient with dignity, respect and humanity. Rather than being seen as two separate and incompatible styles, it is better to think of them as two approaches working in parallel, so that the doctor is skilled in both approaches. The importance of being able to work with both approaches is well illustrated by Kinmonth et al. (1998), who reported evidence of poorer disease management of people with type 2 diabetes by doctors who had received extra training in the patient-centred approach.

The research evidence for the practice of patient-centred care is complicated by different definitions of and methods of measuring patient-centred care. Similarly, definitions of and methods of measuring the outcome of care are not precise. Not all studies have reported a positive association between the practice of patient-centred care and the outcome of that care (Mead et al., 2002), but the weight of the evidence is that patients are more satisfied when they receive patient-centred care (Kinnersley et al., 1999; Little et al., 2001).

This judgement is confirmed by a review of longer consultations (Freeman et al., 2002). Patient-centred consultations generally take more time (Howie et al., 1992), and the review reported that longer consultations were associated with:

- Less prescribing (judged as desirable)
- More advice on lifestyle and health-promoting activities
- Better recognition and handling of psychosocial problems
- Better patient enablement (Howie et al., 1998)
- Better clinical care of some chronic illnesses
- Higher patient satisfaction.

A patient-centred consultation still involves taking a systematic history of the patient's presenting and underlying problems, but it differs from the more traditional paternalistic relationship by integrating it with an enquiry into the patient's ideas, knowledge, beliefs, concerns and expectations (see pp. 38–39). In their study of doctor–patient relationships, Tuckett et al. (1985) showed that consultations were most likely to break down and patients were most likely to be dissatisfied and non-compliant (see pp. 94–95) when doctors failed to elicit and respond empathetically to patients' beliefs and expectations. Of course, patients will sometimes hold unrealistic or inappropriate expectations. In such cases it is important that the doctor and patient are clear what the patient's expectations and beliefs are, and that the doctor explains in a manner that does not make the patient feel stupid or defensive why the belief or expectation is inappropriate. In some cases this will involve negotiation. Some of the strategies that patients and doctors use to control consultations are summarized in Table 1. Working-class people may sometimes express themselves rather directly, which doctors may interpret as a demand for a particular test or treatment. On occasion, no resolution may be found, and both patient and doctor are likely to feel dissatisfied with the consultation.

Table 1 **Negotiation strategies**	
Patients	**Doctors**
Disclose	Physical setting of room
Suggest	Language
Demand	Technical/non technical
Leading question	Open/closed questions
Non-verbal behaviour	Tone of voice
Hesitation/silence	Clarifying/functional uncertainty
Delaying tactics	Listening/interrupting
'While I'm here…'	Picking up/ignoring cues
See a different doctor	Non-verbal behaviour
	Interest/uninterest
	Calm/haste
	Prescription

It is also important to remember that a single consultation between a patient and a doctor does not occur in isolation, particularly in general practice. A 5- or 10-minute consultation may be but one of a series of consultations during which patient and doctor may negotiate the diagnostic and treatment possibilities, and the implications for the patient's general well-being. Continuity of care is important for many patients.

Lack of time may frequently constrain a doctor from being as person-centred as he or she would like, and this puts pressure on the doctor and on the patient. Figure 1 illustrates the surgery of a patient-centred doctor who has a personal commitment immediately the surgery is due to end at 6.10. She uses the first hour to see three patients but, despite trying to catch up, she reaches 5.45 with only 15 minutes available for three patients who have each waited almost an hour past their appointment times.

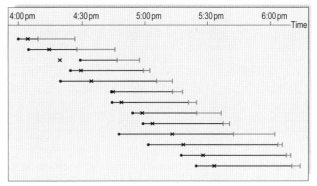

Fig. 1 Afternoon surgery with appointments booked every 7.5 minutes. X indicates appointment time. Red line indicates waiting time, green line the actual visit.

Patients themselves are very conscious not only of their responsibility not to consult with trivia (see pp. 88–89), but also not to take up too much of the doctor's precious time. Patients often feel intimidated by doctors and are reluctant to ask questions, mention anxieties or voice other things (agendas) they want to raise. Barry et al. (2000) describe a qualitative study of 35 patients who had revealed in preconsultation interviews that they had a total of 188 agendas they wished to raise. Only four voiced all their agendas and, in total, 73 agendas were never mentioned. Agenda items that weren't mentioned were associated with negative outcomes, particularly major misunderstandings.

Given that people frequently have anxieties that relatively minor symptoms may mask something more serious, and given their reluctance to present with mental health problems (Pollock & Grime, 2002; and see pp. 88–89), it should not be surprising that they often feel unable to mention their worries lest the doctor think that they are wasting the GP's time with trivia or taking more than their 'fair share'.

 STOP THINK
- Not all studies have found that patients prefer patient-centred care. Why might this be?
- Will the consumerist model become the dominant type of patient–doctor relationship, and if so, how will this affect the patient-centred approach?

Seeing the doctor

- Doctors and patients have different knowledge, beliefs, wants and expectations, and consultations often involve negotiation.
- The process and outcome of care differ not just between patients but between doctors and especially in doctor style.
- Patient-centred doctors are more likely than disease-centred doctors to identify patients' psychosocial problems, and to deal with their anxieties.
- Patients are often reluctant to voice their ideas and anxieties in case they are thought of as inappropriate, stupid or time-wasting.

Placebo and nocebo effects

A remedy without any direct action on a disease, given to keep the patient happy, or to persuade the prescriber that he is doing something positive and useful, or both
(Penguin Medical Encyclopaedia)

The placebo effect (from the Latin 'I will please') is important to understand because it can have a great effect on the treatment of patients. Placebos are used and abused, but often little understood.

The emergence of placebo effects

Until recently there could be no neat distinction between drugs whose mode of action for a specific disorder was known and understood, and any other drug (Fig. 1). With the development of scientific medicine, people then began to identify active ingredients and to become more suspicious of drugs whose action was not understood. This introduced the notion that there were drugs that would treat a particular condition by a particular route and other substances that might be placebos.

However, placebos have been shown to bring about clinical improvement in many branches of medicine: surgery, the treatment of cancer, dentistry, psychiatry, paediatrics and numerous others. They can produce the same phenomena observed with other drugs:

- Habituation (a tendency to increase the dose over time)
- Withdrawal symptoms
- Dependence (an inability to stop taking them without psychiatric help)
- Inverse relationship between severity of symptom and efficacy of placebo.

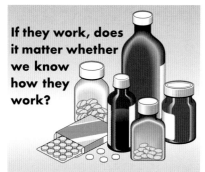

If they work, does it matter whether we know how they work?

Fig. 1 Drugs and mode of action.

The nocebo phenomenon

It is also possible for a drug or procedure to produce adverse effects that are not the result of any known pharmacological mechanism. These are called nocebo effects, from the Latin 'I will harm'. In one study women who believed they were prone to heart disease were nearly four times as likely to die as women with similar risk factors who did not believe this (Eaker et al., 1992). Another large study in California found that Chinese-Americans who had a combination of birth year and disease which Chinese astrology and medicine consider ill-fated died younger than matched white controls (Phillips et al., 1993). Although effects can be severe, reported nocebo symptoms are more usually generalized and diffuse, such as drowsiness, nausea, fatigue and insomnia. In clinical trials these nocebo effects can be severe enough to lead to non-adherence, discontinuation and drop-out.

Placebos and clinical trials

In order to demonstrate the efficacy of any new treatment now, clinical trials include a placebo for comparison so that such effects can be separated from the effects of the experimental compound. These are often double-blind trials, i.e. neither the patient nor the member of staff who gives it knows which is the experimental drug and which is the placebo. This ensures that nothing can influence a patient's expectations about the drug and, therefore, the response.

Types of placebo
- Pure placebo: thought to contain no active ingredient, for example, a sugar pill.
- Impure placebo: contains an active ingredient, but one which is not known to have any effect on the condition being treated, e.g. a vitamin C tablet being given for headache.
- Placebo procedure: a procedure, for instance taking blood pressure, which is not known to produce any clinical change.

What makes one susceptible?
The literature on personality traits as a way of predicting who will and will not experience placebo or nocebo effects has failed to show any reliable predictors. Interpersonal factors such as the therapeutic relationship with the caregiver appear to be more important. However, circumstances and presentation appear to be the most influential. For example, people's perception of pain depends on the situation: people injured in combat appear to tolerate pain better than those with similar injuries in hospital. In war, an injury means evacuation to safety and thus brings great relief; this is not the same in civilian life. With placebos, experiments have demonstrated a number of factors that produce a response, for instance:

- The physical appearance of the placebo; for example, green tranquillizers reduce anxiety more than yellow or red ones (Shapira et al., 1970).
- Branding: products that have been marketed or are branded rather than generic will produce greater effects than unbranded products or placebos.
- The reputation of the setting, e.g. a university research unit will enhance treatment more than a back-street clinic.
- The patient's perception of staff attitudes affects response. For example, where doctors are judged as more interested and enthusiastic, the results are more positive.

The nocebo phenomenon has been found to be more common in women than men, and although cultural and ethnic factors are thought to be important, there is little empirical evidence (Barsky et al., 2002). Nocebo effects are more likely to be found in:

- People who expect to experience side-effects
- Patients who have been previously conditioned to experience side-effects
- Patients with certain psychological characteristics, such as anxiety, depression or neuroticism.

How do they work?

The placebo and nocebo effects are simply a part of a wider field linking social and meaningful processes with human biological processes. This has been termed *sociomatics* (Kleinman, 1986). Consequently, there are various possible contributory mechanisms:

Case study

Levine and colleagues (1978) hypothesized that placebo effects that relieve pain are mediated by endorphin release. If that were the case, then naloxone (an opiate antagonist) would block them. They gave medication to patients after surgery in a double-blind trial (Fig. 2). The patients had all had wisdom teeth removed. Group 1 were given morphine, group 2 had naloxone and group 3 got a placebo. Of those initially given a placebo (group 3), half were given another placebo 1 hour later (group 3a), and half were given naloxone 1 hour later (group 3b). Our interest lies in these two groups of patients. When they were initially given the placebo, 39% reported a significant decrease in pain, but if they were in group 3b, those given naloxone, the pain increased again. For those who had not responded to the placebo, the naloxone made no difference. So it appeared that some patients obtained significant pain relief from a placebo, but this was reversed by an opiate antagonist. The experiments concluded that endorphin release must have occurred with the placebo.

	First dose	Second dose		Levels of pain reported	
				First dose	Second dose
Group 1	Morphine	Morphine			
Group 2	Naloxone	Placebo			
Group 3a	Placebo	Placebo	Responders		
			Non-responders		
Group 3b	Placebo	Naloxone	Responders		
			Non-responders		

Fig. 2 Levels of pain reported in a double-blind trial of naloxone/placebo (from Levine et al., 1978, pp. 654–657, with permission).

- Social influence – doctors are perceived as people in authority and, therefore, their direction and expectations are followed.
- Role expectation – the doctor's role is to organize treatment, and the patient's role is to get better, so he or she plays that role.
- Classical conditioning – for a patient, past experiences of taking drugs led to improvement, so the administration of a new drug is more likely to produce the same response (see pp. 22–23).
- Operant conditioning – the doctor rewards the patient who shows any sign of improvement, thus increasing the probability that the patient will continue to report improvement (see pp 22–23).
- Cognitive influence – the patient has firm beliefs about medical treatment, such as: 'modern medicine is based on scientific evidence, therefore this drug will be effective'. Of course, the opposite would also be true: if the patient believes modern medicine to be harmful, he or she may be less likely to respond and may, in fact, experience adverse effects.

STOP THINK Many people in prison are vulnerable and have in the past been dependent on drugs or alcohol. They feel the need to continue to take something 'to help with nerves'. Part of this dependence is psychological rather than chemical and they frequently come to the medical officer asking for medication.
- Should a medical officer prescribe a placebo in this case, 'to keep the patient happy, or to persuade the prescriber that he is doing something positive or useful, or both'?

What are doctors' attitudes to placebo effects?

Many doctors have strong feelings about the use of placebos in medicine: some are positive, but many are negative, perhaps because the placebo effect is similar to faith-healing, when many doctors prefer to see medicine as a science. Although most health professionals are aware of the therapeutic aspect of placebo, fewer are aware of the nocebo phenomenon. Views about placebo effects can range widely:

- Placebo effects are a nuisance that interfere with the understanding and practice of medicine.
- Placebo effects are powerful, but to use placebos in practice is a betrayal of trust between doctor and patient.
- Placebo effects are powerful and should be usefully incorporated to enhance treatment.

Placebo and nocebo effects

- Placebo effects have been demonstrated in many branches of medicine.
- Nocebo phenomena are usually generalized and diffuse adverse symptoms.
- Placebo effects ought to be controlled in experimental trials of medical procedures.
- There are no established personal characteristics that will predict a therapeutic response to placebo.
- Nocebo phenomena are more likely among people who expect to experience adverse effects or have been previously conditioned to experience adverse effects.
- Effects are influenced by context: culture, expectations and beliefs.
- There are ethical issues involved in the clinical use of placebos.

Patient adherence

Adherence refers to following advice given by health care professionals. This includes taking preventive action (e.g. reducing alcohol consumption), keeping medical appointments (e.g. screening or follow-up appointments), following self-care advice (e.g. caring for a wound after surgery) and taking medication as directed (e.g. in relation to dose and timing). Non-adherence is usually defined as a failure to follow advice, which will lead to a harmful effect on health or a decrease in medication effectiveness. Most medical interventions rely on patient adherence: ordinarily diagnosis and prescription only have an impact on patients' health through their own action. The term 'adherence' is used instead of 'compliance' because the latter implies a need for patient obedience, rather than informed decision-making.

Patients' reports, pill counts and analysis of blood or urine samples can be used to measure adherence. Patients consistently overestimate their adherence when self-report measures are compared to objective measures (Myers & Midence, 1998) but some simple self-report measures can provide good estimates of adherence (Morisky et al., 1986).

How good is patient adherence?

Adherence varies across behaviours but about 40–45% of patients are non-adherent (Ley, 1997). This implies that: (1) almost half of all prescribed medication has a reduced health impact; (2) doctors may only be effective with 55–60% of their patients; and (3) patients are becoming ill unnecessarily due to non-adherence. It has also been suggested that 10–25% of hospital admissions are due to non-adherence. Even when patients' lives depend on taking medication as directed, as is the case with heart and liver transplant patients, between 5% and 33% of patients have been found to be non-adherent (Rovelli et al., 1989).

Why do patients not follow advice?

Patients may be non-adherent for different reasons and in different ways (Donovan & Blake, 1992).

Some patients may intend to take recommended medication but forget to do so or find it difficult. Others may disagree with the diagnosis or the medication regimen and decide not to take the medication, or take more or less than was advised. In addition, as Conrad (1985) noted, patients may test their health or improvement by suspending medication or stop taking medication temporarily to avoid side-effects that could impinge on important social events. Others may be reluctant to take medication for fear of dependence.

How can doctors increase adherence?

Adherence is most likely when patients understand what they are being asked to do and why. Patients must remember what they are told if they are to act on it later and, finally, satisfaction with the doctor and the consultation makes adherence more likely (Fig. 1).

Patients are more likely to feel satisfied and to understand advice when doctors find out what they think is wrong and discuss this. The doctor should seek to reach an agreement with the patient about what is wrong and what should be done about it. The importance of such cooperation has been underlined by the proposal that, instead of encouraging adherence, doctors should seek to establish *concordance* in their consultations (Mullen, 1997). If doctors can facilitate joint negotiated decision-making, or concordance, about treatment, then patients are more likely to intend to adhere. For example, if a drug and regimen are jointly agreed then the patient is likely to be committed to taking the drug as recommended. This implies that the feasibility of any particular regimen needs to be assessed for each patient. For example, in interviews of type 2 diabetic patients

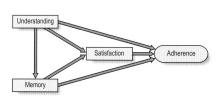

Fig. 1 Key determinants of patient adherence (adapted from Ley, 1997, with permission).

of Pakistani origin, Bissell et al. (2004) found that some patients felt they could not discuss emotional, familial and financial factors which undermined their attempts to follow a diet appropriate to their condition. Thus these patients were unable to discuss key barriers to achieving adherence, so limiting the possibility that their doctor could offer them advice about how to approximate the recommended diet most closely within the constraints they experienced. If doctors are to ensure that their advice is clearly understood and also consider difficulties the patient may have in following an agreed plan, time must be allowed for discussion and negotiation in consultations. This is especially important because studies suggest that patients with less social support are less likely to be adherent.

If patients feels that their doctor is not interested in their problem or has not understood it, this will undermine confidence in the doctor's advice. For example, in a well-known study of paediatric consultations, Korsch et al. (1968) found that mothers who were very satisfied with their doctor's warmth, concern and communication were three times more likely to adhere than dissatisfied mothers. Satisfaction depends upon the patient's perception of the doctor's sensitivity, concern, respect and competence. Reducing waiting time, taking time to greet the patient in a courteous manner and engaging in friendly introductory exchanges are all likely to increase satisfaction. Asking open-ended questions which cannot be answered 'yes' or 'no' and allowing patients time to express their worries is also likely to make them feel satisfied with the consultation (see pp. 96–97).

Using simple words to describe the body or treatments and encouraging patients to express their views is essential to patients' understanding. Clear communication depends upon knowing what others already know and what they expect from us. The doctor's task is like giving directions. Deciding upon the most effective directions involves establishing common understanding of local geography. Similarly, the doctor may need to assess the patient's health knowledge, beliefs and expectations before deciding how to explain the problem and treatment. Assessing health beliefs (see pp. 38–39) and clarifying any misunderstandings regarding, for example, symptom severity, treatment effectiveness or side-effects may motivate patients to follow an agreed treatment plan (see Case Study). Assessing how motivated patients are and what others may think of their illness or of the suggested treatment may also help identify problems that could lead to poor adherence.

Telling someone what you are about to tell them makes it more likely they will remember because this assists with the process of encoding in memory (see pp. 98–99). Such labelling of information is called *explicit categorization*. For example, a doctor might say, 'I'm going to tell you what I think is wrong with you' or 'I'm going to remind you when you should take your tablets and how many you should take' before conveying these important pieces of information. Instructions may also be remembered more easily if the doctor stresses that they are important and repeats them. Specific advice, for example, 'cut the number of cigarettes you smoke by half' or 'make an appointment for 2 weeks' time', is easier to remember than general suggestions such as 'cut down the amount you smoke' or 'come in again soon'. Similarly, simple advice and regimens are easier to understand and remember. Where possible, doctors should negotiate regimens that suit the patient. For example, the progestogen-only pill may not be an appropriate contraceptive for a woman who thinks she is unlikely to remember to take it at the same time every day. Encouraging patients to take notes in consultations and providing printed information can ensure that patients have accurate information. Using such techniques has been shown to improve the amount of information remembered by patients in general practice (Box 1).

Understanding why patients do not adhere is important to promoting adherence. Key questions that influence patients' decisions to adhere, or not, are:
- Do I really need this treatment?
- Am I at risk of symptoms without doing what was advised?
- How effective/beneficial is the recommended action? What side-effects will it have?
- Will adherence conflict with other things I want to do?

If consultations with health care professionals result in

Case study

Janice uses bronchodilator inhaler to control her asthma symptoms. She also has a preventive steroid inhaler but is reluctant to use it because she worried about the potential side-effects of taking steroids. When she asked her doctor for her usual repeat prescription, she was asked to make an appointment.

Her doctor explained that she should be using the preventive steroid inhaler every day to control her symptoms and that she was relying too heavily on the bronchodilator. The doctor asked her if she understood. Janice understood and confirmed this. The doctor wrote the prescription and Janice, who was worried about missing her driving lesson in 15 minutes' time, left without asking any questions.

Janice started taking the preventive steroid inhaler morning and night as advised. Then she watched a television programme about the side-effects of steroids on body builders and, again, began to worry about potential long-term effects of using the steroid inhaler. Combined with her concerns about oral thrush, this was enough to discourage Janice. She stopped using the steroid inhaler and reverted to controlling her asthma by using the bronchodilator. Three months later Janice got a repeat prescription without seeing a doctor.

Box 1 **Helping patients remember in general practice**

Ley et al. (1976) assessed the amount of information that the patients of four doctors remembered. The researchers then developed a brief manual for the doctors, which explained how they could simplify information, use explicit categorization and repetition and give specific rather than general advice. The amount of information patients remembered after their doctors had read the manual increased from an average of 56% to an average of 71%, suggesting that memory-enhancing communication increased the amount patients remembered.

Information remembered by patients		
	Before (%)	After (%)
Doctor A	52	61
Doctor B	56	70
Doctor C	57	73
Doctor D	59	80

misunderstandings regarding illness or treatment, this may also lead to non-adherence.

Finally, adherence may be especially difficult to enhance among some patients with chronic conditions where the behaviour changes required are long-term. In a systematic review of randomized controlled trials of adherence interventions, Haynes et al. (1996) found that 7 of 15 interventions led to improvements in adherence. However, long-term interventions tended to involve a series of techniques requiring additional attention and supervision from health care professionals and even these did not lead to substantial improvements. Thus a different approach

to enhancing adherence in longer-term care may be required, including a deepening of the concordance reached in relationships between health care professionals and their patients.

 STOP THINK A patient taking antihypertension medication returns for a routine check-up. You find that his blood pressure is high. What do you do – increase the dose, change the medication, refer the patient for further tests or talk to the patient about the medication and any problems which may be involved in taking it?

Patient adherence

- Up to 45% of patients are non-adherent.
- Adherence is more likely when patients understand advice, remember it and feel satisfied with the consultation.
- Doctors can increase satisfaction by being friendly and considerate.
- Adherence is more likely when doctors consider and discuss the patient's perspective, including his or her understanding, motivation and any perceived barriers to following advice.
- Doctors can increase understanding by simplifying information and by discussion of patients' health beliefs.
- Doctors can increase patients' recall by using explicit categorization, stressing and repeating instructions and giving specific advice.

Communication skills

A doctor must integrate four components to achieve a successful consultation: (1) clinical knowledge; (2) problem-solving; (3) physical examination; and (4) communication skills. There is no point in having excellent factual knowledge if you cannot identify the reason why your patient attended, or help that patient understand a treatment plan.

If doctors are poor at doctor–patient communication there is increased risk of:

- Failing to identify the patient's main problem (Stewart et al., 1979)
- Poor management (Kaplan et al., 1989)
- Poor adherence with treatment (George et al., 2005), which is in turn associated with increased mortality (Simpson et al., 2006)
- Patient dissatisfaction (O'Keefe et al., 2001)
- Patient complaints (Audit Commission, 1993).

The centrality of communication skills in clinical practice is recognized by the General Medical Council in policy documents, including *Good Medical Practice* (2006). Doctors whose performance is seriously deficient in communication skills can have their registration removed or restricted in the UK. One factor emphasized in *Medical Students: Professional Behaviour and Fitness to Practise* (http://www.gmc-uk.org/students/index.asp) is the importance of not allowing your personal views about, for example, a patient's religion or sexual orientation to influence the professional relationship or prejudice patient care.

The consultation

A consultation involves several key communication tasks which can be summarized as follows: (1) building a relationship with the patient (rapport); (2) gathering information (history-taking); (3) giving information (e.g. test results); and (4) carrying out these tasks in a coherent, logical way (Kurtz et al., 2004). The last factor is increasingly important with short appointment times (see pp. 90–91).

Gathering information is not just a matter of discovering the biomedical facts, but also an opportunity to assess the patient's perspective of his or her illness, as well as relevant social and economic factors (e.g. does the patient have support at home?).

Factors affecting doctor–patient communication within the consultation

These can be considered under three broad headings: (1) preparation and planning; (2) non-verbal communication (NVC); and (3) verbal communication.

Preparation and planning

- Have the right information ready before you see the patient (read the notes!).
- Seating: remove barriers such as tables and desks. Sit at an angle of about 45° to the patient rather than directly facing. Don't stand if the patient is sitting or lying down – sit on a chair next to the bed or the patient.
- Privacy: unless patients know they won't be overheard, they are unlikely to talk freely.
- Noise and interruptions: try to make sure you won't be disturbed, particularly if talking about a sensitive subject or breaking bad news.

Non-verbal communication

NVC refers to behaviour other than speech which influences social interaction. NVC is not normally under conscious control but you can adapt your NVC to send the signals that you want the patient to receive. Among the most important aspects of NVC are:

- First impressions do count. Does your greeting convey warmth and caring, or that you are pressed for time? Think about your body language, clothes and manner.
- Proximity: sitting a comfortable distance from a patient assists communication. Being too distant makes the doctor seem aloof, whereas being too close may feel threatening. Remember that different cultures have different boundaries for personal space.
- Posture: sitting upright but relaxed, with arms and legs uncrossed and leaning slightly toward the patient, conveys attentiveness.
- Eye contact: this is very powerful for initiating, maintaining and ending communication. The doctor's gaze should be in the direction of the patient without staring. Don't look at a computer screen when the patient is in the room!
- Facial expression: you can show interest, compassion and concern by your facial expression – or embarrassment or confusion, but these tend not to inspire confidence in the patient!
- Head nods convey understanding and encouragement to say more. However, don't overdo it – vigorous nodding may be interpreted as impatience.
- Touch: touch can be facilitative (e.g. establishing a friendly relationship with the patient by shaking hands on meeting), functional (e.g. physical examination) or therapeutic (e.g. touching a distressed patient on the hand to console).
- Paralinguistic features: this refers to aspects of verbal messages that serve to modulate their meaning, such as tone, pitch and volume. Paralinguistics can determine whether the same words, e.g. 'You took all the tablets', are expressed as a statement of fact, surprise, or as a question.
- Silence: allow the patient time to respond, or think how to answer a question, without jumping in with another question too quickly.

Used skilfully, non-verbal behaviours offer powerful tools with which to encourage a patient to talk, and to demonstrate interest in, and understanding of, the patient's predicament.

Verbal communication

Language is critical to getting and giving information effectively. Different aspects of verbal clinical communication can be identified.

Questioning

Three broad categories can be distinguished:

1. Opening question. So called as it encourages patients to tell you why they presented today. It is important not to interrupt patients early on so you grasp the problem: listening to their story at this point in the consultation is a useful investment of time.

2. Open questions. These are useful early on for encouraging patients to describe fully their problems. These questions are also good for eliciting beliefs, opinions or feelings, for example:
   - What's been troubling you?
   - How do you feel about the operation?
3. Closed questions. These are so called because they tend to limit the patient to one- or two-word answers. They are useful for obtaining or clarifying details and allowing functional enquiry. Examples include questions which invite:
   - an item of detail – When did the pain start?
   - yes/no response – Is the pain still there?

Typically a consultation will start with open questions, then narrow to closed ones as you gather specific information. It is also important to avoid asking more than one question at once, as this is confusing to the patient, and to avoid leading questions.

Reflecting
When you think patients have more to tell you, often about their worries, reflecting means encouraging them to continue by repeating back to them part of what they have said. For example, 'So, your daughter said …?'

Summarizing
When you think patients have told you all they are going to tell you, and you have gathered all the information you need, a summary draws together the significant aspects of what has been said. For example, 'let me just go over everything to check I've got it right…' Summaries are very useful for showing the patient you've been listening, to clarify any misinterpretations or to remind patients that there is something else they want to tell you.

Giving information/diagnosis
Moving on to the second part of the consultation, delivering lucid, coherent explanations *that the patient understands* is critical to providing patients with an understanding of their illness, diagnosis, investigations or treatment. When giving an explanation it helps to:

- Check what the patient knows already – so you can gauge how much information you need to give, and any misunderstandings you need to correct.

Case study
Peter was a 26-year-old physiology PhD student with a recent history of passing blood following mild exercise. At a busy outpatient clinic he had just undergone an intravenous pyelogram to X-ray his kidneys and was called to see the consultant, Mr Brown.

Mr Brown (looking at X-ray on screen): *Well, Peter, I can find nothing wrong with your kidneys. I think you have a touch of long-march haematuria, which sometimes happens to people who exercise a lot.*

Peter (in a hesitating voice): *Oh? I … I've read a bit about that condition and I don't think it fits with what happens to me.*

Response 1
Mr Brown (turning to stare at Peter with an expression of disbelief and annoyance): *Oh, you don't (pause)! Well, in that case you've just talked yourself into a cystoscopy! We'll send you an appointment for a few weeks' time* (walks off briskly).

Peter (looking very anxious): *Oh dear. Thanks.*

Response 2
Mr Brown (turning with an expression of surprise but interest): *What makes you say that, Peter?*

Peter: *Well, the blood I pass is bright red and in this condition I believe it's usually a dark brown colour.*

Mr Brown: *I see! That's possibly significant (pause). Well, we could do a cystoscopy to have a look in your bladder. That would mean giving you a general anaesthetic and passing a fine optic fibre up through your penis. How would you feel about us doing that?*

Peter (looking apprehensive): *Well … OK, if you think it will help find out what's wrong with me.*

How successful is the rapport and information exchange between doctor and patient in each example? Which would you prefer if you were the patient, and why?

- Ask how much the patient wants to know, e.g. 'Do you want me to explain a bit more about…?'
- Tell the patient what you are going to do, e.g. give test results, explain diagnosis, then explain treatment options.
- Use a series of logical points and give the patient time to ask questions after each piece of information.
- Avoid or explain any jargon.
- Repeat and emphasize key points.
- Use examples and diagrams; write the key points down for the patient to take away.
- Give specific rather than vague advice.
- Ask for feedback on understanding.

 STOP THINK Patients often complain that doctors do not ask about their feelings or emotional responses to illness. But some doctors argue that their job is just to treat disease, not deal with how people cope with it.
- What's your opinion on this view of medical practice?

Communication skills
- Doctor–patient communication is central to effective medical practice and can affect quality of care.
- Effective rapport, information-gathering and giving and carrying out a structured consultation are key tasks in medical interviewing.
- Three factors which influence the effectiveness of doctor–patient communication are:
  1. Preparation and planning
  2. Non-verbal communication
  3. Verbal communication.
- Effective clinical communication requires the ability to use the relevant skills flexibly in response to the needs of different patients.
- Good resources include the website www.skillscascade.com and Jackson (2006).

Breaking bad news

What is bad news?

Bad news has been defined as 'any news that drastically and negatively alters the person's view of her or his future' (Buckman, 1994). Bad news may be giving a terminal or life-changing prognosis, e.g. metastatic cancer or multiple sclerosis, but it could also be news of sudden loss, e.g. telling a young wife that her husband has died after a massive heart attack or parents that their teenage son has been killed in a motorbike accident. It may also be about something seemingly much less dramatic for patients but no less distressing, for example, telling the young man keen to be a pilot that he has diabetes. The impact of the news will have not only medical but also physical, social, emotional and occupational consequences, which health professionals often fail to appreciate (Fallowfield & Jenkins, 2004).

Why is it difficult?

There are several reasons why breaking bad news is an especially difficult task for doctors, irrespective of their age, speciality or professional experience. These may be personal (related to their own personality or past experience), social (to do with society's attitudes), professional (influenced by role or peer values) or legal/political (Buckman, 1994). Some of these are listed in Box 1. In addition, it may be made more difficult if family members want to protect the person from bad news and distress (Kaye, 1996). Under these circumstances, the doctor may be asked to collude with the relatives in order to maintain a conspiracy of silence. This situation often puts strain on a previously healthy relationship both with the doctor and within the family, and can lead to feelings of mistrust and isolation on the part of the patient.

Though traditionally doctors withheld bad news from patients, believing this to be in patients' best interest, studies now show that most people want the truth about their diagnosis but the depth of information sought will vary according to individual needs (Meredith et al., 1996; Yardley et al., 2001). Despite these findings, truth-telling, particularly with cancer patients, is still not universally practised (Surbone, 2006) and 'doctors

> **Box 1** **Difficulties involved in breaking bad news**
>
> **Personal**
> - Fear of own illness/death
> - Fear of expressing own emotions, e.g. crying
> - Recent bereavement
> - Identification with own experience (for example, victim may be the same age)
> - Embarrassment/distress/discomfort
>
> **Social**
> - Removal of death from home to institution makes death unacceptable and taboo
> - Sickness stigmatized
>
> **Professional**
> - Lack of experience or training
> - Fear of eliciting a difficult response, e.g. anger
> - Fear of being blamed by person or superiors
> - Failure to provide cure
> - Fear of causing pain/emotional damage
> - Fear of destroying hope
>
> **Political**
> - Fear of litigation
>
> (From Buckman, 1994, with permission.)

still frequently censor the amount of information they give to patients about prognosis on the grounds that what someone does not know cannot harm them' (Fallowfield & Jenkins, 2004). Research has also shown that doctors find the breaking of bad news so stressful that they adopt a variety of strategies to make the task easier for themselves (Taylor, 1988). The use of these strategies in turn can affect the amount and type of information doctors give to patients, i.e. their policy of disclosure. For example, some use medical jargon and statistics to explain a prognosis and focus on survival rates while others explain the diagnosis with complex euphemisms to soften the blow.

Reactions to bad news

People react to bad news differently. The impact will depend partly on the gap between what the person hopes for and the medical reality (Buckman, 1994). Reactions may also be dictated by the person's past experiences, personality and coping strategies. They may be unrelated to the type or stage of the disease. Reactions may vary from calm or resigned acceptance to acute distress, anxiety, anger, shock and denial.

However, the way a doctor breaks news of this kind can also affect how patients later adjust to and cope with their illness as well as influence their treatment choices (Fallowfield & Jenkins, 2004). This knowledge as well as studies of patients' preferences has led to the development of numerous guidelines which describe ways in which doctors can manage this situation to make it easier for themselves and those receiving the news (Buckman, 1994; Faulkner et al., 1994; Kaye, 1996; Twycross, 1999; Watson et al., 2006).

Preparation

Check the person's physical ability to take in news

Before attempting to give any information of this kind it is important to make sure that the patient or relative is physically and mentally able to understand (Faulkner et al., 1994). In the case of a serious diagnosis, such as cancer, patients may already be experiencing symptoms that are preventing them from thinking clearly, such as confusion or drowsiness. It is necessary, therefore, to treat any condition that will prevent the person from comprehending the news, before attempting to impart the news.

Check own appearance and readiness

How doctors present themselves during consultations can also help patients to accept the news more easily. Making sure that you appear comfortable, relaxed and not rushed will communicate to patients that you have the time to spend with them and feel at ease with the task. Appearing in a blood-stained coat and/or looking tense and harassed will only serve to heighten patients' stress. Doctors should also have familiarized themselves with the patients' notes and made a rough plan of what they want to communicate.

Setting the scene

The context of where the news will be broken is as important as how it is broken. The most appropriate place will be a quiet side room on the ward to ensure the person's privacy and concentration. Bleeps and phones should be switched off to minimize the possibility of interruption. People will absorb the news better if they feel as relaxed and comfortable as possible. Most doctors find it helpful to be accompanied by another member of staff, e.g. a nurse, social worker or chaplain, as well as allowing the person to be joined by a relative or friend. The presence of other people can often help to clarify information that was given by the doctor after the interview, as well as providing emotional support when the news is broken.

Breaking the news

Step 1 It is essential before breaking the news to find out what patients already know and understand about their illness. This will inform the doctor of the degree of insight and provide a baseline on which to build. Sometimes a patient will indicate that he or she already suspects that something is seriously wrong. This may be especially true of people who have been experiencing difficult symptoms or have known a relative or friend who has had the same illness.

Step 2 Before continuing, the doctor should find out what the person wants to know about his/her illness. This can be done by asking the person directly, and should leave the doctor in no doubt about how much information to give. For example, some people will only want to know about their treatment without wishing to speak about their diagnosis or prognosis. Others will require much more detail.

Step 3 The news should be broken simply and clearly but avoiding bluntness and euphemisms. To begin with, some information should be given by the doctor to warn the person that the news is not good. For example, 'The results of the tests are more serious than we thought'.

Step 4 Leave silence and allow time for news to sink in. Seek the patient's permission to continue.

Step 5 You can keep giving information as long as the person is asking for it and understands what is being said. Diagrams or drawings can sometimes help patients to understand more clearly. Check if the person wants more information before continuing or stopping.

Step 6 Encourage patients to express their concerns and feelings. This will show that you empathize with them and increase their satisfaction with the consultation.

Step 7 Plan the treatment programme or the next set of actions with the patient or relatives (for example, with

Case study

Case study

John is a 34-year-old man who is engaged to be married next year. For the past 2 years he has periodically experienced pins and needles in his arms and legs. Although his fiancée and family urged him to go to the doctor he had shrugged the symptoms off. In the last few weeks, however, an episode of blurred vision and a temporary loss of power in his right leg precipitated his referral to a neurologist by his GP. A series of tests confirmed a diagnosis of multiple sclerosis. Unfortunately, the neurologist was unable to give the news himself because a prior commitment to present a paper at a conference meant that he had to be absent from the ward for a few days. He therefore asked his house officer to break the bad news in his place. This worried the house officer because he had never had to do this before. To minimize his anxiety, he decided he would do it while taking blood from John as this would give them both something to concentrate on. On hearing the news, John was devastated. He began to cry and then became angry with the house officer and demanded to see the consultant. Not knowing how to respond to this reaction, the house officer fled to find the ward sister.

bereaved relatives, this may be viewing the body). Asking them to summarize the main points of the consultation will inform the doctor about how much of the news they have understood. It is also vital that the doctor arranges to see the patient at a follow-up interview in order to help clarify any misunderstandings or anxieties the person may have about the news. Follow-up plans should be documented in the patient's notes and shared with colleagues.

No news is bad news

An important part of communicating news to patients is conveying the results of tests. It can be difficult to reassure patients who have been anticipating bad news that the news is good. Studies show that patients who are experiencing symptoms but have negative test results may remain anxious long after the consultation and continue to experience the same symptoms, often leading them to consult again. Reasons for this anxiety may be a misunderstanding of what the doctor has said or disbelief. Doubt may also be fuelled by conflicting evidence from an individual's personal circumstances – for example, knowing someone with the same symptoms who has died or who has had a false-negative result. In these circumstances direct discussion of the patient's concerns is advocated rather than referring the patient on for further tests (McDonald et al., 1996).

Sudden bad news

In cases of trauma, the task of breaking bad news may be even more difficult because of the suddenness and unexpectedness of the death, illness or accident. In addition, there will usually have been no time to establish a relationship with the person beforehand or warn him or her that the

news is serious. Often the situation is complicated by the fact that the victim may be young, the next of kin may be difficult to establish or to contact and it may be less easy to control the context in a busy accident and emergency department or intensive care unit (McLauchlan, 1990). In these situations the police may be a useful source of help in contacting and supporting relatives.

Conclusion

Giving sad and bad news in medicine will always remain a part of the doctor's role. Good training and guidelines can help you do this better (Fallowfield & Jenkins, 2004).

- How would you have broken the news to John?
- What factors might have caused John to react the way he did?
- If you were the ward sister, what would you do to help John now?

Breaking bad news

- Ensure the person is physically able to take in the news.
- Find a quiet room where the news can be broken in privacy and undisturbed.
- Allow the person to be accompanied by a friend/relative/staff member.
- Check what the person already knows, understands and requires to know further.
- Give warning to alert the person that the news is serious.
- Continue giving information if the person is understanding and responding positively to it.
- Monitor the person's reaction and respond.
- Plan next course of action with the person and always arrange follow-up.

Self-care and the popular sector

People experiencing physical discomfort or emotional distress do not always turn to a doctor for advice and treatment. In all societies there is a range of ways in which people either help themselves or seek help from others. Kleinman (1985) has suggested that health care systems are composed of different sectors or arenas – the popular sector, the folk sector and the professional sector – although they may partly overlap with each other (Fig. 1). In western industrialized societies, the professional sector is predominantly that provided by biomedicine. However, doctors certainly do not see all the illness and disease that occurs in a community. Indeed, they only see what has been called the tip of the iceberg of both symptoms and disease (see pp. 88–89). This means that there is a considerable amount of unmet need in the community, where people may be experiencing health problems that would respond to medical treatment. However, it also means that many people are dealing with a range of both self-limiting and chronic illness themselves, by using self-care (the popular sector) or complementary treatments (the folk sector – see pp. 146–147). We can begin to understand self-care by looking at the popular sector in more detail.

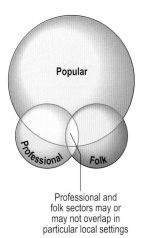

Fig. 1 Three sectors of health care (from Kleinman, 1985, with permission).

Professional and folk sectors may or may not overlap in particular local settings

The popular sector

The popular sector is where ill health is first recognized and defined by people themselves. It is also where much ill health is treated, through self-care, and where various health maintenance activities take place (for example, ensuring healthy diets, taking vitamin supplements). It includes all the therapeutic options that people use without consulting either medical or folk/complementary practitioners. Three components of the popular sector are important: (1) the lay referral system; (2) self-care; and (3) self-help.

The lay referral system

Most people discuss their symptoms with someone else, whether this is a member of their family or a friend. Indeed, some people in the community have an important place in these lay networks – those with experience of an illness, those with experience of raising children and those who are or were health professionals. This system of lay referral may influence health and illness behaviour. For example, if the network or subculture is incongruent with doctors, in terms of beliefs and situation, there may be a low rate of uptake of medical services (McKinlay, 1973; Freidson, 1975). Alternatively, friends and family may encourage attendance at a doctor's surgery or hospital.

Self-care

How people deal with illness themselves will depend on their beliefs, attitudes, resources and access to formal health care. Self-care, and specifically self-medication, is a large and important part of the popular sector of health care. Self-care can include both over-the-counter medicines and home remedies. In research conducted in Scotland involving three generations within a family, the older generation were found to be the most likely to use home remedies, and the younger generation over-the-counter remedies (for themselves and their children) (Blaxter & Paterson, 1982). Other research involving mothers with young children (Cunningham-Burley & Irvine, 1987) found that self-care was the most common response to children's symptoms. In this study, mothers were asked to complete health diaries and participate in an indepth interview: 42 women completed health diaries, and the results showed that the mothers closely monitored their children and often noticed changes which may indicate illness. Something was noticed on 49% of all recorded days. On 65% of these days the mothers took some kind of action in dealing with their children's symptoms, yet they made contact with a health care professional on only 11% of these days.

The mothers thought that you could 'catch an illness early', thus obviating the need to go to the doctor for a prescribed medication. They also knew from their own experience that many illnesses were self-limiting – they would thus try something first, and only go to a doctor if symptoms did not clear up. They also did not want to bother their doctors when they could attempt to treat the child themselves. The main ways in which mothers dealt with the symptoms that their young children were experiencing were through home nursing and home remedies (some of these activities may have been previously recommended by doctors), and by providing over-the-counter remedies, particularly analgesics and cough medicines. Using the pharmacist was an important part of the lay referral system and self-care activities amongst this group. The extracts from interviews, shown in Figure 2, illustrate this.

There has been a rise in the range of over-the-counter medicines available to consumers due to drug deregulation. Some drugs formerly only available

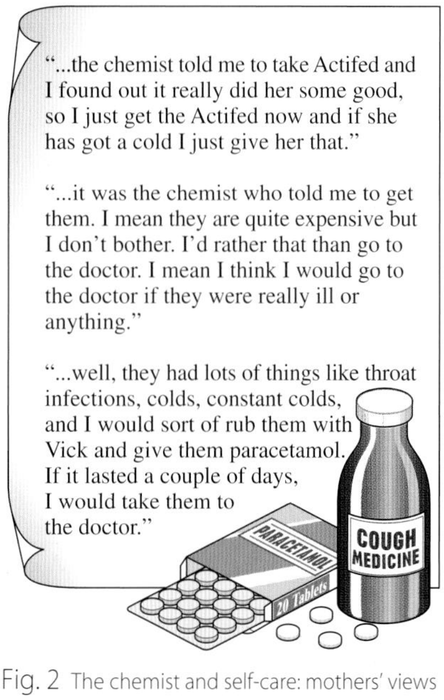

"...the chemist told me to take Actifed and I found out it really did her some good, so I just get the Actifed now and if she has got a cold I just give her that."

"...it was the chemist who told me to get them. I mean they are quite expensive but I don't bother. I'd rather that than go to the doctor. I mean I think I would go to the doctor if they were really ill or anything."

"...well, they had lots of things like throat infections, colds, constant colds, and I would sort of rub them with Vick and give them paracetamol. If it lasted a couple of days, I would take them to the doctor."

Fig. 2 The chemist and self-care: mothers' views (from Cunningham-Burley & Irvine, 1987, with permission).

on prescription from a doctor are now available from a pharmacist. This has led some to suggest that there is now greater consumer choice in relation to medicine taking, and greater autonomy in self-care. However, others suggest that the efficacy of some traditional formulations, such as expectorants, is not well proven (Bates, 2001).

An extended role for the community pharmacist is being emphasized by the profession and by governments. The community pharmacist operates on the boundary between the popular and professional sector. The pharmacist may give specific health advice, but consumers may also use the pharmacy (or indeed supermarket) to purchase a specific product that they have used before for a similar symptom (Williamson et al., 1992). Research suggests that people like the convenience of the pharmacist, and may use the pharmacist as an alternative to the doctor or as a stepping stone to the doctor; in both cases some form of self-care occurs (Cunningham-Burley & Maclean, 1987; Hassell et al., 1998). However, some customers have experienced a lack of privacy (Hassell et al., 2000), and other research suggests that, although pharmacists are held in high regard, there is not a high expectation of their diagnostic and therapeutic role. Pharmacists, however, do offer something different from doctors: the purchase of over-the-counter medicines, along with advice about these and the minor symptoms for which they are intended, seems to form an important part of self-care.

Recent evidence suggests that people want to be more active self-carers and would welcome more guidance from professionals or peers to increase their confidence in self-care, and Box 1 identifies a range of interventions that have been found to be effective at encouraging self-care.

Box 1 **Effective interventions to encourage self-care**
- Self-care education and skills training for adults with asthma
- Individually tailored self-care skills training, including relaxation for people with rheumatoid or osteoarthritis
- Group and family therapies for people with bipolar disorder
- Cardiac rehabilitation involving exercise training, psychosocial and educational interventions
- Pulmonary rehabilitation involving exercise, breathing exercises, psychosocial support and self-care training, including coping with stress and use of medicines
- Computerized information on glucometer data transmission, computerized diet assessment and computerized diet counselling for adults and children with diabetes (insulin-dependent and non-insulin-dependent diabetes mellitus).

(from Department of Health (2007) Self care support: the evidence pack)

Self-help
A third component of the popular sector is self-help (see pp. 142–143). Self-help groups in relation to health have grown in recent years, often providing an alternative to

STOP THINK People may well be experts about their own illnesses, and they certainly may well have self-treated before contacting a GP about symptoms.
- Why is it important for a GP to ask a patient: 'What have you done so far?'

formal medical care. They are important both for the individual members of the group, but also at a more collective level, where they may lobby for a change in attitudes or in the provision of health care. Some groups emphasize the former and are 'inner-focused', and some the latter and are 'outer-focused' (Katz & Bender, 1976). There are different reasons why self-help groups have developed to be an important part of the popular sector of health care. Firstly, existing services sometimes fail to meet the needs of people with a particular condition; secondly, self-help groups provide a panacea to the isolation many feel when experiencing a chronic illness. Self-help groups have several characteristics that give mutual support and help. Members have a common experience of the problem, and there is no distinction made between helper and helped. Reciprocity is an important part of self-help, and the sharing of problems. Groups may provide important information to members, and may help people overcome stigma or feelings of being different.

Practical application
Recognition of the vast amount of health care which takes place in the popular sector is important both for doctors working in the community and for those planning health care services. When self-care represents appropriate treatment, doctors should respect this expertise when someone does eventually consult them. Reassurance that the initial response to symptoms is appropriate is one way of doing this; and education about other options helps to develop a patient's own resources for care. It is also important for doctors to recognize the value of self-help, to be aware of groups in their area, and to alert patients to them. This may be particularly important for people living with a chronic illness, although other problems and conditions are also relevant. Working with other professional and lay groups should be an important component of a doctor's approach, thus bridging the divide between the different sectors of health care.

Case study
Kelleher (1994) investigated self-help groups for people with diabetes. These reflect grass-root activities and recognition of need. They are affiliated to the British Diabetic Association, which is a large national organization, but are small locally run groups. They meet to discuss problems around managing diabetes. This provides an important forum for people to express their worries, to learn from others about how they manage and to admit to temptation. Members begin to feel less guilty about how they manage their condition as part of their everyday lives, and become more confident.

Self-care and the popular sector
- Most illness does not come to the attention of doctors but is dealt with by people themselves through self-care within the popular sector of health care.
- The community pharmacist is an important figure in self-care strategies.
- Self-help is a growing area of health care, based on mutual aid and support.

The experience of hospitals

More and more people visit hospital at some point in their lives (Fig. 1) but hospitals are changing from places where one goes to die to places for acute conditions and specialist care. In the past there was a greater risk of dying in hospital, so it is not surprising that for many older people hospitals are places with negative associations. Modern hospitals may appear quite different, and offer cafés and shops to serve patients, visitors and staff.

Nearly all first births in the UK take place in maternity hospitals. This means that about 90% of women will experience a stay in hospital, and nearly everyone will have known a relative who has stayed in hospital. Elderly people are more likely to be admitted than younger people, although efforts are made to care for them in the community (see pp. 16–17 and pp. 156–157).

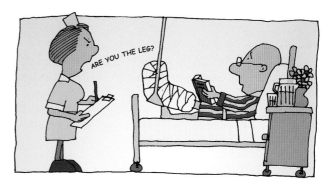

Fig. 2 The person may become invisible on admission, and be identified only by the condition.

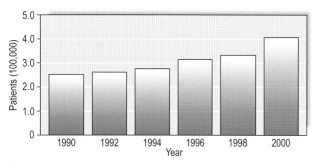

Fig. 1 Hospital outpatient visits in Scotland 1990–2000 (from Office for National Statistics, 2000b).

The experience of being a patient

When someone is admitted to hospital, even if only for a day or overnight stay, then they enter the role of a hospital patient. Goffman (1968a) suggested that the person becomes invisible, leaving only the illness visible. Doctors and nurses may talk about patients as if they were not present (Fig. 2). Being a patient also carries certain expectations. They must move parts of their body on command, respond to probes in parts of their anatomy with declarations of pain and answer questions about the name of the current Prime Minister.

Patients may also resent their loss of freedom. They may wear night clothes throughout the day, and be dependent on others for basic functions. They may have little or no choice about the timing of meals or visits. Lights will go off at a set time and they may be forbidden to get out of bed, or not allowed to stay in bed. They lose their familiar social roles at work and at home.

Not all patients are perceived in the same way by medical and nursing staff. The patients who obey instructions, make no demands, do not ask questions and never complain may be labelled as 'good patients'. 'Good patients' are appreciated by staff and may be easier to manage, but their health may actually suffer. Taylor (1986) points out that 'good patients' may not ask for information and may not report important clinical symptoms. The hospital environment may actually encourage patients to become helpless. The more that patients feel they cannot control the environment around them, the more they will feel helpless.

The patients who ask questions, demand attention and complain may be labelled as 'bad patients'. 'Bad patients' who are not seriously ill may be perceived as difficult patients. However, they may be angry and demanding because they are anxious. These patients may assert their sense of control and independence by breaking the rules. Being a 'bad patient' could be good for health. If more questions are asked, more information will be given, and if symptoms are reported, they may help the diagnosis and treatment.

Control

The feeling of losing control is unpleasant. Taylor (1986) divides control into behaviour control, cognitive control, decision control and information control.

- Behaviour control involves being able to influence procedures in some way. Allowing a patient to control the progress of a painful procedure such as an enema can reduce anxiety. If anxiety before an unpleasant event can be reduced it will be more tolerable.
- Cognitive control is used in cognitive therapy and is very effective. The idea is to think about something neutral or irrelevant (distraction technique) or to concentrate on the positive aspects of the procedure. In childbirth the pain of contractions can be borne by learning to apply distraction techniques such as recalling a tune, or a poem.
- Decision control – if patients can choose when to have an unpleasant procedure, e.g. an injection, then they will experience less discomfort.
- Information control – it is often assumed that the more information the patient receives the better, but this is not so for everyone. Information may be reassuring because it may reduce fear of the unknown and enable people to adopt coping strategies.

Stressful aspects of hospitals

Medical students may quickly get used to hospitals, but patients and relatives may find them stressful. In a study in France symptoms of posttraumatic stress disorder (see pp. 122–123) were found in a third of family members of those whose close relatives were admitted to intensive care units (Azoulay et al., 2005). Medical and nursing staff may also have to cope with stressful events in the hospital. A major road traffic accident, a fire or outbreak of infection can cause disruption and additional stress on all grades of staff. In 2003 there was an outbreak of severe acute respiratory syndrome (SARS) in Canada and a qualitative study looked at the psychosocial reactions of patients, relatives and staff (Maunder et al., 2003). Patients with SARS were treated in isolation units and recent contacts required quarantine. This aroused feelings of guilt, anger and fear for the welfare of friends and family. Patients had to spend many hours alone and those with mild symptoms complained of boredom and loneliness. Staff members were discouraged from interacting outside the hospital, causing further stress.

Privacy

In a single-bedded ward patients have more control over their own activities, but a multiple-bedded ward can be a friendly place.

The ward environment

Patients and visitors may find noise, smells and elaborate instruments stressful.

The professional role

In a joint report (Royal College of Physicians and Royal College of Psychiatrists, 1995) it was emphasized that medical patients also need psychological care. Health professionals may find it difficult to discuss psychological problems with patients in hospital and may avoid this by offering false reassurance or by switching the discussion to a safer topic. Nurses, junior doctors and medical students have different social identities and roles. Each social role has role-related rights such as being allowed to inflict pain, to administer drugs or to ask intimate questions. Each role also has obligations to be respectful, to be caring and to preserve confidentiality.

 ■ In what ways may a hospital's teaching and research interests conflict with the interests of patients? What could be done to reduce this conflict?

Stressful medical and surgical procedures

Many people undergo minor, but potentially stressful, medical procedures in hospitals as inpatients. A diagnostic procedure such as a laparoscopy may be the cause of anxiety because of the fear of what might be found. Some procedures can be very painful, e.g. pelvic floor repairs, and in most surgical procedures an anaesthetic is given. However, although this alleviates the pain, it also means that there is a loss of control.

Some studies of preparation for stressful procedures in adults have shown benefits (Mathews & Ridgeway, 1984). Information given about the procedure beforehand can reduce anxiety. In a study of cervical screening, anxiety was reduced by giving information, reassurance and the opportunity to ask questions (Foxwell & Alder, 1993). Many women find the procedure of taking a cervical smear distressing and do not fully understand the meaning of a negative result. One group of 30 patients (the study group) was given routine care plus an extra 10 minutes of information, reassurance, and an opportunity to ask questions. The control group was given brief information and a leaflet. The two groups were no different in anxiety scores before the smear was taken; however, when they received the results 3–4 weeks later, anxiety levels were significantly reduced in the study group, but not in the control group. Fears and worries about staying in hospital may be increased by media reports of meticillin-resistant *Staphylococcus aureus* (MRSA) and *Clostridium difficile* infections and the cleanliness of wards.

Research into anxiety

Janis (1958) suggested that people differ in their approach to surgery. Some people worry a great deal, feel very vulnerable and have difficulties sleeping. A second group show moderate levels of anxiety. They are somewhat anxious, worried about specific procedures but ask for information. The third group are unconcerned about the operation. They sleep well and deny that they feel worried.

Although these early studies claimed a curvilinear relationship between fear level and outcome, this has not been confirmed by other studies. There is more likely to be a linear relationship between anxiety and recovery. The greater the level of fear before surgery, the poorer was the recovery. Those who are anxious beforehand have more pain, more medical complications and slower recovery (see pp. 104–105).

Case study

Mrs McNab, aged 75 years, had never been into hospital before. Her two children had been born at home, delivered by the local midwife. She was frightened by the ambulance ride from her remote croft into the city, although the paramedical staff were kind and gentle. On arrival she was undressed and given a hospital nightgown. The hospital bed was in a large ward full of strangers. Mrs McNab had never before slept in a bed outside her own home. The operation to remove her appendix was explained to her and she signed a consent form, although she had not brought her reading glasses with her. Following the successful operation she experienced great pain but did not ask for pain relief because she thought this would damage her brain. She missed her family intensely and was frequently found weeping.

■ What could be done to alleviate her distress?
■ How might her distress affect her recovery?

 ■ Talk to someone who has been a patient recently or has visited someone. How do their experiences relate to the Case study?

■ Do you think there are gender differences in patient behaviour? What are they?
■ Contrast your experience of hospitals with a recent television drama.

 ■ In what ways may a hospital's teaching and research interests conflict with the interests of patients

The experience of hospitals

■ Hospitals are changing as more medical care takes place in the community.

■ The experience of being a patient may be stressful, and not all patients react in the same way.

■ Stressful aspects of hospitals include lack of privacy, the ward environment, identification of professionals, worry about surgery, worry about the outcome and anxiety about the family at home.

■ Many medical and surgical procedures are stressful, but the stress can be alleviated by preparation.

Psychological preparation for surgery

Psychological preparation for surgery is important because it has been shown to reduce patients' anxiety and to improve recovery in the postoperative period.

Anxiety

Anxiety is an unpleasant emotion associated with threatening situations or thinking about threat. People differ in the degree to which they experience anxiety when facing challenges such as surgery. High anxiety makes it more difficult for the patient to understand information and to cooperate fully with instructions and can interfere with a psychological and physiological recovery processes, including wound healing (see pp. 126–127).

Anxiety in surgical patients

Patients are anxious before surgery for a number of reasons: they have an illness requiring surgery; they have to undergo the surgical procedure; and there may be uncertainty about the outcome and the likely speed of recovery. In addition, patients worry about being away from home and how their family is coping, as well as continuing to worry about their usual preoccupations, such as money and relationships.

Using standard measures of anxiety which have been developed to deal with the problems of subjective reporting, patients are found to have high levels of anxiety both before and after surgery. For example, Figure 1 shows daily anxiety levels from 4 days before to 14 days after major gynaecological surgery. Compared with normal levels of anxiety as measured 5 weeks after surgery, patients show high levels both before and after surgery. Anxiety before surgery has been found to relate to many postoperative outcomes, including: distress, pain, use of analgesics, and physiological functioning, return to normal activities and length of hospital stay.
Therefore methods of reducing anxiety are likely to improve patient outcomes.

Methods of psychological preparation

A variety of methods of preparing people for surgery have been developed. They are typically administered on the day before surgery, although some have been used in outpatient visits prior to admission. Some of these methods can be delivered to groups of patients, and others incorporate the use of booklets, audio and video tapes. Methods used include:

Information-giving

Procedural information
Patients are informed about the procedures they will undergo, when they will happen and where they will be. E.g. they might be told about waking in the recovery room and the possibility of having a drip or catheter.

Sensation information
Patients are additionally informed about the sensations they are likely to experience. E.g. they might be told that premedication will not necessarily make them feel drowsy or that following major abdominal operations they may experience pain due to wind.

Behavioural instruction
Patients are instructed and may be encouraged to rehearse things they can do postoperatively to reduce pain and facilitate recovery. For example, they may be taught how to cough without pulling on the wound incision or how to turn over in bed without causing unnecessary pain.

Cognitive coping
Based on the assumption that patients' thoughts about what is happening may serve either to raise or reduce their anxiety, interventions have been designed to encourage more adaptive cognitions. For example, patients may be trained to reinterpret events in a more positive manner, e.g. a patient thinking that a doctor passing the end of her bed is a sign that her condition is causing concern may, after training, propose that this is a sign that she is making progress. Or she may be trained to use cognitive coping techniques that she has found useful in other situations, e.g. if she reports that distraction has been useful in previous anxiety-provoking situations, she may be advised on how to use such a technique before and after surgery.

Relaxation/hypnosis
Patients can practise a variety of relaxation and hypnotic techniques before surgery, even when in bed, sometimes using taped instructions.

Emotion-focused/ psychotherapeutic discussion
Patients are invited to discuss their worries, either one to one with a therapist or in groups including other patients. There are no clearly specified instructions for this type of intervention.

Modelling
This method, which is most commonly used with children, involves showing the patient a film of a similar-aged patient going through various stages of the surgical procedures. The method communicates a considerable amount of procedural information and may demonstrate use of any of the other methods.

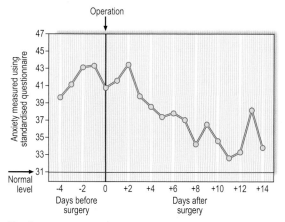

Fig. 1 Anxiety levels before and after surgery (from Johnston, 1980, with permission).

Results of psychological preparation

The first properly controlled trial of presurgery anxiety reduction randomly allocated 97 patients to special preparation or normal care (Egbert et al., 1964). The specially prepared group had less pain, used fewer analgesics postoperatively and their hospital stay was on average 2.7 days shorter than for patients in the control group.

Since then, there have been more than 40 controlled trials involving comparison of groups randomly allocated to psychological preparation versus normal care. The results of these studies have been aggregated using meta-analysis and clear benefits for patients have been demonstrated (Johnston & Vögele, 1993). Figure 2 shows the mean difference between the psychologically prepared and control groups, expressed in units of standard deviations, and the 95% confidence intervals, for each outcome.

The group receiving psychological preparation showed statistically significant benefits where the mean difference is greater than zero and where the confidence interval does not pass through zero. Thus there is evidence of benefit on measures of distress, pain, use of analgesics, physiological indices such as heart rate and blood pressure, and behavioural indices, including resumption of normal activities and length of hospital stay. Clinical ratings of recovery did not show a reliable difference. One might have expected to find improved patient satisfaction, but too few studies had examined this variable to draw conclusions.

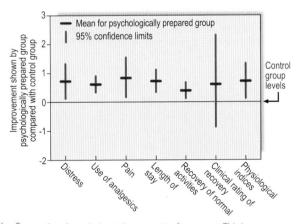

Fig. 2 Benefits of psychological preparation for surgery. This is a summary of 40 clinical trials (data from Johnston & Vögele, 1993).

Preparation for the postdischarge period

It is important that information covers not only the immediate surgical procedure but also the postsurgery recovery process. Many surgical procedures, for example elective inguinal hernia repair surgery, are now carried out with a minimal stay in hospital for the patient – some even undergo such procedures as day-case patients. This means that many patients are discharged very quickly to their home environment where they do not have immediate access to professional medical support. Some postsurgical experiences such as swelling and extensive bruising may be seen as part of the normal recovery process by medical professionals but if the patient is not aware that such symptoms are normal, further concern is likely to result and further medical help to be sought (Fig. 3). Thus, providing patients with a good understanding of what is to be expected after surgery can minimize anxiety and conserve health care resources (see pp. 102-103).

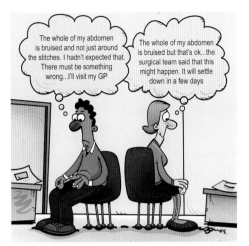

Fig. 3 Preparation for postdischarge recovery – impact of worry on health service use and the benefits of sensory information.

Case study

Mr Jones was admitted to a surgical ward for abdominal surgery. He was anxious about the procedure and particularly concerned about undergoing anaesthesia. On the morning of surgery, he could not contain his anxiety and discharged himself. He returned to his GP as a patient who required surgery but could not tolerate the procedures.

The GP referred Mr Jones to a psychologist who used psychological preparation procedures involving relaxation training and cognitive techniques. Mr Jones was trained to use relaxation as a distraction technique, especially when experiencing worrying thoughts. He was taught to recognize negative thoughts such as: 'What if I die during surgery?' and to deal with them by thinking of counteracting thoughts, e.g. 'I've never heard of that happening to anyone I know – why should it happen to me?'

Mr Jones was able to return to the surgeon and to proceed with treatment without further interruption.

 STOP THINK Although the benefits of psychological methods of preparing patients for surgery have been known for at least 20 years, they have not been widely implemented. Why might this be?
The limitations in implementing these techniques may be due to the lack of appropriately trained staff. The development of booklets or taped instructions may facilitate the use of these techniques but such approaches need to be fully evaluated.

Psychological preparation for surgery

- Patients are anxious before and after surgery.
- High preoperative anxiety is predictive of poor postoperative outcome.
- A variety of methods has been developed for preparing patients for surgery (e.g. information-giving, behavioural instruction, cognitive coping, relaxation, emotion-focused discussion and modelling).
- These methods have been shown to improve postoperative outcomes in well-controlled clinical trials.

Heart disease

Coronary heart disease (CHD) describes a number of conditions, including angina pectoris and myocardial infarction (MI). Angina pectoris refers to a sensation of tightness or chest pain caused by a brief obstruction or constriction of a coronary artery and MI refers to death of heart muscle (myocardium) as a result of blockage of a coronary artery that prevents oxygen reaching the myocardium.

The main medical interventions are: (1) pharmacological (medications to reduce blood pressure, prevent clotting and reduce serum (blood) cholesterol); (2) revascularization: percutaneous coronary interventions (PCI), coronary artery bypass grafts (CABG); (3) coronary care; (4) cardiac rehabilitation; and (5) risk factor reduction (primary and secondary).

Causation and prevention

CHD is the commonest cause of premature mortality and a frequent cause of morbidity in western societies. Major well-established risk factors are smoking, hypertension and high serum cholesterol. Additional lifestyle risk factors include physical inactivity (leading to obesity) (see pp. 86–87), hostility and stress.

The type A behaviour pattern (hard-driving, time-urgent and hostile) was identified in the 1960s as typical of the coronary-prone individual. Subsequent research has indicated that high hostility alone is the factor most associated with greater risk of CHD (see pp. 126–127). In surveys, patients and healthy populations believe stress to be the commonest cause of MI (see pp. 62–63). The challenge for health professionals is to educate the population about the importance of behaviours such as smoking in heart disease (see pp. 66–67).

Experimental studies can provide definitive evidence, and strong evidence that stress causes heart disease comes from animal studies. Figure 1 shows cross-sections of coronary arteries of monkeys subjected to different living conditions. Greatest occlusion of the coronary artery was found in dominant monkeys subjected to the stress of having the group they lived with broken up regularly (c). Less occlusion was found in those living in stable groups (a and b) or in subordinate monkeys in unstable social groupings (d).

CHD is related to socioeconomic disadvantage (see pp. 44–45). This may be due in part to patterns of smoking, diet and work experience, as working-class groups smoke more, have a poorer diet and are more likely to have jobs where they have little control and high demands compared with those in the middle classes. CHD is also the major cause of death for both women and men in western countries. However, evidence shows that both women and their doctors may not pay enough attention to this fact. Women fear breast cancer much more that heart disease, although women are about 10 times more likely to die of heart disease than breast cancer over their lifetime (Ulstad, 2001). Similarly, symptoms which doctors attribute to cardiac conditions in men are sometimes attributed to other conditions when presented by female patients. This effect is more common when doctors are working in stressful, time-pressured settings. There has been extensive professional attention recently to address this gender bias in symptom perception.

There have been substantial positive changes in population behaviour and lifestyle in many western countries in recent years. The most important changes have resulted in decreased smoking, blood pressure and serum cholesterol. Coupled with improvements in cardiovascular medications and interventions, these are associated with significant reductions in mortality from CHD. The trend of declining CHD mortality, and factors contributing to it, are shown for the UK (England and Wales) in Figure 2. CHD mortality has halved from 1981 to 2000, meaning there were 68 230 fewer deaths than expected in 2000, based on 1981 prevalence projections. More than half of the decline is due to lifestyle change to reduce cardiovascular risk factors and half to treatments – medications and interventions. Of concern for the future is the negative impact of increasing physical inactivity and obesity and diabetes (both linked to physical inactivity and diet), particularly in younger groups. The first

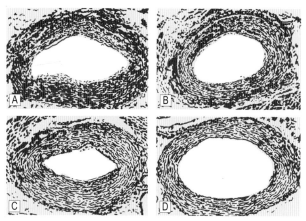

Fig. 1 Effects of social stressors on the coronary artery in monkeys. The diagrams show cross-sections of coronary artery of monkeys subjected to different living conditions. (Drawing based on photograph in Manuck et al., 1983).

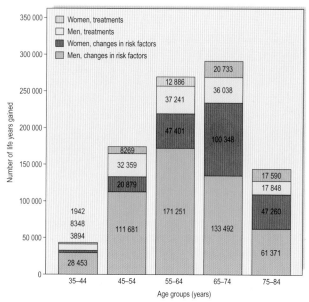

Fig. 2 Life years gained from changes in treatments available for coronary heart disease (CHD) and population changes in CHD risk factors: data from England and Wales 1981–2000. For men, 4665 deaths were prevented or postponed by reductions in risk factors and 574 by treatments. For women 672 deaths were prevented or postponed by reductions in risk factors and 219 by treatments (from Ünal et al., 2005, with permission of the American Public Health Association).

evidence in slowing the progress in managing CHD is now emerging in the UK with, for instance, CHD death rates for young men (aged 35–44 years) rising for the first time in two decades (O'Flaherty et al., 2007). These risk factors are the major behavioural challenges in the coming decades.

Response to symptoms and myocardial infarction

Individuals may misinterpret symptoms. A large number of patients referred to cardiology departments present with non-cardiac chest pain, probably due to anxiety about physical symptoms. Equally, many patients experiencing an MI do not recognize the symptoms and delay seeking help (see pp. 88–91). Given the importance of early thrombolysis and allowing greater oxygen supply to the heart by means of percutaneous coronary intervention (PCI) procedures, such delays may critically determine the patient's treatment and survival (see Case study). A rapid response ensures more effective treatment and therefore better outcomes.

MI is a sudden life-threatening event and many patients experience high levels of anxiety and depression following MI. Close family members may be even more distressed than the patient in the early period, while the patient is in hospital. These high levels of distress are unrelated to the severity of the MI and may persist for months or years. Depression is also associated with higher mortality rates. In a study of 222 MI patients, depressed patients were over three times as likely as non-depressed patients to die within 18 months. This remained true even when other factors, such as severity of MI, were controlled for. In addition, patients who were socially isolated were more likely to die in this period (Frasure-Smith et al., 1995).

Cardiac rehabilitation

Cardiac rehabilitation programmes have been shown to:
- reduce psychological distress for patients and their families
- improve cardiovascular fitness
- reduce mortality (by at least 20%)
- increase rate of return to paid employment
- reduce health service costs.

Benefits from such programmes persist for years. Programmes may involve education, exercise, dietary and vocational counselling, and psychological components such as stress management. The addition of psychological components to exercise- and education-based programmes results in greater patient benefit.

Patients and their families are often anxious about resuming physical activity following a cardiac event or intervention. Routine testing and rehabilitation classes can promote patient self-efficacy (i.e. belief in their own ability to complete behaviours successfully). For instance, a study where spouses were allowed to observe routine treadmill testing to assess cardiovascular fitness increased both patient and spouse self-efficacy in the patient's ability to engage in energetic activities. Assessed at follow-up, those with higher self-efficacy (and not necessarily those who did best on the exercise text) were more physically active, in line with doctors' advice, in the weeks following the test.

Response to stressful medical procedures

Medical procedures may be stressful due to the discomfort or pain experienced as well as the uncertainty about

the outcomes. Psychological preparation can reduce the stressfulness of procedures and improve outcomes (see pp. 104–105). These principles can be applied in coronary care settings when patients are being prepared for CABG surgery and PCI. Research has also shown that patients can provide important role models for other patients in ways that can speed recovery. Preoperative cardiac surgery patients randomized to share a double room with a postoperative patient having the same surgery were found to be less anxious before the surgery and to recover more quickly following the procedure. They also became more active more rapidly postoperatively and were discharged earlier than control patients (Kulik et al., 1996).

 STOP THINK Psychological factors are involved in many aspects of CHD. How might a psychologist contribute to the work of a cardiology department?

Case study
Delay to treatment for symptoms of a myocardial infarction
On the way home from their wedding anniversary meal, Mrs MacDonald feels pressure in her chest. She thinks it unlikely to be anything more serious than indigestion at her age (51). She does not like to mention it as it would spoil the evening. Going upstairs to bed the pain intensifies and she comes out in a cold sweat, so she lies down to see if she feels better. Her husband worries that it is a heart attack, but Mrs MacDonald says: 'I don't think so – women don't have heart attacks. It's more likely to be the menopause!' After some hours of increasing symptoms, she calls an ambulance. Unfortunately, by the time she gets to hospital, she has already had substantial damage to her myocardial (heart) muscle and so will not benefit as much from available cardiac interventions as she might have by presenting earlier.

Heart disease
- CHD may be prevented or delayed by changes in behaviour and lifestyles.
- Socioeconomic disadvantage and stress are associated with higher incidences of CHD.
- Patients may fail to recognize the symptoms of MI, with resulting delays in seeking medical treatment.
- Anxiety and depression are common responses to MI of both patients and their spouses.
- Depression following MI is an independent predictor of mortality.
- Cardiac rehabilitation, including psychological components, enhances patient outcomes and survival.
- Psychological preparation for medical procedures reduces their stressfulness and improves postoperative recovery.

HIV/AIDS

Human immunodeficiency virus (HIV) appeared at a time when it was widely believed that science had brought infectious diseases under control, and it seemed that all of a sudden a new incurable disease presented itself. Until recently it was only possible to treat some of the secondary effects of HIV and acquired immune deficiency syndrome (AIDS – the disease stage of most infected people) and since the infection is currently not curable, the main remedy still lies in prevention. Since the virus can be transmitted in different ways (Box 1), prevention requires targeting different types of behaviour.

Although HIV is widespread (40 million cases were reported worldwide by 2006), it is clear that the infection is not equally spread amongst members of society or between societies. Even within the UK (Fig. 1), we see great differences in the proportion of people infected through sexual intercourse between men and intravenous drug users (IDU). The figure for women as a percentage of the total number of people diagnosed with AIDS differs considerably between Scotland and the UK as a whole (Fig. 1). The proportion of IDU among the people diagnosed with AIDS in Scotland (31.8%) is six times higher than in the UK (5.5%). Thus certain groups of people have a far higher infection rate than others, depending on different parts of the country.

The disease has distinct social aspects. At a social level it involves several taboos, such as sex, drugs, and death and dying; consequently it is heavily stigmatized. Secondly, at a personal level, the acceptance of being diagnosed as HIV-positive can be very difficult. People can feel isolated, shocked, frightened, panicked and/or guilty, profess denial and become depressed, but some also display a sense of coming to terms with themselves, and even acceptance. Such emotions are understandable, as people have to accept that they have a long-term illness (in high- and middle-income countries) and/or become more aware of their own mortality (in many low-income countries). Treatment using antiretroviral drugs is expensive, which is particularly a problem in sub-Saharan Africa (see pp. 158–159).

Double stigma

HIV has what is called a double stigma attached. Stigma refers to the identification and recognition of a bad or negative characteristic in a person or group of people and the treatment of them with less respect or worth than they deserve due to this characteristic (see pp. 60–61). The double stigma refers to terminal illness and sexually transmitted disease. The former stigma is also applicable to cancer and other terminal diseases. The latter refers to stigma attached to 'deviant', 'unnatural', or socially undesirable activities, such as men having sex with men (MSM), injecting drug use or prostitution. Alonzo & Reynolds (1995) explain that stigma is the 'identification of some sort of moral contamination that causes others to reject the person bearing it'. Thus people living with HIV are regarded as 'dangerous, dirty, foolish and worthless' in comparison to descriptions of cancer or stroke patients.

Experiencing stigma (stigmatization) may lead to low self-esteem in the infected person, reduced willingness to seek medical and social help, and increased difficulty in sharing worries with friends, relatives and neighbours. At a societal level, widespread fear of HIV/AIDS still exists, despite the fact that it has been scientifically demonstrated that AIDS is not communicable by day-to-day social contact. This fear and stigmatization can easily be translated into discrimination and victimization of people with HIV. HIV/AIDS is branded a plague, which implies that people living with HIV are threatening and dangerous rather than threatened, because they carry the potential to contaminate the healthy through transmission of a contagious disease. This has led to some dentists and doctors refusing treatment in the past even when safe procedures were available.

Society also often makes a distinction between 'innocent' and 'guilty' victims. It is believed that the people with HIV bring it on themselves through their own doing, and they are blamed for their disease, and as a result are branded as 'guilty' victims. In contrast, 'innocent' victims are infected through mistakes by the medical profession or infected blood. Babies of HIV-infected mothers are included as innocent, whereas their mothers may be seen as guilty.

The use of the phrase 'risk group' reinforces the idea that HIV can only happen to certain people. The idea of stressing risk behaviour is far more meaningful both in terms of reducing the stigma attached to being HIV-positive and in terms of preventing the spread of the infection. It is not what people are that gives them a higher risk, but what people do.

HIV and the media

The media are a major source of information for people, as well as influential in forming or at least confirming people's opinions (pp. 52–53). Many people in industrialized countries will not personally know anyone who is infected with HIV; consequently, the perception of the disease is likely to be mediated or even formed by mass media. This includes 'facts' in, for example, newspapers and television news programmes, and 'fiction' in soap operas and cinema films.

In an interview with *The Independent* newspaper (3 November 1993, p. 23), Suzanna Dawson, who in a soap opera played the wife of a character who had AIDS, said:

> *I've had some terrible experiences of the kind of prejudice HIV-positive people face ... I've been slapped and spat at in the street, booed off the field in a charity match ... it makes you feel so alone, so scared ... I've picked up the phone at 2 a.m. to hear some*

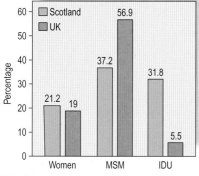

Fig. 1 Percentage of women, men who have sex with men (MSM) and intravenous drug users (IDU) among cumulative number of AIDS cases in Scotland and the UK as a whole (March 2007) (from HPS eWeekly Report 18 April 2007: http://www.hps.scot.nhs.uk/ewr/index.aspx, with permission).

guy screaming: 'You're a dirty bitch, spreading disease throughout the world'.

Ms Dawson suffered this level of abuse even though she was merely the actress playing that role.

Psychological issues

One key set of psychological issues centres on the question: 'Who do you tell?' Being diagnosed HIV-positive may involve having to adapt one's behaviour and outlook on life. Telling a partner or family could mean having to admit to injecting drugs, or having sex with another man, or being sexually unfaithful. Telling your employer might mean losing a job, not necessarily because the employer wants to get rid of you, but because your colleagues do not want to work with you any longer. Bringing up the issue of using safer sex methods can also be problematic. It is a difficult enough issue for most, especially at the time of first sexual intercourse. However, people with HIV might find suggesting the use of condoms with prospective sexual partners difficult, because of the fear of being rejected, both emotionally and physically (see pp. 62–63).

Health promotion and HIV

HIV health-promotion activities have often focused on the sexual transmission of the virus. Since: (1) people with HIV are generally not recognizable until the end-stages of the disease; and (2) the virus has a long incubation time, the health promotion message had to be aimed at all men and women who are sexually active, not just the high-risk groups.

Figure 2 shows one of the posters/postcards with a safer sex message targeting the general population. The

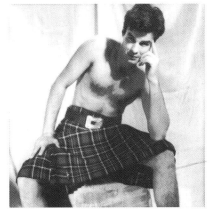

Fig. 2 One HIV health promotion in Scotland. The slogan read: 'What should a real Scotsman wear under his kilt?' Answer: 'A condom!' (Courtesy of Scottish AIDS Monitor and Lothian Health.)

message is clearly aimed at men, unlike previous health promotion activities for condoms, when condoms were 'only' contraceptives, and often seen as a woman's responsibility (see pp. 6–7).

Despite all the health promotion messages over the past two decades, talking about condom use and sexual desires still proves to be difficult for many people. Moreover, there is growing evidence that young people in the UK are less aware of the risk of HIV.

HIV/AIDS in developing countries

The majority of people with HIV live in developing countries (see pp. 158–159). In Africa HIV is mainly transmitted by heterosexual contact; in Europe and the USA MSM is still a leading factor, although heterosexual transmission is increasing. Many areas of Africa do not have the resources to screen blood consistently, which means that HIV is still being transmitted through blood transfusions, and very few medicines or social services are available for people living with HIV/AIDS. It is worth remembering that, for some African nations hit hardest by AIDS, the

entire national health budget is only equal to that of one large US hospital. Consequently many developing countries cannot afford to offer the kind of treatment that has made long-term survival of HIV patients common in industrialized countries.

People living with HIV/AIDS in developing countries can also experience discrimination and stigma, leaving them isolated and deprived of social care and support. The death of parents in several countries, especially in sub-Saharan Africa, has led to a large number of so-called AIDS orphans, whose life changes are drastically reduced compared to children with a living parent.

Box 1 **Routes of transmission of HIV**

- Unprotected penetrative sex (vaginal, oral or anal)
- Unsterilized needle/syringe previously used by someone infected with HIV
- Mother to child during pregnancy, labour and breast-feeding
- Infected blood or tissue transfer
- Receiving semen from an infected man for artificial insemination

Case study

Andrew (age 20 years) is a third-year medical student. He took an HIV test with his new partner when they started a sexual relationship. He felt it was a waste of time, a fashion, and really went along to please his partner. Although he was counselled at the time, he was very shocked to be told that he tested HIV-positive. His thoughts jumped back and forth between his partner and what would happen to the relationship, his study and career. He wondered: 'Who gave me the virus?' and 'Which private habits do I have to disclose, and to whom? Will I die young and horribly?'

STOP THINK

- What other issues might this medical student face after his recent diagnosis?
- Why is society's reaction to people with HIV generally negative?

HIV/AIDS

- People living with HIV/AIDS often suffer from a double stigma.
- Mass media have played an important role in influencing public perception of the disease.
- We should move away from thinking in terms of risk groups to risk behaviour. It is not important who you are, but what you do.

- The majority of people with HIV live in the developing world, where much less funding is available for prevention and (often expensive) care (www.unaids.org/hivaidsinfo/index.html).
- Prevention is the main, or even the only, approach to stop the spread of HIV/AIDS.

Cancer

Despite differences in the progress of different cancers and the increasing effectiveness of medical treatments, cancer continues to be the most widely feared group of diseases. It creates greater anxiety than coronary heart disease, which has approximately double the fatality rate. Psychological and social factors are involved in the aetiology and response to the disease and its treatment.

Aetiology

In a review of the preventable causes of cancer, behavioural factors were implicated in the majority of cancers (Doll & Peto, 1981): smoking (involved in 30% of cancers); diet (35%); reproductive and sexual behaviour (7%); and alcohol use (3%). Thirty-five per cent of the 7 million global deaths from cancer in 2001 have been attributed to nine behavioural or environmental risk factors. The lead risk factors were smoking (596 000 deaths), alcohol use (88 000), overweight and obesity (69 000), low fruit and vegetable intake (64 000) and physical inactivity (51 000 deaths) (Danaei et al., 2005).

Communication about cancer

Cancer is associated with many social and clinical taboos. In popular language and in medical settings euphemisms such as 'growth', 'tumour', 'lump', 'shadow' and 'the big C' are used to avoid the word 'cancer' (see pp. 98–99). These communications may arise from the fears and misconceptions surrounding cancer, but in turn they also give rise to such fears. Thus patients with benign disease sometimes suspect that they have malignant disease but that their doctor is withholding the information. On the other hand, such language may lead patients who do have a malignant cancer to misunderstand the full implications of their condition.

Research shows that members of the general public are much more likely to say that they want to be informed of a terminal diagnosis than doctors estimated they would (Jenkins et al., 2001) and want to be told personally, rather than have other people (such as relatives) told first.

Health care staff sometimes worry that giving patients with cancer information about their condition or treatment may increase anxiety. However, a systematic review of interventions to improve information given to advanced cancer patients found positive results (e.g. improved satisfaction with communication) in six of eight trials. The other two trials showed no difference between groups (Gaston & Mitchell, 2005).

Communications about cancer are fraught with problems due to negative attitudes of patients, their families, health professionals (including doctors and nurses), other hospital personnel and the wider lay community. Doctors rate the quality of life of cancer patients significantly worse than the patients' own ratings.

Providing patients with information enables them to decide whether or not they would like to participate in decision-making (rather than leave the decision-making to medical professionals) and, if they wish to be involved in decision-making, helps them to arrive at the optimal decision for their personal situation.

Delay

People may not seek medical help when they experience potential cancer symptoms and may not choose to participate in cancer screening programmes. Screening for the detection of precancerous cells or for the early diagnosis of treatable cancers has often had poor uptake rates (see pp. 68–60).

Patient delay in seeking help when a symptom is noticed has four components: (1) appraisal delay (deciding the symptom indicates an illness); (2) illness delay (deciding that the illness merits a consultation with a doctor); (3) behavioural delay (making the appointment); and (4) scheduling delay (the time between making the appointment and actually seeing the doctor) (Andersen et al., 1995; Fig. 1). Appraisal delay can form a major part of the delay time. For example, a person with a cough might initially ignore or not notice the cough, until it becomes clear that it is persistent. Even so, if that person were a smoker, he or she might attribute the cough to 'smoker's cough' rather than an illness and therefore not realize that it could be a symptom of a serious condition, such as lung cancer, early enough to obtain the most effective treatment.

Response to diagnosis

Even when the term 'cancer' is used in giving the diagnosis, patients may subsequently report that they have never received such a diagnosis. In order to ensure that patients can recall the full description of their condition and the potentially reassuring communication about treatment and prognosis, some clinicians have provided patients with an audiotaped recording of the diagnostic consultation. Evidence suggests that many patients find such recordings useful both for aiding their recall of the consultation and for helping them to communicate information about their condition and its treatment to their families.

Patients have varied ways of coping with a cancer diagnosis. Kübler-Ross (1969) proposed a sequence of staging of the response to a poor prognosis ranging from shock and denial, through anger, depression and, finally, to acceptance. While there is considerable doubt about the actual sequence of stages, this range of responses is commonly observed in patients with cancer. Researchers have investigated whether some coping methods may result in better adjustment. In general, coping strategies that focus on emotional aspects of the response are associated with poorer emotional adjustment. By contrast, patients whose strategies focus on thinking about the issue in a different way, e.g. on reaching acceptance of the condition or on seeking solutions to problems, show better subsequent adjustment (e.g. Carver et al., 1993).

Early research suggested that coping strategies e.g. 'fighting spirit' influence prognosis and survival (Greer et al., 1979; Spiegel et al. 1989) but this has not been consistently supported (Petticrew et al., 2002; Coyne et al., 2007)., These authors emphasize the role of psychological factors in morbidity and quality of life rather than mortality.

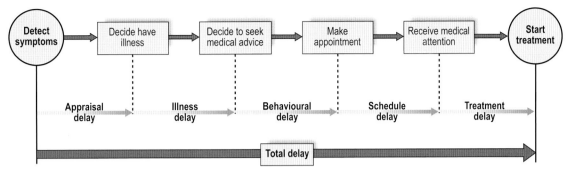

Fig. 1 Stages of delay in obtaining treatment (adapted from Andersen et al., 1995).

Response to treatment

Where two medical treatments are thought to have a similar prognosis, patients may be offered a choice of treatment. For instance, in patients with advanced prostate cancer, orchidectomy (surgical removal of testicle) or bimonthly hormonal injections (synthetic luteinizing hormone) with minimum side-effects have similar survival rates. Yet, when given the choice of treatment, a large proportion – 23 out of 50 men – opted for the mutilating surgery rather than the minimally invasive injections (Chadwick et al., 1991). It may be that people have more confidence in a surgical procedure which allows them to feel that the cancerous tissue has been physically removed.

Two studies of patients receiving chemotherapy examined the impact of side-effects on participants (Nerenz et al., 1982; Love et al., 1989). Some side-effects (e.g. vomiting and tiredness) were associated with distress and disruption, others were not. For example, hair loss was not, by itself, associated with emotional distress, perhaps because it is less debilitating than other side-effects that affect how patients physically feel and what they are able to do or because they understood hair loss to be due to the treatment while other side-effects might be interpreted as due to cancer itself (Fig. 2). People who had more side-effects or felt they had failed to cope with side-effects were more distressed.

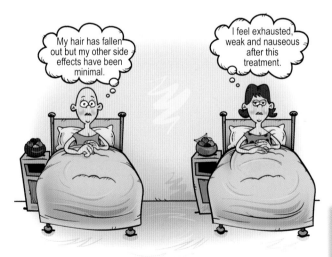

Fig. 2 Which patient is likely to be more depressed – A or B? Which patient is the observer likely to think is more depressed?

Many patients experience anticipatory nausea and vomiting as chemotherapy progresses. For the initial treatments, nausea is experienced during and after the treatment. With later treatments, the nausea can occur before treatment, on arrival at the hospital or even on the journey to hospital. This effect has been explained in terms of classical conditioning (see pp. 22–23) – the patient learns to associate the visit to hospital with the administration of chemotherapy and therefore responds as if to chemotherapy, with nausea and vomiting. Considerable success has been achieved in training patients to practise relaxation techniques in anticipation of and during chemotherapy, thus reducing the need for antiemetic drugs (Carey & Burish, 1988; Burish & Jenkins, 1992).

 STOP THINK Patients with lung cancer in the UK have poor survival rates compared with those in other developed countries.
- Why do you think this might be the case?
- How much do you think this is caused by patient behaviour and how much by doctor behaviour?

Case study

Providing test results in an oncology clinic

Doctor: *The tests on your breast lump are negative …*

Alison : *So there's nothing you can do …*

Doctor: *Oh yes. Don't worry; we don't leave things like this. We'll be proceeding with local excision of the necessary tissue.*

Alison : *That means I'll have to have the operation after all. What's the point?*

Doctor: *That's how these lumps are always managed. Everything will be fine. Try not to get upset. We'll fix a date for doing this as soon as possible. What about Wednesday next, coming in on Tuesday evening. OK?*

- What did the doctor understand by the word 'negative'?
- What did Alison understand?
- What is Alison likely to think when she comes into hospital for surgery?

Cancer

- Cancer is the most widely feared of all diseases.

- Behavioural factors are important in the aetiology of cancer and therefore offer opportunities for prevention.

- Communication about cancer may be limited by social taboos, concern to avoid upsetting patients and undue pessimism about the impact of the disease.

- Delay in reaching treatment can negatively affect prognosis and there are a number of stages where this can be addressed.

- Patients' coping strategies can affect subsequent adjustment.

- Patients' choice of, and response to, treatment may be unexpected from a medical point of view, but may be psychologically meaningful.

Anxiety

Anxiety is part of everyday life. It is adaptive: it provides the motivation to study for exams and prompts the rush of adrenaline that gives a certain sparkle to a public performance, whether this is sport or presenting a seminar paper. Most of us have experienced episodes of unpleasant anxiety. Usually these are time-limited and resolve themselves. But even when they do not warrant treatment, their physiological effects can interfere with health by making other conditions worse (e.g. asthma or eczema), or by confusing the clinical picture (e.g. in the diagnosis and management of heart disease). Anxiety can also affect health by its influence on health risk behaviours such as comfort eating, smoking and not using condoms.

Anxiety in health care situations

Many aspects of health care are anxiety-provoking in themselves. Waiting to see a doctor may make patients anxious because they are already feeling ill and therefore vulnerable, or they are worried about what the doctor may say or do. They are dependent on the doctor for help, do not know what to expect and may find it difficult to say exactly what they want to say. Coming into hospital may produce the same effect, but has the added stress of being taken into a strange institution and having control taken away from them (pp. 102–103). It is easy to underestimate the degree of anxiety that patients feel when faced with a doctor. They may react in maladaptive ways: by not giving the right information, or by being defensive, hostile or tearful. They are frequently too anxious to understand, think about or remember what is said to them. They may show clinical signs of anxiety that may be mistakenly attributed to some other illness. Every effort should be made to reduce anxiety in order to get the most out of a clinical encounter (see pp. 96–97).

What is anxiety?

Anxiety refers to an emotional state that can usefully be divided into three components:

1. Thoughts – these often act as the trigger for creating the state of anxiety, e.g. 'What if my foot slips off this ledge and I fall down the rockface?', 'What if I can't answer key questions at the interview?' or 'What if we split up and I'm left on my own?'
2. Physical symptoms – these are numerous; most commonly they include an increased heart rate, increased blood pressure, feelings of tension in the muscles, sweating, nausea or indigestion, trembling, blushing, tightness or dryness in the throat and dizziness.
3. Behaviour – this is what you do in order to reduce anxiety, for example, refusing to go on up the rockface, or avoiding interviews or doing deep breathing in order to ease the physical symptoms of anxiety in an interview. Behaviour that reduces anxiety without damaging health or welfare is adaptive, but many of the ways in which we respond to anxiety are maladaptive, e.g. avoiding social occasions or using alcohol for relief (pp. 126–127).

How is anxiety maintained?

The three components listed above can interact to maintain anxiety and can also make it worse. The case study illustrates how anxiety can escalate. Whatever the initial cause of Andrew's symptoms, he had interpreted the sensations as potentially threatening (the risk that he would faint in the shop and how embarrassing this would be). These anxious thoughts set off further symptoms (through the release of adrenaline and noradrenaline). Escaping reduced symptoms and avoidance prevented them.

Types of anxiety problem

High anxiety that interferes with everyday functioning may be categorized as follows (Davison & Neale, 2001).

Phobias
A phobia is a fear that is out of proportion to the potential threat posed by a particular object or situation. Being afraid of a pitbull terrier dog would not be classed as a phobia, but being afraid of a moth would. There is a significant objective risk to your safety in the first, but not in the second.

Common specific phobias are to blood and injections, enclosed places such as lifts, animals and aspects of the natural environment, such as heights and water. Phobias to blood and injections are characterized by a decrease in heart rate, often causing fainting, whereas other phobias are associated with an increased heart rate. Social phobias may develop from the common social anxieties experienced in adolescence. They can be debilitating, leading to acute embarrassment in the company of others and avoidance of social situations.

Generalized anxiety
Generalized anxiety refers to the experience of all-pervasive anxiety, not apparently linked to any specific situation, event or object. The person experiences a high state of arousal for much of the time and a general sense of dread. He or she is likely to experience uncontrollable worry, a variety of somatic complaints, tension and restlessness.

Case study

Andrew was recovering from flu when he went into a supermarket on a Saturday afternoon to stock up on food. He was dressed in warm clothing to combat the winter weather outside. Inside the shop it was hot and crowded, and he had to wait in a long queue for the checkout. While waiting he began to feel very hot himself, slightly faint and nauseous. He broke out in a sweat and thought that he might actually pass out in the shop. He put down the basket and went straight to the entrance for fresh air. He began to feel better, but decided just to go home.

The next time he went to the supermarket, he thought about his last visit and wondered if it might happen again. He thought that people might notice if he looked flustered or nervous, and this would be embarrassing. Thinking and imagining the scene was accompanied by a quickening heart rate, and then sweating and a feeling of dizziness and nausea. He thought again that he might faint and that this would be terrible. He made straight for the door and on getting outside began to feel better again.

Panic attacks

Panic attacks are sudden waves of intense anxiety that seem to come out of the blue. People may be overwhelmed by feelings of loss of control, going mad or even dying. Panic attacks that occur in public places and involve feelings of being trapped are called agoraphobia. They may be associated with fear of shopping, crowds or travelling.

Obsessive-compulsive disorder (OCD)

People with OCD suffer from obsessional ruminations, which are intrusive and recurrent, and often distressing thoughts or images, e.g. about contamination or harming others. They may also experience compulsions to perform certain repetitive behaviours, such as checking and rechecking, and lengthy cleaning rituals.

Posttraumatic and acute stress

This is an extreme response to an extreme stressor, such as assault, environmental disaster or war. Its symptoms form three categories: (1) frequently re-experiencing and being distressed by the traumatic event (e.g. nightmares); (2) avoiding or forgetting or feeling numb towards the trauma; and (3) being highly aroused (e.g. sleep and concentration problems, feeling jumpy).

Treatment

Methods of preventing or managing anxiety depend on the nature of the anxiety, its impact on everyday functioning and the individual's preference. Evidence-based guidelines produced by the National Institute for Health and Clinical Excellence (NICE) provide recommendations for diagnosing and treating panic disorder, agoraphobia and generalized anxiety disorder (NICE, 2004).

Drugs

These work by reducing the physiological symptoms of anxiety. The most commonly used group of drugs are the benzodiazepines, but these can cause dependence. Beta-blockers, which control heart rate, are sometimes used to reduce symptoms for a one-off occasion, e.g. a musician giving an important performance. For generalized anxiety and OCD, antidepressants may be used.

Psychological therapies

Behavioural approaches are effective treatments for anxiety problems. For a simple phobia, graded exposure to the feared object is combined with learning to use relaxation techniques (called systematic desensitization; see pp. 22–23). In this way, the patient learns that the feared object is tolerable (Fig. 1). Exposure-based treatments are also effective in reducing agoraphobia and posttraumatic stress disorder (PTSD). For PTSD, exposure is to the traumatic images, and therapy seeks to help people gain control over the images and their emotional responses to them. As a general principle, cognitive-behavioural techniques aim to identify the situations and thoughts that cause and maintain anxiety problems, and then break the cycle of anxious thoughts, physical and

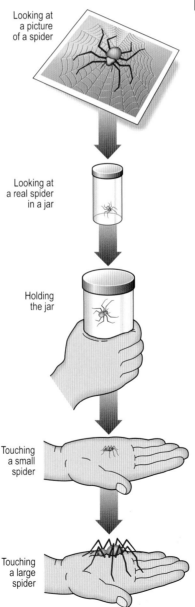

Looking at a picture of a spider

Looking at a real spider in a jar

Holding the jar

Touching a small spider

Touching a large spider

Fig. 1 Graded exposure to a spider (from Puri et al., 1996, with permission).

emotional symptoms and maladaptive behaviour (see pp. 138–139).

Learning social skills may help social phobics to feel confident and to behave appropriately in social situations. Modelling, or observational learning (see pp. 22–23), is another effective technique in which someone demonstrates a non-anxious response to situations feared by the anxious person. Relaxation and cognitive therapy may also be used for panic attacks and generalized anxiety. Recent developments in cognitive therapy for depression and anxiety are mindfulness-based approaches which train people in acceptance rather than challenging beliefs (see pp. 138–139).

STOP THINK

■ Think of the last time that you sat a difficult exam. When did your anxiety peak? Was it a week before, the day before, the morning of the exam, waiting outside to go in, sitting down at the desk, looking at the paper or answering the questions? It differs from person to person, but commonly the anxiety peaks at some point before the exam, rather than during it. This is a common feature of anxiety: anticipation of an event is often worse than the actual event. Anxiety-provoking thoughts initiate and maintain the anxiety while waiting, but are replaced by the thinking necessary to tackle the feared situation itself. It may help to remind yourself of that when you are next anxious.

Anxiety

■ Anxiety is common and usually time-limited.

■ Persistent anxious thoughts, physical symptoms and maladaptive behaviour can interfere with healthy functioning.

■ Anticipation of anxiety and avoidance of feared situations can maintain and increase anxiety in a feedback system.

■ Behavioural and cognitive therapies are used either with or without drug treatments, which may run the risk of dependence.

■ The prevalence and effects of anxiety among patients are underestimated.

Depression

Depression is a common and serious disorder. At any one moment in time, about 1 in 20 individuals suffers from a significant depressive disorder, and it is estimated that 17% of the population will suffer from a major depressive disorder at some point throughout their life (Hammen & Watkins, 2007). Depression can be a disabling condition, and patients may be unable to function effectively for several months. According to the World Health Organization, depression is currently rated the fourth leading cause of disability throughout the world, and it is predicted to rise to second leading cause by the year 2010. It is becoming increasingly recognized that children and adolescents can suffer from depression, and that this is often not diagnosed or treated.

What is depression?

The major features of depression are outlined in Box 1. Typically patients have a systematically biased negative view not just of themselves, but also of their world and their future (the *negative cognitive triad*). Depression can be a chronic or recurring condition. Suicidal thoughts and attempts are the most worrying and disturbing features of depression. It has been estimated that between 11 and 17% of individuals with a diagnosis of major depression eventually die by their own hands. A startling fact is that, currently in the UK, suicide is the leading cause of death in men under the age of 35.

Box 1 **Diagnostic criteria for a major depressive episode as defined by the *Diagnostic and Statistical Manual*, 4th revision (DSM-IV) (American Psychiatric Association, 2000)**

A Five or more of the following over the same 2-week period, representing a change from previous functioning and featuring either 1 or 2
1. Depressed mood
2. Loss of interest or pleasure in activities
3. Significant weight loss or gain
4. Insomnia or hypersomnia
5. Psychomotor agitation or retardation
6. Fatigue or loss of energy
7. Feelings of worthlessness or guilt
8. Diminished ability to think or concentrate
9. Recurrent thoughts of death

B The symptoms do not meet criteria for a mixed affective episode

C Symptoms cause clinically significant impairment in social or occupational functioning

D Symptoms not due to direct effects of drug or general medical condition

E Symptoms not better accounted for by bereavement

Gender

Studies throughout the world report approximately a 2:1 rate of depression for women compared to men (Hammen & Watkins, 2007). However, this may partially reflect a greater readiness on the part of women to admit distress and to seek help from health professionals. Men may present their distress in a disguised manner, e.g. presenting with somatic complaints such as pain. However, similar data on sex differences in rates of depression have also been derived from community surveys. Men may be more prone to self-medicate in response to depression, e.g. by alcohol abuse.

Social support

A crucial environmental factor that markedly affects the risk of depression is the availability of good-quality support from friends and family. This seems to offer protection in helping individuals deal with stressors that may otherwise precipitate a depressive episode. The lack of an intimate or confiding relationship, is a good example of lack of social support increasing the risk for depression.

Genetic factors

Some types of depression tend to run in families. McGuffin et al. (1996) reported concordance for lifetime major depression of 46% for monozygotic twins compared with 20% for dizygotic twins, with both rates being higher than lifetime depression in the general population. Evidence such as this suggests a strong genetic contribution to the development of major depression. However, genetics cannot be the whole story; if it were, the concordance rate would be 100% for monozygotic twins.

Treatment

A particular problem with depression is that many patients are reluctant to seek treatment. They may be concerned about the stigma of being labelled as having suffered from a psychiatric disorder. Some patients do not recognize themselves as being depressed, but rather believe that they are lazy, wicked or simply undeserving of treatment. Of those who do seek treatment (often following persuasion by friends and family), many will be treated by their GP, using antidepressant medication such as selective serotonin reuptake inhibitors (SSRIs). It usually takes some time before patients note any benefit, and they may need to be encouraged to persist with treatment. Many antidepressants have side-effects, particularly in the early stages of treatment, and this can lead to patients discontinuing treatment. The SSRIs are as effective as the older tricyclic antidepressants and are less likely to be discontinued because of side-effects. Many patients may be reluctant to take antidepressant medication because of fears regarding dependence and toxicity. Such fears should be elicited and addressed during the consultation.

Cognitive-behavioural therapy (CBT) (see pp. 138–139) and interpersonal psychotherapy are structured, time-limited psychological treatments and have also been shown to be effective treatments for depression (Luty et al., 2007). They are useful for patients without psychotic symptoms who are able to engage in the learning process involved. CBT strives to help patients see the link between thinking, mood and behaviour. Patients are helped to develop the ability to evaluate evidence regarding their beliefs objectively, and this leads to improvement in mood. CBT is clearly more expensive than drug treatment in the short term, but there is accumulating evidence that CBT reduces the risk of future depressive episodes (NICE, 2007). For many patients, a combination of antidepressants and psychotherapy may be most helpful (Keller et al., 2000). This may be because the drug treatment provides a boost to increase activity and aid concentration, enabling the patient to take an active part in a psychological intervention, which in turn may reduce the risk of future relapse. Many other forms of psychotherapy, counselling and alternative treatments are currently available; however few have a strong evidence base regarding their efficacy (see NICE website at http://www.nice.org.uk/CG023).

Electroconvulsive therapy (ECT) is a controversial treatment for severe depression. ECT has been shown to be effective in controlled clinical trials (Geddes, 2003). It should be used only to achieve rapid and short-term improvement of severe symptoms after an adequate trial of other treatment options has proven ineffective, and/or when the condition is considered to be life-threatening, in individuals with a severe depressive illness. Patients often complain of memory loss following ECT (Rose et al., 2003), but the evidence for this is inconclusive, as depression itself is often associated with both subjective and objective cognitive impairment.

There is no perfect treatment for depression and many have high drop-out rates. This is likely to be due to a number of reasons: depressed patients lack energy and concentration and will find the effort of attending clinics difficult. They are also likely to have a pessimistic view of the treatment (one of the common symptoms is a sense of hopelessness). No treatment is immediately effective, so patients receive little positive reinforcement for attending initial treatment sessions.

Depression in the general medical setting

Many patients who suffer from general medical conditions also suffer from depression. In a recent study of 300 consecutive new attenders at a neurology outpatient clinic, 27% met diagnostic criteria for major depressive disorder (Carson et al., 2000). Comorbid depression may also be associated with poor prognosis in medical conditions, e.g. following myocardial infarction, patients who were depressed have significantly increased mortality rates (Frasure-Smith et al., 1993). This may be because they see the future as bleak and pointless, and do not have the motivation or energy to engage in cardiac rehabilitation programmes, change unhealthy behaviours (e.g. smoking, exercise, diet) and may not adhere to prescribed medication. Unfortunately, many medical patients do not get their depression diagnosed or treated, yet even in terminal disease states such as metastatic cancer, treating an underlying depressive illness can markedly improve the patients quality of life.

Health and social policy implications

It is important to consider possible preventive measures at individual, family, community and population levels. Increased social support, income support, employment

opportunities and good housing could all potentially help reduce psychosocial stressors. Giving health professional resources and training to identify depression may help to reduce the high rate of untreated depression. A simple protocol involving telephone follow-up and review by the practice nurse resulted in markedly improved outcomes when treating depression in general practice. At 2-year follow-up, 74% of patients treated with this 'enhanced care' approach were in clinical remission, versus 41% of those who received 'treatment as usual' (Fig. 1) (Rost et al., 2002). Depression is largely effectively treated in primary care, but accessible and speedy referral pathways to specialist mental health services are vital, particularly for treatment-resistant, recurrent, atypical and psychotic depression, and those at significant risk. Greater public awareness and understanding could help remove the stigma attached to seeking help for mental health problems. Optimal intervention involves early detection, the use of evidence-based treatments (both pharmacological and psychological), systematic patient follow-up and monitoring of response, and modifying treatment as necessary.

Case study

Diane, a 33-year-old bank clerk, has been married for 12 years and has three children all under the age of 10. In the past 3 years both her parents died and she was promoted at work to a more demanding position. The family moved to a new home 6 months ago. Two of the children had problems settling in at their new school. For 6 weeks, Diane was wakening at 4 a.m. and was unable to get back to sleep. She worried constantly that they had made the wrong decision moving home, and she also regretted taking up her promoted post. She became increasingly convinced that she was failing in her job, and as a wife and mother. She felt that she could not confide in her husband as he had enough on his plate with work-related stress. She lost her appetite and 12 lb in weight in 1 month. She felt constantly exhausted and irritable. She felt joyless and saw the future as bleak. She was convinced that her husband and children would be better off without her. Her husband became increasingly concerned about the changes in his wife, and this made her feel even guiltier for causing concern. Eventually, her husband persuaded her to go to her GP, who diagnosed a major depressive episode. She was treated with a combination of antidepressant (paroxetine) and cognitive-behavioural therapy. Diane reduced her working hours and joined a gym and this also enabled her to meet new people. Over a 3-month period she gradually improved and felt that she was slowly getting back to her 'old self'. The GP recommended that she stay on her medication for a further 6 months.

Depression

- Depression is a common and serious illness, which can prove fatal.
- Symptoms lie on a continuum from mild to severe.
- Vulnerability factors and stressful life events increase the risk of depression.
- Effective treatments include antidepressant medication, cognitive-behavioural therapy and interpersonal psychotherapy.
- Primary prevention includes alleviating material and emotional deprivation.
- Optimal intervention involves early detection, the use of evidence-based treatments, systematic patient follow-up and monitoring of response, and modifying treatment as necessary.

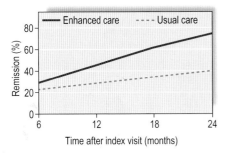

Fig. 1 Improved outcome in the treatment of depression 2 years after presentation with enhanced care versus treatment as usual (from Rost et al., 2002, with permission).

Inflammatory bowel disease

Inflammatory bowel disease (IBD) illustrates how social and psychological processes have an impact on the response to and the experience of illness, and some of the issues which these processes generate for medical care. Ulcerative colitis (one type of IBD) will be used to demonstrate this (Kelly, 1992).

Clinical features

Ulcerative colitis is a disease of the lining layer of the large bowel. It can occur at any age. Its principal symptoms are chronic unpredictable diarrhoea accompanied by heavy anal bleeding, weight and appetite loss and abdominal pain. Its causes are unknown. There is presently no medical cure. For the moment the mainstays of treatment are rectal and systemic 5-aminosalicylic acid derivatives and corticosteroids, with azathioprine in steroid-dependent or resistant cases (Ghosh et al., 2000).

The complications of colitis can be severe. There may be perforation of the bowel, and the effects on the overall health of the patient can be extremely serious. Where the disease is present for more than 10 years there is a very greatly enhanced risk of the development of bowel cancer. At present, the best treatment option available in the face of unremitting symptoms and grave deterioration in the patient's health or the development of cancer is the surgical removal of the bowel. This involves either creating an internal pouch to collect the waste matter of digestion with normal anal evacuation, or simply redirecting the faeces through the abdominal wall via a stoma, a procedure called panproctocolectomy and ileostomy. The operations are major and in the case of ileostomy have profound effects on appearance because the small bowel protrudes externally, and although patients are cured of the colitis, they are incontinent of faeces. They will always have to wear a bag to collect the products of digestion.

Onset

When the first symptoms – usually diarrhoea – appear, the typical response by the sufferer is to minimize or ignore them. Diarrhoea is quite common, so the sufferer often makes the assumption that the symptoms will remit of their own accord, as diarrhoea usually does. This response may continue until such time as blood appears in the motion. This is usually regarded by the patient as very significant and frightening. Whereas diarrhoea is common, anal bleeding is not. Contact with the medical profession is frequently made some time after the appearance of blood, although some patients do seek help for their diarrhoea. When the symptoms of diarrhoea are presented they are sometimes misdiagnosed.

I was working. I had two children …
I began to feel, y'know, unwell. Went to my GP. Didn't examine me at all, and told me I was suffering from piles, haemorrhoids, and gave me some medication. The piles wouldn't go away, and I was back there. And by this time it was terribly painful. And I started to get really worried because I was losing blood. So I made another appointment with another doctor in the practice, and she took me into the examination room, examined me straight away, and within a week I was up at St George's Hospital
(38-year-old teacher: Kelly, 1992).

The important social–psychological concept involved here is help-seeking (see pp. 88–89). Diarrhoea comes well within the range of the normal experience of most people. They generally wait and to see whether it passes in a day or two (temporizing behaviour). The observation of blood in their motion signals something out of the ordinary and acts as the trigger for them to consult the doctor. From a medical point of view rectal bleeding is something requiring investigation. It is however quite unlikely to engender the same degree of anxiety as experienced by the patient. As far as colitis is concerned, bleeding does not necessarily indicate an exacerbation of the illness. Thus the patient's estimation of the seriousness of the symptom may not necessarily correspond to the doctor's. However, in order to manage the patient's symptoms and anxieties successfully the doctor must be aware not only of the physical symptoms but also how they are being interpreted by the patient. The fact that the patient believes a symptom to be grave is what is important in understanding why the patient has consulted.

Diagnosis and treatment

Confirming the diagnosis will involve inspecting the patient's colon with a colonoscope or a sigmoidoscope. Barium enema can provide radiological confirmation. From the patient's perspective these procedures are undignified, uncomfortable, frequently painful and often highly stressful. One patient described barium enema:

So I got the appointment for the X-ray department, went in, without a care in the world. I came out absolutely devastated … it was terrifying … And you go into this place, which had this revolving table and everything and this room, and they pump all this stuff into you. It was ghastly
(33-year-old female school teacher: Kelly, 1992).

Most X-ray departments have little or no time to prepare people for these procedures, and the fear and anxiety that may be generated are considerable because the patient is uncertain as to what is happening. The stressfulness of these kinds of experiences has been shown to be significantly reduced if patients have been well prepared in advance (Fig. 1) (see

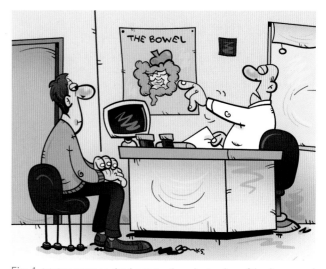

Fig. 1 It is important to check a patient's understanding of the disease, and of any procedures before they happen, in order to manage stress and anxiety (http://www.nacc.org.uk).

pp. 102–105). Furthermore, recognizing the indignity of the procedures can also be reassuring for the patient.

Diagnosis is not always straightforward and determining whether it is colitis or some other form of IBD is sometimes difficult. However, having made the diagnosis, the physician faces a dilemma. If the disease can be brought under control, all well and good. However, what the physician also has to convey is that this may offer only temporary respite and that the patient may face a long period of chronic illness of varying degrees of severity. Although the patient would be entitled to receive a full description of the likely prognosis and the treatment options available, for many patients this raises more problems and questions than it solves. Discussions of cancer, surgery or long periods of severe ill health may terrify patients and cause them to lose hope and certainly may lead to raised levels of anxiety. And the treatment options are not necessarily clear-cut. The disease process is uncertain; phases of exacerbation and remission are unpredictable. The long-term risk of cancer and sudden and major acute deterioration must also be borne in mind. From a lay point of view this is a large amount of unwelcome and irresolvable information with no easy options. Moreover it is usually the case that the patient enters treatment for this disease in the expectation of a cure. Eventually patients will come to realize that they are not going to recover fully.

This is further complicated by the fact that, in spite of all the problems, many patients try to live as normal a life as possible in the face of the illness. If patients are trying to live a normal life, they face a tension between the demands of fulfilling usual social responsibilities and accepting the limitations imposed upon them by the illness.

Although this is not easy, people do manage to cope with their illness in spite of the difficulties it presents. Doctors can help here, by encouraging patients to live as normal a life as they can, but also by helping them to recognize the limitations the illness can produce.

Living with the illness

Many aspects of life are likely to be affected by the illness. The chronic, unpredictable diarrhoea means that things like travel, shopping, walking, eating and socializing are interrupted as the sufferer has to go off and find a toilet. The nature of the symptoms are such that the patient usually has very little warning (perhaps less than 30 seconds) of the need to evacuate. Sufferers become highly skilled in breaking off from social interaction, arranging journeys and trips so that toilets are always within easy reach and carrying a change of clothes for the occasions when they self-soil.

I didn't enjoy shopping or anything.
I was always wanting to be near a toilet; I, well, always felt nauseated with it.
I didn't have the energy to go shopping like everybody else … we couldn't plan anything …
(46-year-old housewife: Kelly, 1992).

It is sometimes remarked that patients suffering from colitis exhibit odd behaviour, such as obsessive attention to detail and concerns about personal cleanliness. However, the general consensus is that this behaviour is an adaptive product of the struggle with the illness, rather than a cause of it, which allows them to survive and function in the world in spite of their illness.

Surgery

For some patients with colitis the prospect of surgery has to be confronted. There are two important behavioural issues. Firstly, patients have to deal with the prospect of major body-altering surgery which, with some operations, will leave them with a stoma. Secondly, the patient now faces a new psychological threat. Although the medical decision may be relatively straightforward, it is not automatically viewed in that way by the patient. Some will refuse surgery, believing that the threats arising from the illness are preferable to the threats arising from the surgery. Helping the patient adapt to surgery is, therefore, a key problem in this procedure. Preparations for surgery should not involve trying to make patients 'accept' their illness or the fact that they need an operation. Helping patients to prepare for surgery should be about allowing them to acknowledge the psychological pain and distress and the associated feelings of loss that this surgery engenders. It should aim to help them work through their feelings of hurt. This is a difficult and traumatic procedure from the patient's perspective and one which requires considerable social and psychological skills on the part of the people caring for that patient (see pp. 104–105).

■ To what extent might there be a conflict between the medical and psychological management of colitis? Is the refusal of some patients with colitis to have surgery adaptive or maladaptive?

Case study

Gillian is 52. She was first diagnosed as having colitis when she was 46. She is married with two teenage children. Her doctor has just told her she needs to have a total colectomy and ileostomy. She is completely distraught at the prospect. She thinks of herself, and always has, as an attractive woman. She is horrified at the prospect of wearing a bag. Yet she is very ill. She has not had a proper night's sleep for nearly 3 years. She has to get up in the night three or four times to go to the toilet. During the day it is even worse. She usually cannot go for longer than an hour before she has to open her bowels. Her work as a secretary is becoming increasingly difficult. Her boss is very understanding but the fact that she constantly has to leave the office has made things very awkward. Her appetite is poor, and when she does eat she sticks to a diet of minced breast of chicken and white bread. She and her husband used to go out a lot, but they stay at home all the time now. Her doctor has told her that the operation will make her better. Gillian, however, is resolute in her refusal to have the operation.

Inflammatory bowel disease

■ The process of making decisions about seeking help are governed by social and psychological factors as well as the degree of medical seriousness of the condition.

■ Symptoms which are regarded as critical by the patient will not necessarily be the same ones as those identified as medically serious.

■ In a disease like colitis, social and psychological symptoms may be evident, but they are usually a consequence rather than a cause of the illness.

■ As with many illnesses, the treatments for colitis are frequently viewed as more psychologically threatening by the patient than the illness itself. These threats condition patient behaviour as much as the threats from the disease and its symptoms.

■ The surgery performed to cure colitis is often associated with very powerful feelings of distress and loss.

Physical disability

Physical disabilities are limitations in the ability to perform activities and can be the result of such diverse conditions as cerebral palsy, rheumatoid arthritis, stroke, multiple sclerosis or accidental injury. As shown in Figure 1, the commonest disabilities in western industrialized countries are in locomotion, personal care activities (such as dressing, washing, feeding and toileting) and hearing. Approximately 21% of adults and children in the UK report at least one limiting long-standing illness. The prevalence of disability increases with age; approximately half of those over 75 years have locomotion limitations.

Activity limitations can result in social disadvantage. Disability present from birth, e.g. in cerebral palsy or cystic fibrosis, may disadvantage individuals throughout their lifetime and affect school, employment, marital, parenting and other social opportunities. By contrast, an injury as a young adult, a myocardial infarction in middle age or a stroke after retirement will have very different impacts on both the individual and his/her family.

Assessing disability

In research or clinical practice, levels of disability are assessed to ascertain the severity of the condition or to evaluate improvement or deterioration. Clinical assessments may be used to make decisions about medical care, referral to rehabilitation services (especially physio-occupational and speech and language therapists), provision of aids or adaptations to the home or recommendations for absence from work, pensions or welfare benefits.

Disability is typically assessed by measures of activities of daily living (ADL), which assess the person's ability to perform everyday self-care or mobility activities. These measures assess activities that virtually everyone would wish to perform and, therefore, do not include activities that may be important for particular individuals. For example, the Barthel index (Johnston et al., 1995) includes personal toilet (wash face, comb hair, shave and clean teeth), feeding, using toilet, walking on level surface, transfer from chair to bed, dressing, using stairs and bathing.

There are two main methods of assessment: self-report and observation. The first requires individuals to describe difficulties experienced, and in the second they perform defined activities while a trained observer notes successes and failures. Self-report has the advantage of allowing the assessment of a wide range of activities, occurring in home and private situations, covering all times of day and night and over days, weeks or months. Observational methods are restricted to what can be assessed in the limited setting of the hospital or in the limited period available for a home visit; patients who can use the toilet independently in the hospital setting may not be able to do so at home if there is less space to manoeuvre or no support to lean on, and they may be even more disabled if they need to go to the toilet during the night if this involves additional flights of stairs. Also, electronic monitors e.g. pedometers, can record activity through the day, in the individual's normal environment.

Models of disability

Three models of disability have each contributed to a broader understanding: medical, social and psychological. These have been combined in the World Health Organization's *International Classification of Functioning, Disability and Health* (ICF) model (World Health Organization, 2002b), an integrative model appropriate to the multidisciplinary management that disability necessitates. For example, a stroke patient may require neurologists to address the underlying brain damage; rehabilitation staff deal with activity limitations; psychologists address dysfunctional beliefs and enhance mood; and social services work to adapt patients' living space, e.g. by providing ramp access to their home. The ICF identifies three components of disabling conditions: (1) impairments to body structures and functions; (2) activity limitations; and (3) participation restrictions, each of which are affected by personal and environmental factors (Fig. 2).

Medical model

The traditional medical model regarded disability as a direct consequence of an underlying disease or disorder. From this perspective reductions in disability can only be achieved through the amelioration of the underlying pathology. However, pathology is a poor predictor of disability: for example, the degree of joint degeneration is a poor predictor of mobility disability in people with osteoarthritis (Dieppe, 2004). This traditional model also engenders stigmatizing language (see pp. 60–61), and does not recognize social and psychological factors. By contrast, the ICF recognizes a role for impairment in disability but also incorporates social and environmental factors.

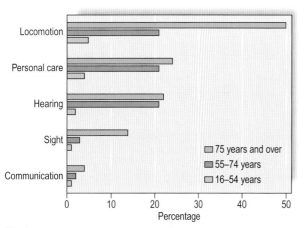

Fig. 1 Prevalence of disabilities by age (percentage reporting each disability) (adapted from Bajekal et al., 2001, with permission).

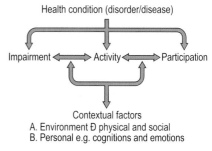

Fig. 2 International classification of functions (adapted from World Health Organization, 2002b).

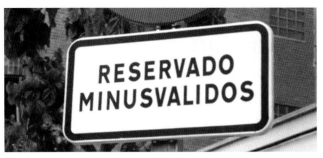

Fig. 3 Social values. Would disabled individuals feel valued by a society that offered this 'special' car-parking space ('reservado minusvalidos' means 'reserved for the disabled')? Or would they feel that they were 'minus validity'? English uses similarly stigmatizing vocabulary, e.g. 'invalid' (with two pronunciations) or 'handicap' (derived from the 'cap in hand' of the person begging).

Social model

A social model of disability emphasizes that activity limitations and participation restrictions result from social and environmental constraints. So individuals are limited not by their medical condition per se, but by the behaviour of other people towards them and by environmental barriers, such as the inaccessibility of buildings or poor sound systems, that make it impossible for them to participate fully. A person may be less disabled when activity is supported than in a protective social environment; there is evidence that compassionate attention to activity limitations can increase levels of disability (Romano et al., 1995). In Figure 3 we see an attempt to overcome problems of access for individuals with locomotion impairments, but the language used reflects the stigmatizing attitudes that can make participation difficult (see pp. 60–61). The inclusion of a role for contextual factors as well as impairments enables the ICF to reconcile social and medical models of disability. In addition, it incorporates the possibility that social participation may affect activity limitations and impairment, e.g. joining a social club may result in increased physical activity, thus reducing joint stiffness.

Psychological model

A psychological model of disability emphasizes that activities performed (or not performed) by someone with a health condition are influenced by the same psychological processes that affect the performance of these behaviours by non-disabled people. So individuals will be motivated to engage in the activity because it results in things they like, because they believe that other people who are important to them would like them to do it and because they believe they can (see Case study 1). Thus, two people with identical medical conditions, living in identical social and environmental situations, may face very different activity limitations because of their cognitions, emotions or coping strategies (see Stop and Think box and pp. 38–39). Depressed or anxious people are likely to be more limited because of their cognition. For example, individuals who believe that they can overcome their disability, who find the activity more rewarding or see family and friends as being more supportive will be more likely to engage in the activity than someone with different beliefs.

There is ample evidence that psychological factors predict disability outcomes. For example, stroke patients with a stronger belief that they can influence their recovery are found to do more than patients with less belief in personal control, and this difference persists for at least 3 years following stroke (Johnston et al., 2005). Interventions that enhance perceived control beliefs have resulted in reduced activity limitations (Fisher & Johnston, 1996). The role of psychological process in disability is accommodated in the ICF through the recognition that personal factors, such as individual beliefs, act to influence the relationships between impairments, activity limitations and participation restrictions.

> ### Case study 1
>
> Following a road traffic accident, Miss Lopez did not resume eating and drinking when she was physically capable. She only regained normal ingestive activity following a behavioural programme which socially reinforced taking sips of water and enabled her to have the confidence that she could do it.

STOP THINK Mr Harrison, was disabled as the result of a spinal-cord injury after falling from a lorry but reported that his quality of life had improved because he was studying for a degree rather than being a manual worker. The clinical team believed that Mr Harrison could learn to walk again but seemed unmotivated. What factors are likely to be influencing Mr Harrison's degree of disability? What should the clinical team do?

STOP THINK
- Elizabeth Edison uses a wheelchair to get around. What image comes to mind when you picture Elizabeth Edison? Is she elderly and frail in appearance? Or, is she a young, fit paraolympic basketball champion?
- Social stereotypes can affect how we think about age and disability and how we behave toward people with disabilities. How well are the needs of young people with disabilities accommodated in our society? How valid is the assumption that to be old is to be disabled?

> ### Physical disability
>
> - Disability is assessed by ADL measures, using both self-report and observational methods.
> - Disability and its impact can be explained in terms of disease and social and psychological factors.
> - Disability is influenced by impairment due to disease or disorder, the physical environment, the social environment, emotions, cognitions and coping strategies.
> - The World Health Organization's ICF provides a comprehensive model.

Learning disability

The implications of a learning disability for the health of individuals who are affected and their families can be far-reaching, and they may need considerable clinical care and psychological and socioeconomic support.

What is learning disability?

'Learning disability' is the term currently used in UK legislation and policy for a range of conditions that fit within the World Health Organization criteria of:

- A state of arrested or incomplete development of mind
- Significant impairment of intellectual functioning
- Significant impairment of adaptive/social functioning
- Present from childhood.

This means that somebody with a learning disability will have difficulties in understanding, in learning new things and generalizing these to new situations, and difficulties with social tasks like communication, self-care, awareness of and responses to danger. These difficulties will be present in differing permutations and will vary in severity depending upon the extent and nature of the disability. Learning disability fits the social rather than the medical model of disability: it cannot be cured nor in any real sense can it be treated, although in some cases it can be avoided by prompt medical intervention or by improved antenatal care, and in many cases its impact can be mitigated by appropriate responses across a range of disciplines. UK & USA studies have confirmed that mild learning disability is more common among socially disadvantaged families. They have also shown that preventive strategies targeting children with mild learning disability are effective in preventing developmental delay and have long-term benefits. Moderate to severe levels of disability show little correlation with social class. Although their impacts can also be moderated by prompt and appropriate supports, significant levels of disability will remain.

Prevalence

There are no reliable figures for the number of people with a learning disability in the UK but estimates suggest a prevalence rate of 25 per 1000 population with a mild to moderate learning disability and a further 3 per 1000 with severe disabilities. In 2000 it was estimated the numbers would grow by approximately 1% per annum to 2010 but this is now thought to have been an underestimation.

Antenatal screening, with access to abortion if the fetus is shown to have significant disabilities, has reduced the number of babies with Down's syndrome born to older mothers. However, there has been an overall increase in numbers due to better survival rates for very-low-birth-weight babies or others born with severe impairments; and both children and adults are living longer because of better health and community care.

Causes

The commonest causes of inherited disability are fragile X syndrome and Down's syndrome. Birth-related disabilities are mostly caused by insufficiencies in the oxygen supply, or prematurity. After birth the most common causes are early childhood illness or physical accident.

The cause of mild learning disability is generally multifactorial and the precise mechanisms are not clear.

However there is a statistical correlation with factors associated with poverty and deprivation (nine times higher in working-class families than in other social groups).

Health implications of learning disability for the individual

The incidence of ill health in people with learning disabilities is higher than in the general population. The most common coexisting health problems are mental ill health, problem behaviour, epilepsy and sensory impairments. For the parents of a child with learning disabilities problem behaviours and sleep disorder are frequently mentioned as having the greatest impact on family life.

Allocation of health resources is increasingly driven by targets focused on the major causes of morbidity and mortality. However, because these causes are different for people with learning disabilities, prevention and treatment campaigns are of lesser benefit to them and may only widen the existing gap in health and longevity.

Today people with learning disabilities are less likely to be denied certain treatments because of assumptions about their quality of life or life expectancy. However communication difficulties, atypical responses to pain or problem behaviour being regarded as either 'just part of the condition' or a manifestation of mental illness can often mean considerable delay in diagnosing physical, treatable, conditions.

On the other hand, there is a high rate of medication and much prescribing is not evidence-based. Studies have found that between 20% and 50% of people with learning disabilities are prescribed psychotropic medication, yet 'the reason for its use is often unclear and sometimes it is used in the management of problems for which there is little reliable evidence of effectiveness due to lack of research' (NHS Report, 2004). This is a population that is typically denied control over many basic aspects of daily living, subjected to higher than average experience of bullying and denigration and with limited opportunity for self-expression or fulfillment – all factors recognized as having an impact on levels of stress, depression and mental illness in the general population. Reducing inappropriate prescribing might help to focus attention on factors related to the social conditions of people rather than their learning disability.

Health implications of learning disability for the family

Although there is now a greater awareness of the importance of how to communicate any diagnosis, it is still the case that many new parents feel inadequately supported when their child is diagnosed as having a learning disability. Nor do they feel well prepared for what this will mean for their family, or feel well supported through the early years. Where the disability is not immediately obvious, it can take parents years to achieve a diagnosis and their efforts can have them labelled as anxious, neurotic or worse. Achieving a diagnosis may still leave parents having to fight for effective help or support. This situation tends to worsen when the child reaches 16 and makes the transition to adult services. The period around transition can be a time of great anxiety for parents and of renewed battles for support.

Added to the pain of having to let go hopes and ambitions

for their child, parents will also have to adjust to a child who will require basic care for a protracted (or indefinite) period, who may have very disturbed sleep patterns and other problem behaviours and who may have coexisting conditions such as epilepsy, cerebral palsy, sensory impairments, eating problems and others.

In such situations parents are at risk of exhaustion, of neglecting their own health and well-being, and of stresses affecting their own relationship and their relationships with other children. There is also good evidence that having a child with a significant disability affects the earning power of a family, thus adding a further stress.

Because learning disability is a lifelong condition, and because there is a shortfall in appropriate and acceptable provision, many parents remain carers into their 70s and beyond, and only become known to social services when they become too frail to continue caring. Given the universal coverage of general practice, GPs are well placed to identify earlier these so-called hidden carers.

Implications of learning disability for the health services and society

In 1969 there were nearly 60 000 people with learning disabilities living (permanently) in hospital. By 2005 most of those hospitals had closed and the residual population was in the hundreds. Officially, no children now live in hospital. The paradigm shift from medical to social model of disability helped this movement but has also been consolidated by it. Thousands of people who were previously invisible now live in our communities and neighbourhoods. Their health care is now the responsibility of general practice with a few specialist clinics, e.g. for epilepsy. Social services now have statutory responsibility for their welfare but in practice families still carry most of the burden of care.

The social model has prevailed over the medical model. Policy continues to follow the route of individualizing services and transferring control to the patient or client, but disputes over resources and affordability mean service delivery is still far from personalized or user-controlled. *Valuing People* (Department of Health, 2001) and *Same as You* (Scottish Executive, 2000) have set goals for change but the future is uncertain (Box 1).

Box 1 **Principles of service delivery to people with a learning disability**

- People with learning disabilities should be valued. They should be asked and encouraged to contribute to the community they live in. They should not be picked on or treated differently from others.
- People with learning disabilities are individual people.
- People with learning disabilities should be asked about the services they need and be involved in making choices about what they want.
- People with learning disabilities should be helped and supported to do everything they are able to.
- People with learning disabilities should be able to use the same local services as everyone else, wherever possible.
- People with learning disabilities should benefit from specialist social, health and educational services.
- People with learning disabilities should have services which take account of their age, abilities and other needs.

(From Scottish Executive, 2000, with permission.)

Case study

John was introduced to his support service by the clinical psychologist when he was 10 years old. He lived in the family home but was mainly restricted to one room. Most of the furnishings had been progressively damaged and removed. At home, John would not stay clothed, eat at a table or from a plate, use cutlery or use toilet facilities – he resisted bathing, had few settled nights, engaged in little play and frequently hit out and bit. There was little support going into the home and the family resources were exhausted. Transfer to a specialist residential school, out of area, was under active consideration but the family was not keen to have him sent away.

Intensive cooperation involving health, social work, education and housing services working with the support service saw John and his family carer, 18 months later, in a new home. He still did not have full run of the house but his bedroom and sitting room were furnished and he had games, materials and activity equipment indoors and in the garden. He was experiencing more engagement in activities in and around the home, and at the local parks and beach. He now slept in his bed, with sheets and duvet, bathed twice a day, had settled nights and ate with appropriate equipment at the table. In addition he was using signs and symbols to communicate needs and wants, including the sign for toilet, and indicating choices about food and clothes. The threat of removal to a residential school had receded.

Four years on and John has a regular, daily routine including recycling waste from his home and from the local office of his support service. He is home-schooled, growing more competent in using symbols to indicate choices and initiate requests, and taking some independent action, helping himself to food and drink from the kitchen. He smiles, makes eye contact and engages in high-fives and interactive games with his supporters. His mother says she can now enjoy her son. The lynchpin has been the collaboration of the clinical psychologist and the support team but the joint working across the wider group at key points has been crucial to John's progress.

 STOP THINK The healthcare needs of people with learning disabilities are not always looked at well enough in medical education. Nor are the wider issues about how doctors should best communicate with them.
- Why is this the case? What can you do to improve your understanding and communications skills?

Learning disability

- Although the prevalence of people with learning disability is relatively low, the impact on the individual and his or her family is likely to be considerable. Carers of people with learning disabilities may experience exhaustion, stress and poor health.

- The social model of disability has made an important contribution to the individualizing of services and to transferring control to the individual.

- The transition from childhood to adulthood (at age 16) and accessing appropriate support can be a time of considerable anxiety to parents and the individual.

- Doctors can be a great support to a family if they listen carefully and work with the individual, the family and other health and social services to obtain the support that the individual and family want and need.

Posttraumatic stress disorder (PTSD)

What is PTSD?

Posttraumatic stress disorder (PTSD) is a condition where exposure to an intense and frightening emotional experience leads to lasting changes in behaviour, mood and cognition. Often after a life-threatening incident (e.g. a violent assault, rape or wartime experience), the individual re-experiences the event(s), e.g. via intrusive and distressing thoughts, images, flashbacks or nightmares. The individual may exhibit phobic avoidance and/or physiological reactivity (e.g. increased heart rate) to reminders of the trauma. Increased arousal in terms of sleep disturbance, irritability and exaggerated startle response are common. In addition, the individual may exhibit a restricted range of affect, sense of a foreshortened future, and may lose interest in previously rewarding hobbies or activities. The current diagnostic criteria of the American Psychiatric Association are shown in Box 1.

As stated above, PTSD is characterized by intrusive, distressing memories of the traumatic event. Paradoxically, it is also often associated with marked impairments in learning and memory for new material (anterograde memory: see pp. 28–29). Patients often complain that they remember what they do not want to, yet cannot remember what they now wish to. Heightened arousal at the time of encoding may result in modulation (strengthening) of the emotional memory trace, possibly via noradrenaline release in the amygdala. Subsequent anterograde memory impairment may be due to the deleterious effects of prolonged elevated levels of stress hormones (e.g. long-term hypercortisolaemia) on hippocampal functioning. Some magnetic resonance imaging studies have shown that chronic PTSD is associated with reduction in volume of the hippocampus, a brain area critically involved in new learning and memory.

How common is PTSD?

The US National Comorbidity Survey Replication Study consisted of structured diagnostic interviews of 9282 community residents aged 18 years and older (Kessler et al., 2005). The estimated lifetime prevalence for PTSD was 6.8%. The most common precipitating traumas are combat for men and rape and sexual molestation for women. It is important to note however that: (1) most people do *not* develop a disorder after experiencing a stressful life event; and (2) many disorders other than PTSD often develop following adversity, in particular phobias, depression, acute stress reaction and adjustment disorders. It is clear that some individuals are more likely than others to develop PTSD following exposure to trauma. Predictive variables that have been identified include trauma severity, dissociation during the trauma, perceived threat and premorbid vulnerability factors including prior emotional disorder, particularly depression.

Debriefing and PTSD

When disaster strikes there is an understandable desire to try to act quickly to support survivors. With increasing recognition that PTSD can be a debilitating outcome in many individuals who experience trauma, rapid psychological interventions, i.e. critical incident stress debriefing (CISD) became popular during the 1990s. Systematic reviews of controlled trials in this area failed to find any evidence that CISD reduced general psychological morbidity, depression or anxiety; rather a significantly *increased* risk of PTSD has been observed in those who had received debriefing (NICE, 2005) (Fig. 1). This may be because those who did not receive immediate professional treatment instead utilized existing social support mechanisms and gradually came to terms with their traumatic experience over time via discussion with close confidants.

Box 1 **Diagnostic criteria for posttraumatic stress disorder as defined by the *Diagnostic and Statistical Manual*, 4th revision (DSM-IV: American Psychiatric Association, 2000)**

A The person has been exposed to a traumatic event in which both of the following were present:
1. The person experienced, witnessed or was confronted with an event that involved actual or threatened death or serious injury, or a threat to the physical integrity of self or others
2. The person's response involved fear, hopelessness or horror

B The traumatic event is persistently re-experienced in one or more of the following ways:
1. Recurrent and intrusive distressing recollections of the event
2. Recurrent distressing dreams of the event
3. Acting or feeling as if the traumatic event were recurring
4. Intense psychological distress at exposure to cues that symbolise/resemble the event
5. Physiological reactivity on exposure to cues that symbolise/resemble the event

C Persistent avoidance of stimuli associated with the trauma and numbing of general responsiveness as indicated by three (or more) of the following:
1. Efforts to avoid thoughts, feelings or conversations associated with the trauma
2. Efforts to avoid activities, places or people that arouse recollections of the trauma
3. Inability to recall an important aspect of the trauma
4. Markedly diminished interest or participation in significant activities
5. Feelings of detachment or estrangement from others
6. Restricted range of affect (e.g. unable to have loving feelings)
7. Sense of a foreshortened future

D Persistent symptoms of increased arousal as indicated by two (or more) of the following:
1. Difficulty falling or staying asleep
2. Irritability or outbursts of anger
3. Difficulty concentrating
4. Hypervigilance
5. Exaggerated startle response

E Duration of disturbance is more than 1 month

F The disturbance causes clinically significant distress or impairment in social, occupational or other important areas of functioning

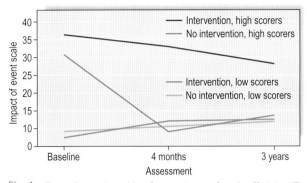

Fig. 1 Effects of immediate debriefing on victims of road traffic injury. Those with high initial scores on the impact of events scale (intrusive thoughts and avoidance) had worse outcomes than untreated controls 4 months and 3 years later (from Mayou & Farmer, 2002, with permission).

Treatment of PTSD

Bisson et al. (2007) recently reviewed the evidence regarding the effectiveness of psychological treatment for chronic PTSD. The most effective treatments were trauma-focused cognitive-behavioural therapy (TFCBT) and eye movement desensitization and reprocessing (EMDR). Direct comparisons of these two approaches did not reveal any significant advantages of one over the other. In PTSD, symptoms may be maintained via overt and covert avoidance of reminders or thoughts about the event. Exposure-based behaviour treatments have consistently been shown to be effective. These involve patients confronting their fears, either via systematic desensitization (imaginal exposure to feared stimuli while in a relaxed state, in a graded, hierarchical fashion) or 'real-life' graded exposure. EMDR is a relatively new technique that consists of imaginal exposure while the therapist waves a finger across the patient's visual field with the patient tracking the finger. EMDR is a controversial treatment as some authors initially made remarkable claims for its efficacy (Herbert et al., 2000). The effective component of EMDR may be due, in part, to the exposure component. The evidence base for drug treatments in PTSD is limited (NICE, 2005). The selective serotonin reuptake inhibitor (SSRI) antidepressant drug paroxetine appears to be helpful, and in many cases the traumatized individual may fulfil diagnostic criteria for both PTSD and comorbid major depression.

PTSD in the general medical setting

A significant number of individuals may be traumatized by their experience of medical events and procedures. This may be particularly so in emergency departments, and orthopaedic and plastic surgery clinics. Shalev et al. (1993) pointed out that modern medicine and surgery often employ invasive procedures for which the patient has little or no preparation. For example, many individuals who previously would have died are now alive due to medical and surgical advances. Although such patients are now discharged as medical 'success stories', some survivors develop PTSD and become markedly disabled. Very often these cases are not identified in the general hospital setting, and appropriate interventions are not offered. Such individuals may subsequently avoid further contact with the medical profession, or show poor adherence with treatment regimes.

 STOP THINK
In a debate in the *British Medical Journal*, Summerfield (2001) proposed that PTSD is a 'social invention' and that, 'it was rare to find a psychiatric diagnosis that anyone liked to have, but PTSD is one'. He also stated that, 'once it becomes advantageous to frame distress as a psychiatric condition, people will choose to present themselves as medicalised victims rather than as feisty survivors'. In reply, Shalev (2001) argued that the diagnostic criteria for PTSD are not built in stone, 'but neither are depression, psychosis or delirium'. He concluded that 'Doctors ... have nothing to gain from claims that the pervasive and interminable personal disaster that is posttraumatic stress disorder is not a disorder'.
■ What do you think?

Case study

Mrs C, a 30-year-old woman, underwent a tonsillectomy. While in hospital her husband brought their baby to visit her. Mrs C went to the baby boy and started to take off his hood. Suddenly, blood spurted out of her mouth all over the floor. Panic ensued and she was rushed in a state of hypovolaemic shock to the operating room where a bleeding artery was ligated. She remembers overhearing a doctor tell her husband that 'she'd had one foot in the grave'. For months following this event, Mrs C lived in a constant state of anxiety. She feared that the pharyngeal scar would open and she would bleed to death. Intrusive thoughts and memories of the event kept her awake at night and disturbed her during the day. She was terrified to make a careless move in case it triggered a further episode of bleeding. She withdrew contact from her baby because of a fear that while hugging him blood would again spurt out of her mouth. Treatment involved controlled exposure, involving visiting the surgeon who had operated on her throat, and receiving accurate information regarding future risk. Gradually she returned to her previous level of functioning (from Shalev et al., 1993).

Posttraumatic stress disorder (PTSD)

■ PTSD is an increasingly recognized, though controversial disorder.

■ PTSD is commonly reported following extreme trauma.

■ Most people do not develop a disorder following a traumatic life event.

■ There is increasing evidence that some medical events (e.g. myocardial infarction) or treatments (e.g. defibrillation) can lead to posttraumatic symptoms.

■ Patients with PTSD following medical events are often not identified.

■ Sufferers may avoid further medical care and show poor adherence with treatment.

■ Improved recognition should lead to appropriate treatment and improved ability to make use of medical care.

■ Effective treatments include trauma-focused cognitive-behavioural therapy and eye movement desensitization and reprocessing.

Diabetes mellitus

The number of people worldwide with the chronic condition diabetes mellitus has increased dramatically over the past 10 years and is expected to go on rising. As a diagnostic category, diabetes includes numerous disorders, but the two commonest are known as type 1 and type 2 diabetes. At least 2 million people in the UK have diabetes and there are probably another 750 000 who have not been diagnosed. Approximately 5–10% of those diagnosed have type 1, and 85–95% have type 2 diabetes. Both types of diabetes share the symptom of raised blood glucose levels. Abnormally elevated blood glucose levels have adverse consequences in both the short and long term.

Type 1 diabetes

Type 1 diabetes is typically diagnosed in childhood or adolescence. As a result of a combination of genetic and environmental factors, an autoimmune process progressively destroys the cells in the pancreas that produce the hormone insulin. Insulin is necessary to facilitate the uptake of glucose from the blood by body tissue. In the absence of insulin, blood glucose levels continue to rise, leading to the characteristic symptoms of type 1 diabetes: frequent urination, thirst, fatigue and weight loss. If untreated, there is a risk of ketoacidosis leading eventually to coma, which can be fatal. Type 1 diabetes is treated by replacing the insulin no longer produced by the body with exogenous insulin delivered by injection or pump. The complex treatment regimen requires the patient to use the results of blood glucose monitoring to balance food consumption, insulin administration and energy expenditure. Imbalance can lead to hyperglycaemia (abnormally high blood glucose levels) or hypoglycaemia (abnormally low blood glucose levels), both of which have negative health consequences. The aim of treatment is to achieve good glycaemic control: that is, keeping blood glucose levels within the normal range.

Type 2 diabetes

Type 2 diabetes is predominantly a disease of the middle-aged and elderly although, with increasing levels of juvenile obesity, it is now beginning to be seen among children and adolescents. Blood glucose levels are abnormally high because of both impaired insulin production and insensitivity to insulin. The symptoms are similar to type 1, but often are less pronounced, so that type 2 diabetes can go undiagnosed for years. Type 2 diabetes has a stronger genetic component than type 1. The lifetime risk of developing type 2 diabetes is increased 40% by the presence of a first-degree relative with the disease. Being overweight and having a sedentary lifestyle are also risk factors for developing type 2 diabetes. The treatment of type 2 diabetes involves modifications to diet and exercise, and tablets for reducing blood glucose levels. If these measures are not effective then insulin will be necessary.

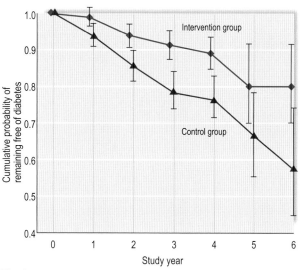

Fig. 1 Results of a trial to prevent type 2 diabetes by improving lifestyle. The proportion of subjects who developed diabetes was significantly higher in the control group than the intervention group from the second year of the study onwards (adapted from Tuomilehto et al., 2001, with permission).

Prevention of diabetes

Tuomilehto et al. (2001) demonstrated that type 2 diabetes can be prevented by changes in lifestyle. Participants were middle-aged, overweight and had impaired glucose tolerance (a diabetes risk factor). All received individualized counselling aimed at reducing fat consumption and increasing physical activity. The risk of developing diabetes in the intervention group was reduced by 58% over the period of the trial in comparison to the usual care control group (Fig. 1). Currently, there is no known intervention to prevent type 1 diabetes, but trials are under way in the USA to test the effectiveness of orally administered insulin for those at risk of type 1.

Complications of diabetes

Abnormal blood glucose levels increase the risk of diabetic complications resulting from damage to the small and large blood vessels. As a result, diabetes is a leading cause of blindness, kidney failure, amputation and coronary artery disease. People with type 2 diabetes have 3–5 times increased risk of cardiovascular mortality. Recent trials have demonstrated that some of these complications can be prevented or delayed by improvements in glycaemic control (DCCT research group, 1993; UK Prospective Diabetes Study Group, 1998), which underscores the importance of good self-management of diabetes.

Depression and diabetes

It is well established that people with diabetes are more likely than people without diabetes to have depression in addition (Eaton, 2002). Depression adversely affects glycaemic control and depressed people engage in less self-management of their diabetes (Lustman & Clouse, 2002). Therefore, it is important to treat depression in people with diabetes. However, antidepressive medications must be used with caution because they can have adverse effects on glycaemic control.

Self-management of diabetes

For both types of diabetes, the person with the disease plays the central role in controlling the illness (Holman & Lorig, 2000). The treatment regimen includes medical elements (blood glucose monitoring and medication – tablets, insulin or both) and lifestyle elements (diet and exercise). People with diabetes find the lifestyle elements more difficult and more damaging to their quality of life than the medical elements (see Case study). Diabetes self-management presents different challenges depending on a person's age (Snoek & Skinner, 2000).

Ways to support diabetes self-management

Patients benefit from education and support from health care professionals to improve their self-management (Clement, 1995). Dose Adjustment For Normal Eating (DAFNE) teaches people with type 1 diabetes how to match their insulin dose to their food choices to maximize blood glucose control. In a UK trial, this approach improved blood glucose control without adversely affecting quality of life (DAFNE Study Group, 2002). For the far larger numbers of people with type 2 diabetes, a tailored approach which focuses on the individual's most pressing self-management problems is effective and efficient (Glasgow et al., 1997). Such an approach has been successfully adapted for the UK setting (Box 1).

Box 1 Tailored self-management intervention for people with type 2 diabetes

A tailored intervention that was brief, patient-centred and supportive was evaluated with 100 people with type 2 diabetes. Compared to the control group, the intervention group reduced their intake of high-fat foods and achieved a reduction in waist circumference (Clark et al., 2004).

- Brief – basic information about the person's eating habits and physical activity levels was obtained using questionnaires. This information was used to guide the 20-minute session with the interventionist.
- Patient-centred – together, the patient and interventionist agreed upon specific goals (e.g. 'I will snack on raw vegetables instead of crisps when watching television'), discussed anticipated barriers to achieving this goal, and agreed on strategies the patient would use to overcome these barriers.
- Supportive – progress was monitored and supported by follow-up telephone calls (a cost-effective way to increase the likelihood of successful behaviour change) and a follow-up appointment.
- Diabetes is more common among ethnic minorities in the UK, particularly among South Asians and African-Caribbeans. In what ways could health care for diabetes be made more culturally sensitive?

Case study

Part 1: self-management for a teenager with type 1 diabetes

Tracey is 16 and enjoys going clubbing. When Tracey stays out late dancing and drinking she misses her evening snack, and the alcohol and exercise lower her blood glucose levels. Her blood glucose levels drop while she is asleep and she is often hypoglycaemic by the time she gets up. Her very low blood glucose makes her bad-tempered and uncooperative, or worse. Tracey has been rushed to hospital unconscious on several occasions. How can her health care team help Tracey to take better care of herself?

Part 2: how can we help Tracey?

- Encourage Tracey to attend sessions specifically for groups of teenagers with diabetes where they can discuss how to overcome the lifestyle challenges posed by their self-management.
- Tracey's doctor may be able to suggest an adjustment to her insulin injections on evenings when she is going out.
- The dietician may be able to recommend certain foods Tracey should eat before going out, and snack foods or soft drinks that she could have while clubbing.
- Tracey or her mother could leave a favourite snack conveniently by her bed for when she returns home late.
- Parents should not relinquish responsibility for their teenage children's diabetes too soon.

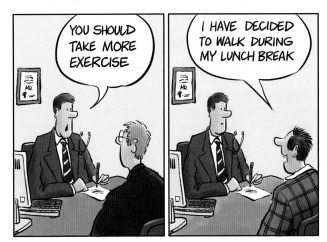

Fig. 2 Which patient is more likely to increase exercise levels – A or B?

Diabetes mellitus

- Diabetes is an increasingly common chronic illness, in part because of the ageing of populations in developed countries and the rise in obesity.
- Type 2 diabetes can be prevented by changing diet and exercise patterns.
- The onset of complications of both type 1 and type 2 diabetes can be prevented or delayed by improved blood glucose control.
- Day-to-day management of diabetes is primarily the responsibility of patients, who need empowering and supporting in their self-management of this disease.
- Interventions to enhance patient self-management are most effective when they are patient-centred and tailored to individual needs (Fig. 2).
- Diabetes occurs in all age groups, from the very young to the very old, and different approaches to providing appropriate health care and support are needed for different age groups.

Stress and health

Anything from major trauma to the experience of working in a noisy room might be described as stressful. 'Stress' is used as shorthand for feeling anxious or suffering physical symptoms and has become a convenient diagnosis for a range of somatic and psychological symptoms. It has proved difficult to define 'stress' precisely, but a widely accepted view is that it arises from a mismatch between our perceptions or appraisals of environmental demands and our assessment of our own resources and abilities to cope with these demands (Folkman et al., 1986). Thus the same event may be stressful to one person but not to another and our experience of stress does not necessarily correspond to others' assessment of the demands we face. For example, gifted students who have always done well in the past may still feel stressed before an examination. Nonetheless, we can characterize events that are related to many instances of stress (Box 1).

Measuring stress

Holmes & Rahe (1967) developed the first life events scale (Miller & Rahe, 1997). This approach involves asking people to list events in their recent past that might be expected to be stressful and adding up the burden. For example, death of a close family member warrants a high score (100), as does losing one's job (47), while trouble with one's boss attracts a lower score (23). This scale also acknowledges that changes in general, even those that seem positive, can increase stress. For example, 12 points are added just after Christmas! Psychologists have also measured the occurrence of more minor daily hassles, such as taking examinations or getting a low grade in a test (Holm & Holroyd, 1992). Measures of work demands, support and control have also been developed (Jackson et al., 1993). An important limitation of such measures is that they do not measure the particular appraisals made by different people. They measure potential stressors, rather than stress. Such measures can be supplemented with measures of individual stress responses, including assessments of anxiety or general psychological well-being. In addition, since stress affects the sympathetic nervous system (SNS), measures of SNS activity can be used as indicators of stress response. These include blood pressure, heart rate and skin conductance (which changes when we sweat), as well as concentrations of corticosteroids (e.g. cortisol) and catecholamines (e.g. adrenaline and noradrenaline) in the blood.

Factors influencing the experience of stress

Our experience of stress depends on objective, demanding situations and on our individual reactions. When we feel confident in our abilities and resources and perceive demands as challenges rather than burdens we are better able to cope. We are also less likely to experience stress if we are familiar with an event or well prepared for it. For example, a doctor who has previous experience of preparing a patient for surgery (pp. 104–105) or has been well trained in breaking bad news (pp. 98–99) is less likely to feel stressed. Patients are also likely to experience stress if they are unsure of their diagnosis and treatments. Ensuring patients have the information they require (pp. 96–97) and that they have their questions answered can reduce the stress of undergoing medical procedures.

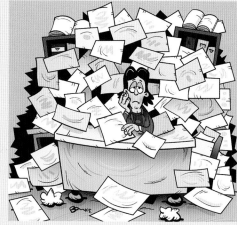

Fig. 1 Work-related stress is common.

Impact of stress – cardiovascular system

Stress is a risk factor for cardiovascular disease. Those with lower levels of control at work are particularly at risk because they cannot control the demands of their job or delegate to others. Stress may influence heart disease by increasing known risk factors, such as hypertension or smoking, by accelerating atherosclerosis or by precipitating earlier myocardial infarction amongst those with underlying disease (Schnall et al., 1994).

Personality affects stress reactions. Type A personality refers to people who are very ambitious in relation to the amount they try to get done in a given time, and are more likely to be competitive and hostile towards others. This may result in strong, frequent stress responses, which results in considerable wear and tear on the cardiovascular system. Hostility (e.g. thinking 'It's safer to trust nobody') appears to be the most dangerous aspect of the type A personality, with those scoring highly on hostility measures being more likely to suffer coronary heart disease (Miller et al., 1996).

Impact of stress –immune functioning

Stress is associated with weaker immune responses and slower wound healing (Kiecolt-Glaser et al., 1995). For example, medical students report higher stress during examinations and also show reduced immune response. This includes lower T-helper (CD4) counts, less rapid proliferation of these cells in laboratory tests as well as reduced natural killer cell activity (Kiecolt-Glaser et al., 1994). Similar evidence of compromised immune functioning has been observed amongst carers of people with Alzheimer's disease and amongst those who have been recently separated, divorced or bereaved. These results suggest that ongoing stress may leave us more susceptible to infection and slow wound healing and inhibit tumour surveillance. Furthermore, divorce and marital conflict increase the incidence of diseases linked to impaired immune functioning. For example, in laboratory studies, couples asked to resolve interpersonal conflict showed reduced endocrine and immune functioning (Kiecolt-Glaser & Newton, 2001).

Evidence suggests that associations between stress and immune function are the result of communication between the nervous and immune systems. People who show strong SNS responses to stress also show the greatest immune responses. By contrast, only small immune effects are observed amongst those who have little SNS response to a stressor (Cohen & Herbert, 1996). The field of research exploring relationships between the nervous and immune systems is known as *psychoneuroimmunology*.

Stress and health risk behaviours

Stress may also increase the likelihood of illness indirectly through stress-induced behaviour. Food, cigarettes, alcohol and other drugs may be used as a compensation for stressful days. Furthermore, those trying to adopt and maintain health behaviours such as diets, exercise regimes or giving up smoking may be unable to keep up the self-control effort required because of stress responses. Stress may also reduce adherence to doctors' advice (pp. 94–95), cause sleep loss and lead to risk-taking that increases the likelihood of accidents, especially in high-risk jobs.

Reducing stress

Stress may be reduced either by limiting people's exposure to stressors or, where this is not possible, helping them to appraise them or cope with them more positively.

Tackling stressors

Reducing stressors is clearly a desirable option where possible. This is often the case in the work situation where stress can be caused not only by job demands (which may be unavoidable) but also by how much decision-making power people have, that is, how much control they have over work schedules and setting priorities (Karasek, 1979). Consequently, giving people more control over work can reduce stress. When people are unclear about their work role or suffer contradictory demands, this will also increase stress. For example, doctors and nurses may experience stress when they are unclear about management priorities or when they feel they have to compromise patient care because of administrative demands. These factors can be modified by good management. Monotonous or isolated jobs can also be stressful. Thus increasing work variety, providing opportunities to learn new skills and increasing social support can be effective.

Unfortunately, some features of modern employment increase stress. Job insecurity is greater than in the past and, apart from the threat to income and standard of living, the loss (or threat of loss) of an identity-linked work role can be very stressful. Poor work–life balance is also an increasing problem as boundaries between work and home are reduced by new technologies such as mobile phones and computers. This can lead to role conflict when the demands of one role (e.g. a work role) prevent one from fulfilling the obligations of other roles (such as friendships or parental roles). Where these stressors cannot be avoided strategies to help people cope may be required.

Helping people cope

Where stressors are inevitable, people need to cope by modifying their appraisals and by developing other coping resources. Social support can serve several purposes. These include providing intimacy that allows people to talk about their problems and fears (pp. 142–143) and providing information and actual resources, including money and time. Social support groups have proved useful for people suffering from chronic diseases such as breast cancer, and internet support groups are a growing resource for many with health problems.

Encouraging people to change their appraisals may also help. This could involve focusing on how they have managed to deal with similar demands in the past or by helping them to see that the stressor is less important than they think. Some employers offer counselling services (see pp. 132–135) to work with stressed employees using therapeutic techniques. Often they employ techniques from cognitive-behavioural therapy (see pp. 138–139), for example, helping people to change what may be unconscious negative appraisals of stressors (e.g. 'If my boss is angry with me it must be because I am useless at my job') to more positive and constructive interpretations looking realistically at what may be potential reasons for the problem and how they can be addressed. People may also benefit from relaxation training so that they can reduce physiological stress responses. Physical activity is also a useful strategy for reducing the experience of stress and its impact on health.

Some workplaces provide stress management courses including these features. Researchers have compared the effectiveness of such interventions and found that, although all approaches are useful, cognitive-behavioural approaches seem particularly helpful (Van der Klink et al., 2001). Similar stress management interventions are used in medical settings. For example, patients facing invasive procedures or recovering from heart attacks may be offered stress management help. Relaxation training is perhaps the commonest approach used to help with medical stressors, but social support and cognitive-behavioural techniques have also been successfully used for those dealing with serious illnesses.

STOP THINK Examinations have been shown to increase students' stress. Which thoughts and perceptions increase this stress? How could you help a friend who says (s)he feels very stressed about a forthcoming examination?

Stress and health

- Stress arises when we think that we may not be able to deal with perceived demands.
- Stress involves negative emotional responses and affects physiological functioning.
- Feeling positive, confident in our abilities and in control will help reduce stress.
- Continued stress responses damage the cardiovascular system over time.
- Stress is associated with weaker immune responses and slower wound healing.
- People suffering from stress may also damage their health through their behaviour.
- Stress management techniques that change stressors or help people cope can reduce stress and its impact on health.

Asthma and chronic obstructive pulmonary disease

Asthma, which is experienced by almost 1 in 10 of the UK population, can occur from infancy to old age and is genetically based. Chronic obstructive pulmonary disease (COPD) is experienced by 8% of UK men and 3% of women and is an adult illness, in most cases the consequence of lung damage caused by smoking (less than 10% is due to occupational illness). Symptoms in asthma and COPD have many similarities, such as breathlessness, ranging from mild to severe, and a pattern of exacerbations that can be triggered by infections (for both) or allergens in the case of asthma. For moderate asthma the most important intervention is inhaled corticosteroid, an anti-inflammatory medication. Used daily, and continuously, inhaled steroids reduce lung inflammation and prevent symptoms in asthma. Higher-dose oral steroids are used in short courses to manage exacerbations. In severe asthma they may be taken daily for regular control.

Bronchodilating medication is the other main medical intervention. It relaxes airways and relieves symptoms, but does not reduce airway inflammation, the underlying mechanism that drives asthma. Patients use this medication when they feel mildly breathless or before exercise. It is usually given through a pocket-sized inhaler. In mild asthma, with only occasional breathlessness, this may be the only medication used. Medical interventions for COPD consists of bronchodilating medication to relieve symptoms, taken daily through a pocket-sized inhaler or an electrically powered nebulizer, and antibiotics for COPD exacerbations resulting from chest infections. Oral or inhaled corticosteroids are appropriate for some patients with COPD.

Quality of life in asthma and COPD

From the patient's viewpoint, the main difference between asthma and COPD is that, for most people with asthma, lung obstruction is reversible. This means that breathlessness in asthma is relieved by regular use of inhaled or oral steroids, and occasional use of bronchodilators. With appropriate medication almost all people with asthma can lead a non-restricted life. In about 90% of patients with asthma, activities need not be limited, and exacerbations can be reduced to a very low level.

COPD has more significant effects on quality of life, because lung damage is non-reversible. A diagnostic criterion of COPD is lung function (FEV_1) that is less than 60% of normal of comparable age. Constant moderate-to-severe breathlessness, cough and phlegm production with periods of acute symptoms triggered by infection are characteristic of COPD. About 15% of all hospital admissions are due to COPD. COPD is a disease of adulthood and old age.

In about 70% of patients with COPD, daily activities are limited by breathlessness, sleep is frequently disturbed and patients have severe attacks of breathlessness, which can lead to hospital admissions. In COPD, pulmonary rehabilitation can help patients cope with constant breathlessness and manage everyday activities.

Adherence in asthma

In mild to moderate asthma, lung inflammation can be controlled by daily use of inhaled corticosteroid, but most patients (60% or more) do not take their inhaled steroid as frequently as prescribed. This is for a variety of reasons. Patients may believe that they only need their medication at certain times of the year (pragmatic adherence) (Osman, 1998). Patients may stop medication in order to test if symptoms reappear (testing) (Osman, 1998). Some patients also express 'steroid phobia', but dislike of taking any medication regularly may be as great an influence on non-adherence as specific dislike of steroids (Osman et al., 1993). Patients who are depressed are more likely to be non-adherent (Bosley et al., 1995). It has been shown that a fact-based approach to persuading patients does not increase adherence (Hilton et al., 1986), but a patient-centred approach based on agreement on self-management is effective in improving outcomes (British Guideline on the Management of Asthma, 2004).

Self-management plans in asthma

In the spread on patient adherence (see pp. 94–95), it was pointed out that adherence is most likely when patients understand what they are being asked to do, and why. Clear communication between patient and doctor and agreement on self-treatment increase the likelihood of adherence. Self-management plans (Fig. 1) are brief instructions on how to use asthma medication and when to vary medication, such as increasing inhaled steroid when symptoms increase, which have been discussed and agreed between the health professional and the patient. Use of self-management plans has been shown to improve outcomes for asthma and COPD patients, to reduce symptoms and to increase quality of life. A simple 'credit card' self-management plan can be used in general practice. Figure 1 shows a self-management plan used before hospital discharge of patients admitted with acute asthma. Patients who were given this plan were significantly less likely to be readmitted.

YOUR ASTHMA DISCHARGE PLAN

These are the asthma medicines you should be taking when you leave hospital

Your GP may change this plan after seeing you

With hindsight, when did your asthma start to get worse and what do you think you could have done to prevent this admission to hospital?

Plans for controlling and preventing future attacks

Prevention inhaler use/oral steroid use/GP contact/trigger avoidance (circle)

YOUR ASTHMA MEDICINES

Your Relief Inhaler is This inhaler quickly helps mild breathlessness It does not prevent bad attacks	When you are well you should not need to use your relief inhaler more than 1 or 2 times a day
Your Long Acting Relief Medicine is This inhaler should be taken every day It does not prevent bad attacks	You should take ___ puffs ___ times every day
Your Prevention Inhaler is This is an inhaled steroid. If you take it every day, it helps you have little or no breathlessness. It also prevents sudden attacks	You should take ___ puffs ___ times every day
Oral steroid course It is important to continue taking your inhaled steroid while you are taking any steroid tablets. See your GP if you are not back to normal after finishing your steroid tablets	You should take every day after breakfast ___ tablets (mgs) for ___ days ___ tablets (mgs) for ___ days ___ tablets (mgs) for ___ days then

Asthma warning symptoms

When you return to your usual level of prevention inhaler you know your asthma is worsening

- if you feel more breathless than usual and need to use your relief inhaler every two hours or more often
- if you wake at night feeling breathless
- AND IF YOUR PEAK FLOW DROPS BELOW

Remember 'What you can do'

- Act early. Don't wait until you are too breathless to do normal activities
- Double your usual inhaled steroid, or start tablet steroids when your peak flow drops
- Do not hesitate to contact your GP for guidance
- See your Yellow Book Plan for details

A GOOD PEAK FLOW FOR YOU IS

SEE YOU DOCTOR IMMEDIATELY IF YOUR PEAK FLOW DROPS BELOW

Fig. 1 Hospital discharge self-management plan.

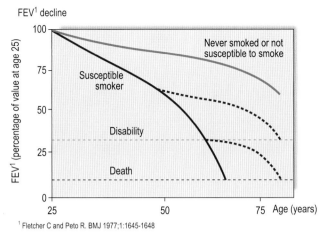

FEV[1] decline

Fig. 2 Smoking and lung function decline: Peto graph.

¹ Fletcher C and Peto R. BMJ 1977;1:1645-1648

Smoking cessation in COPD

Smoking cessation is the main method of controlling further deterioration and early death in COPD (Fig. 2). (In asthma, smoking cessation is important in limiting symptoms and controlling exacerbations and smoking cessation by parents is important in reducing the risk of asthma in children.)

Family and health professional advice are the most important influences in encouraging attempts to stop. Brief doctor advice increases the likelihood that a smoker will stop by about 2–3% and advice plus nicotine replacement therapy leads to increased cessation of about 10% (Fig. 3).

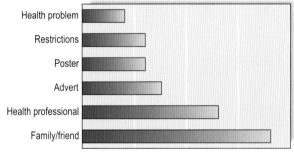

What prompted an attempt to stop smoking?

Fig. 3 Influence on smoking cessation attempts.

STOP THINK
- Do you know the most helpful ways to discuss smoking cessation with patients?

Psychological issues in asthma and COPD

Asthma deaths are uncommon, and psychiatric morbidity is high among the small group of people (less than 1%) with a history of severe life-threatening asthma attacks. A summary of adverse factors associated with near-fatal asthma attacks is shown in Box 1.

Intensive individual management programmes, with one-to-one contact and fast access for patients to doctor or nurse support have been the most successful approach to reducing life-threatening attacks among this small high-risk group. Molfino et al. (1992) followed 12 patients who had had near-fatal asthma attacks, and who had been recommended for closely supervised follow-up. Seven of the 12 agreed, and all survived. Five refused; of these, two died within 6 months of hospital discharge.

Box 1 **Factors associated with near-fatal asthma attacks (Yellowlees & Ruffin, 1989; Campbell et al., 1995; Innes et al., 1998)**

- Depression
- Denial
- Psychiatric caseness
- Alcohol or drug abuse
- Severe domestic stress
- Social isolation, living alone
- Unemployment
- Being female

STOP THINK
- Do you, or does someone you know, have asthma? Does it have a major or minor effect in your/their life?
- Do you know anyone with COPD? What effect does it have on their life?

Case study

Adolescents and asthma (Slack & Brooks, 1995)

In a focus group study 28 teenagers (13–17 years) with asthma talked about their experience with asthma and health care. The teenagers were concerned about adverse effects and the cost of medications and wanted more information about asthma and its treatment. They considered themselves compliant with therapy, but felt that they had had conflicting advice and inappropriate rules from adults about medication use. Members of the group wanted complete responsibility for medication, felt they did not disobey adults and did not believe peers had a negative influence on them.

In 1997 the National Asthma Campaign carried out a national study of UK teenagers' attitudes to asthma. This showed that worries about asthma attacks and about use of inhalers were greatest among younger teenagers, and lessened as teenagers grew older.

Pulmonary rehabilitation in COPD

COPD rehabilitation programmes include physical exercises aimed at building up patients' exercise tolerance, and techniques of managing breathlessness and improving efficient breathing. They are usually run by physiotherapists for small groups of patients, taking place once or twice a week for 6–8 weeks. Rehabilitation programmes can improve patient quality of life and respiratory muscle strength even when objective indicators of exercise tolerance and lung function do not change.

Asthma and chronic obstructive pulmonary disease

- Regular inhaled steroids reduce risk of exacerbations in asthma, but many patients stop taking preventive medication when they have no symptoms.
- In asthma and COPD, agreement on treatment goals between patient and health professional improves outcomes. It is best achieved through developing a self-management plan with the patient.
- Smoking cessation is the most important intervention for COPD.

Death and dying

The medicalization of dying

Dying and death, like birth, are a normal part of everyday life. Over the past few decades, western society has largely removed death and dying to the confines of institutions such as hospitals and hospices. Care of the dying and the dead is still, for the most part, the remit of professionals such as doctors, nurses and undertakers. As a result, death has become marginalized and stigmatized and, some would argue, increasingly medicalized (Clark & Seymour, 1999). More recently, media images of death, dying and mourning, such as the Princess of Wales' funeral in the UK and the events surrounding 9/11 in the USA, have gradually reintroduced this topic to the public arena. Public outpourings of grief on national television have become more acceptable.

Place of death

Paradoxically, though we know that most people would like to die at home, in their own beds, surrounded by family and friends, the majority of people do not. UK data on place of death showed that 66% of all deaths occurred in hospital in the year 2000 (Ellershaw & Ward, 2003). A combination of factors, such as poorly controlled symptoms, lack of family support, the burden on carers, badly coordinated services and changes in people's preferences as their disease progresses, can result in people being admitted to a hospital or a hospice before they die. Thorpe (1993) suggests that improvements in care could enable more people to die at home (Box 1). However, not all patients will want to die at home and to help patients die where they want it is important for doctors to explore patients' thoughts and fears in order to understand the reasons for their choice (Faull & Woof, 2002).

Box 1 **Factors that would allow dying people to remain at home**

- Adequate nursing care
- Good symptom control
- Confident and committed general practitioners
- Financial assistance
- Access to specialist palliative care
- Effective coordination of resources
- Terminal-care education

Attitudes to death and dying

Many doctors find caring for those who are dying a stressful but important part of their workload (Ahmedzai, 1982). This may be because doctors feel guilty or frustrated at their failure to achieve a medical cure or because they have difficulty in knowing how to communicate with the dying and their relatives. In addition to these professional concerns, most doctors will face common human fears when contemplating the inevitability and uncontrollability of death (Faull & Woof, 2002). The more anxious health professionals are about death then the more negative their attitudes and behaviour may be towards people at the end of life.

Stages of dying

Theoretical models have helped us to understand individual psychological responses to death. In her interviews with terminally ill cancer patients, Kubler-Ross (1970) described the dying process as a series of stages that the person passes through before finally coming to terms with his/her imminent death. These stages include shock, denial, anger, bargaining, depression and ultimately acceptance. Similar staged theories have been used to describe the bereavement process (see pp. 18–19). However, not everyone passes through these stages in sequence and individuals may fluctuate between acceptance and denial as they try to maintain hope about their prognosis (Johnston & Abraham, 2000). Carers and health professionals, therefore, need to be prepared for fluctuations in patients' moods so that they do not misinterpret them.

Caring for people from different faiths

The way we care for people as they die and prepare the body after the death should be guided by the person's cultural and religious beliefs. Unfortunately, such beliefs and associated rituals are often compromised by the organizational and bureaucratic barriers imposed by modern health care or by a lack of understanding on the part of health professionals. Yet, respecting these beliefs and ensuring prescribed rituals are adhered to can help patients to achieve a peaceful and dignified death, and facilitate the bereavement process for carers (Firth, 2001).

Viewing the body after the death

Junior medical staff may often be involved in dealing with the relatives after the death. This may involve breaking the news of the death to the relatives and accompanying them to view the body, either on the ward or in the hospital chapel or mortuary where the body has been taken (see pp. 98–99). Although this may be an uncomfortable duty, it is an important part of the grieving process and allows the relative to begin to absorb the loss and to say a final goodbye. It will be especially difficult, however, if the death has been sudden or unexpected.

The good death

Achieving a good death for patients is an important goal for health professionals who work with the dying (Ellershaw & Ward, 2003). Studies of the dying process have led to a debate about the characteristics of a 'good death'. Table 1 describes the perceptions of one group of palliative-care professionals about factors that constitute a 'good' and 'bad' death (Low & Payne, 1996). Good deaths occur when patients accept death and have control over the circumstances of their death, whereas bad deaths occur when patients are unprepared and the dying process is managed badly.

The importance of achieving a good death has led to the publication of guidelines and recommendations to help health professionals improve the standard of care for dying patients. For example, a report by an English charity, Age Concern, identified 12 principles that facilitate a good death in elderly patients (Health and Care Group, 1999) (Box 2).

Table 1 Factors constituting a 'good' and 'bad' death

Good death	Bad death
Lack of patient distress	**Negative effects on family**
■ Family acceptance	■ Unfinished business
■ Dying in presence of close people	■ Relatives' distress
■ At peace	■ Not dying with close people around
■ Continuing previous interests	■ Terrible physical symptoms
■ No physical pain	
■ No anxiety	
■ Dying in place of choice	
Patient control during dying process	**Patient non-acceptance**
■ Following appropriate cultural rules	■ Non-preparation of relatives
■ Dying in place of choice	■ Non-acceptance of illness
■ Cultural perceptions of good death	■ Fighting death to the end
■ Patient control	■ Badly managed death
■ Dying in presence of close people	
Role of staff	**Patient fears**
■ Comfortable process	■ Psychological distress
■ Peaceful death	■ Not dying in a place of choice
■ No anxiety	■ Terrible physical symptoms
■ No pain	■ Fighting death to the end
	■ Not dying with close people around

Box 2 Principles of a good death

■ To know when death is coming, and to understand what can be expected

■ To be able to retain control of what happens

■ To be afforded dignity and privacy

■ To have control over pain relief and other symptom control

■ To have choice and control over where death occurs (at home or elsewhere)

■ To have access to information and expertise of whatever kind is necessary

■ To have access to any spiritual or emotional support desired

■ To have access to hospice care in any location, not only in hospital

■ To have control over who else is present and shares the end

■ To be able to issue advance directives that ensure wishes are respected

■ To have time to say goodbye, and control over other aspects of timing

■ To be able to leave when it is time to go, and not to have life prolonged pointlessly

Social death

The stigmas surrounding death and difficulties in knowing how to talk to those who are dying can mean that terminally ill people experience a type of 'social death' before their bodies fail. This may occur because family, friends and health professionals find it difficult to talk to people who are dying and therefore withdraw from them, or because the dying themselves begin a process of disengaging from people in an attempt to prepare themselves for their death (Johnston & Abraham, 2000; Astley-Pepper, 2005). This process may be initiated or exacerbated by physical symptoms that prevent patients from leading a normal life. Its result, however, may be that patients become lonely and isolated. Hospital staff may unwittingly compound this isolation by moving dying patients to side wards or hiding them behind bed screens. Maintaining good communication with patients at the end of life is essential to reassure them that they are still supported and valued as people, and have a purpose in life.

Ethical issues

Core ethical principles underpinning all clinical practice can be difficult to apply when dealing with those approaching death (Twycross & Wilcock, 2001; Watson et al., 2006). Dilemmas arise when trying to balance the benefits and burdens of life-sustaining treatment, and with the goal of enhancing end-of-life care for patients: promoting a good death may mean withdrawing or withholding treatment (Twycross & Wilcock, 2001). Confusion around the various definitions of euthanasia and assisted suicide and the extent to which they should be legalized is a matter of continuing debate and one in which doctors will always have a central role (Hope et al., 2003). While it has been argued that the emergence of palliative care has precluded the need for these, the discipline's approach to pain and symptom control has sometimes led to criticism and accusations from the public and others who misunderstand the importance of relief of suffering as a clinical goal (Twycross & Wilcock, 2001; Hope et al., 2003; Watson et al., 2006). Similar problems surround the use of cardiopulomonary resuscitation in patients who are dying and discussion with the patient and family about whether or not to apply a do not rescusitate order can be difficult and distressing for the doctor (General Medical Council, 2002b). In addition, cognitive impairment in patients can mean that decisions have to be made on their behalf by either relatives or doctors. Taking time to explore patients' and relatives' wishes and questioning the efficacy of treatments are important to ensuring that interventions are both ethical and legal (Twycross & Wilcock, 2001; Faull & Woof, 2002).

STOP THINK

■ What steps could you have taken to ensure that Mr Ahmed had a 'good' death?

■ How might you have found out more about the rituals that the family wanted to perform?

■ How might this experience affect Mrs Ahmed's bereavement process?

Case study

You are a house officer on a busy medical ward to which an elderly Muslim man has been admitted. The patient's condition is terminal and that his prognosis is short. The consultant has informed the patient's wife that allowing him to die at home would not be advisable. The patient has a large family, who are very distressed by the news. They want to visit every day and insist on bringing special food that they want the nurses to prepare. Their behaviour is causing disruption, but there are no single rooms available. On the night of his death the nurses ask you to tell the family to go home and come back in the morning. You are uncomfortable about this, but do as you are asked. A few hours later the patient dies. On hearing of his death, Mr Ahmed's family are very angry and say that because they were not present at the death to perform special rituals his soul will never be at peace.

Death and dying

■ Our attitudes to death may affect the way we care for dying patients. Most patients want to die at home but most still die in hospital.

■ 'Good' deaths can be achieved if people are in control of the way they die. End-of-life care can pose challenging ethical questions for doctors.

What counselling is

Counselling resembles psychotherapy and life coaching in that similar techniques are used across these interventions, but counselling is more often provided to those who are worried and/or upset about their lives, rather than those suffering from mental illness or those seeking 'personal growth'. Counselling is also provided for patients to help them make medical decisions and cope with illness.

The immediate goal of counselling is to promote and protect individuals' psychological welfare, which generally means promoting an individual's contentment, happiness and life satisfaction. Although influenced by many things, people's happiness crucially depends on how well adjusted they are to the situations and relationships they regularly encounter. Counselling typically involves exploring ways of changing the interaction between situations and people's feelings, actions and thoughts.

The relationship between objective situations, perception of those situations and affective and behavioural responses to those situations is critical to the counselling endeavour. No matter how dire or favourable people's objective circumstances may be, the functionality of their affective, behavioural and cognitive responses will often have a great influence on how well those people suffer or thrive.

Counselling approaches

Most counselling approaches broadly fall within or across three types: (1) psychodynamic; (2) person-centred; and (3) cognitive-behavioural.

Psychodynamic approaches
Psychodynamic approaches suggest that psychological problems start when young children's needs or desires are either excessively frustrated or excessively indulged, usually by a parent and often in ways that infants come to associate with either the presence or the prevention of danger. In later years, reminders of such early events can cause people to regress to functioning in much the same way that they did as children. This usually results in dysfunctional adjustment to their adult circumstances, often with detrimental consequences that further increase their distress. This can lead to a vicious circle of perceived threat–anxiety–infantile response–dysfunctional interaction with situation-renewed, sustained or enhanced perception of threat–further anxiety, and so on.

To illustrate, imagine a young girl tentatively expressing curiosity about her father's penis and then being (or simply feeling) punished by her parents for 'being inappropriate'. Anything that as an adult reminds her of this early trauma may cause her anxiety *and* to react in a relatively immature way. She might feel uncomfortable contemplating sex, for example, and attempt to cope with this by avoidance of and withdrawal from sexually charged situations.

Psychodynamic counselling involves identifying infantile anxieties and defences that are being dysfunctionally manifested in subsequent situations. A major technique for doing this is identifying instances of transference, where clients react to others in ways that seem likely to reflect their emotionally loaded childhood interactions with their parents. Because such interactions are associated with childhood trauma, people are likely to have little or no conscious awareness that this is occurring. Psychodynamic counsellors

will typically interpret what is going on, thus bringing it into people's conscious awareness. As people move towards insight, they re-experience their childhood traumas (i.e. experience catharsis) and come to realize that as adults they have the option of responding in different ways – ones more functional to their current circumstances.

Person-centred approaches
Person-centred approaches to counselling suggest that psychological problems start when people internalize the idea that they are worthwhile only if they behave in certain ways or achieve particular goals. This can lead people to stop having faith in their own sense of what is good and bad or even about what is personally pleasant or distasteful. If this happens, people can find themselves grimly pursuing goals that may be insatiable and which rarely lead to a sense of sustained satisfaction.

Parents frequently set conditions of worth for their children, for example when they insist that children are valued only whilst they are being 'nice' or 'successful' – in whatever ways the parents define such terms. Throughout life, other social influences either reinforce or contradict people's early beliefs about conditions of worth. Laws, political and religious systems, education and the media provide obvious examples. Such messages can undermine people's sense of intrinsic worth. At extremes, people can come to feel that they are valuable or worthwhile *only* to the extent that they make money, achieve status or have successful relationships. As conditions of worth in a society are pervasive and often contradictory, this can lead people to feel confused and irredeemably worthless.

Person-centred counselling involves developing a relationship in which people feel valued for who they are, irrespective of what they do or have. Within such a relationship, counsellors help people uncover and examine their feelings of conditional worth. As people learn to trust first the counsellor and then themselves they become increasingly knowledgeable about and accepting of their own feelings, motives and judgements and thereby re-establish an intrinsic sense of their own value.

Cognitive-behavioural approaches
Cognitive-behavioural approaches to counselling suggest that psychological problems start when people adopt dysfunctional beliefs about or behavioural responses to the world. This may occur through classical or operant conditioning. For example, someone feeling sick after eating prawns might come to believe that eating any fish will make them ill. Dysfunctional beliefs about 'what goes with what' in the world can also arise from observing what seems to happen to other people. If one's closest relatives live to a ripe old age on a diet of cigarettes and alcohol, it might become very difficult to believe that such things genuinely cause ill health.

Regardless of where dysfunctional thoughts and behaviours originally come from, cognitive-behavioural counsellors attempt to identify and change the processes that sustain them. Examples of common dysfunctional thinking patterns are shown in Box 1.

Dysfunctional thoughts and behaviours may themselves be challenged cognitively or behaviourally. Someone terrified about speaking in public can be asked: 'What is the worst that can happen?', for example, or encouraged to overcome

> **Box 1 Common dysfunctional thought processes**
>
> - Jumping to conclusions, e.g. the test will be positive
> - Overgeneralization, e.g. I'm ill now so I'll always be ill
> - All-or-nothing thinking, e.g. either I'm (100%) healthy or I'm (100%) sick
> - Mind-reading, e.g. I can just tell that the doctor thinks I'm dying
> - Tunnel vision, e.g. there is nothing good about this situation
> - Catastrophizing, e.g. having this condition will ruin my life
> - Personalization, e.g. it's all my fault I'm ill
> - Should statements, e.g. I ought to do what my parents suggest
> - Labelling, e.g. I am (nothing other than) an amputee
> - Emotional reasoning, e.g. I feel worse, therefore I must be getting sicker
>
> (see Beck, 1995, for details)

anxiety and actually speak in public. In either case, the hope is that individuals will come to change their beliefs about 'what goes with what' in the world and/or their ability to act functionally in that world (see pp. 138–139).

Counselling and communication

The tasks involved in counselling require highly developed communication skills. Counsellors must notice things about their clients of which the clients themselves are likely to have little conscious awareness, e.g. infantile anxieties, defence mechanisms, transference patterns, conditions of worth, concealed judgements and desires, behavioural responses to environmental triggers and automatic thoughts. This means that counsellors need to be skilled at the receiving side of communication, i.e. eliciting and interpreting information.

Counsellors also need to be skilled at the transmission side of communication, i.e. at imparting information in ways that are understandable and useful to clients. Among other things, counsellors need to be able to increase clients' consciousness of their current patterns of feeling, thinking and behaving. Additionally, counsellors need to bring to clients' attention the possibility of more functional alternatives.

Part of counsellors' skill in transmitting information is making sure that clients have accurately received that information. Similarly, counsellors must be able to let clients know that they have accurately received information that clients want them to have.

Counselling however requires much more than just the transmission and reception of information. It also requires counsellors to communicate to clients that a particular sort of relationship exists between them. The exact nature of this relationship varies across counselling approaches and across time within any given approach, but will always include indications that the counsellor is both trustworthy and caring of the client's welfare. Characteristics that make a counsellor trustworthy are those that promote effective and ethical practice, e.g. competence, humility, resilience and integrity (BACP, 2007).

Counselling in medical settings

Counselling takes two main forms within medical settings. The first involves supporting people facing unusually difficult circumstances or decisions, e.g. whether or not to undergo complex, risky or arduous procedures such as HIV testing, genetic screening, organ transplant or similar. Counselling of this type requires counsellors to be medically knowledgeable but beyond that relies primarily on effective interpersonal

and communication skills such as those involved in eliciting and clarifying clients' assumptions and priorities, providing relevant information and supporting clients throughout the decision-making process.

Counselling is also used in medical settings to promote psychological adjustment. This type of counselling is likely to draw upon psychotherapeutic counselling approaches to a greater extent than counselling to support medical decision-making. This counselling is used when clients seem likely to benefit from help or support when facing challenging life changes. To illustrate, although all patients are likely to be challenged and to benefit from receiving social and decision-making support when receiving a cancer diagnosis, they might additionally benefit from receiving counselling to facilitate their psychological adjustment if they react to the diagnosis with unusual levels of, for example, denial (which may be a psychoanalytic response), suppressed distress (which may result from conditions of worth dependent on 'bravery' or 'stoicism'), or depression (which may stem from dysfunctional but persistent beliefs about the diagnosis and its consequences).

The British Medical Association provides a 24-hour confidential counselling service for doctors in distress or difficulty (tel. 08459 200 169).

> ### Case study
>
> At first Pat's counsellor appeared to do little more than provide a safe space and a sympathetic ear whilst Pat careered between expressing terror, rage, self-pity, despair and a whole host of other intense emotions. Following a diagnosis of testicular cancer, Pat's counsellor was nevertheless hard at work. Having discreetly conducted suicide risk and mental health assessments, the counsellor listened and increasingly probed gently for clues about factors that might be exacerbating the difficulties Pat was having coping with the news of his condition.
>
> Picking up and pursuing such clues, Pat's counsellor explored with Pat various possibilities; some associated with Pat being reminded of how he felt when his father had died of lung cancer; others to do with Pat's worries about being a 'proper' man and husband.
>
> Through counselling, Pat was given the opportunity to vent emotions that were stopping him from thinking and relating to others and to his condition effectively. He was also supported in exploring ways of pursuing more functional alternatives.

 STOP THINK Try to remember in detail something that you have felt anxious about recently. How many of the reasoning errors in Box 1 could have been involved? How else could you have thought about things?

> ### What counselling is
>
> - It uses similar techniques to psychotherapy and life coaching.
> - It is provided to people who are in general the 'worried well'.
> - Counselling explores ways of changing the interaction between people's situations and their thinking, feeling and behaving.
> - It has psychodynamic, person-centred and cognitive-behavioural perspectives.
> - It requires, but is not restricted to, effective use of communication skills.
> - Counselling requires communication of caring and trustworthiness.
> - It can prioritize informational or therapeutic support.

How counselling works

How effective counselling is depends on the resources and abilities of counsellors and their clients. These need to vary according to the challenges faced but some key elements associated with effectiveness can be identified.

Space and time

Counselling usually happens in a particular place and at specific times, e.g. an hour a week over 12 weeks in a dedicated room. This provides clients with respite from the demands of their daily lives and establishes a new and often calming routine. Clients quickly develop an appreciation of having an arena 'just for them'. Counselling provides people with the opportunity to reflect upon how things are and could be for them and allows them to examine themselves and their situations safely and, if necessary, repeatedly. Where change is sought, clients can rehearse and refine new patterns of thinking and behaving with guidance from a sympathetic expert companion. For example, an amputee coming to terms with her or his new physical appearance may find it invaluable to be encouraged to develop new ways of thinking and acting within counselling sessions prior to entering new social situations and re-entering old ones.

A client focus

Whatever their professional style, counsellors seek to serve patients' needs unwaveringly. Counsellors do not have a direct personal stake either in the difficulties clients face or the consequences of decisions clients may make. Counsellors are also trained to monitor their personal reactions during interactions and ensure that wherever possible these are used in the service of clients' needs. An effective counsellor with anxieties about death and dying should be able to differentiate these concerns from those of his or her clients and ensure that addressing the latter remains paramount.

Counsellors work towards increasing their clients' autonomy. This can involve motivating, supporting and even instructing clients. However, wherever feasible, the counsellor's ultimate aim

is always to help each client become increasingly *self*-sufficient. Counselling is most effective when clients are helped to develop and make best use of their own skills. The flip side of this is that counselling can only be effective to the extent that clients are motivated to make it work.

Perhaps above all else, counsellors *care* about each of their clients and sooner or later clients come to *realize* that their counsellor cares about them 'as a person'. The counsellor does not relate to clients primarily in terms of any characteristics that they may or may not have, such as a particular symptom, condition or pattern of behaviour. In the terminology of person-centred counselling, counsellors have a positive regard for – and an attendant warmth towards – individual people that is unconditional. As clients come to realize that someone values them despite whatever may be troubling them at the time, the foundations are laid for clients to increase their unconditional positive regard and warmth towards themselves. Receiving unconditional positive regard from another can thereby promote *self*-acceptance which alleviates psychological distress such as depression and anxiety. This, in turn, can increase clients' abilities to address other challenges more effectively and, if necessary, change their behaviour (see pp. 136–137).

Professional training, supervision and skills

Reputable counsellors belong to professional organizations that demand and certify minimum levels of practical and theoretical expertise. In the UK, these include the British Association of Counselling and Psychotherapy (BACP) and the British Psychological Society (BPS). Competence is assured and maintained through active one-to-one supervision throughout counsellors' working lives. In retaining a client focus, such supervision is invaluable in helping counsellors critically reflect upon their casework and explore with other experts possible modifications to their ongoing practice.

BPS-accredited counsellors must be proficient in the techniques of more than one approach to

counselling (see pp. 132–133). This helps counsellors evaluate situations from more than one perspective and tailor their interventions to the specific needs clients face in their unique circumstances. For example, a counsellor might adopt a predominantly person-centred approach whilst building a working relationship with a particularly anxious client, a predominantly psychodynamic approach when conceptualizing and understanding possible origins of that client's difficulties and a predominantly cognitive-behavioural approach when eventually helping that client alter habitual but dysfunctional thinking patterns. Thus professional counsellors are able to be flexible in matching their approach to people who may face a variety of psychological challenges. For example, Box 1 illustrates some of the various benefits a recently bereaved client could gain from counselling. Moreover, counselling needs may alter as people face new life and health challenges. For example, recent advances in genetic testing mean that counsellors are now employed to: (1) help prospective parents estimate the risks of their children inheriting certain diseases and make decisions based on this understanding; and (2) help patients assess their own risks of developing illnesses and make life decisions based on this knowledge.

Effective counsellors need highly developed communication skills. They must be able to facilitate clients telling their stories; synthesize verbal and non-verbal information; monitor both what is said and what is left unsaid; convince

---

Box 1 **What could a counsellor offer a bereaved client?**

- Enable the client to admit and express his/her loss
- Help him/her to express the range of feelings this gives rise to
- Encourage him/her to explore the prospect of life without the deceased
- Help him/her anticipate and understand his/her feelings over time
- Question potentially dysfunctional coping strategies, e.g. social withdrawal
- Offer support while encouraging the establishment of alternative sources of social support

(see Worden, 1991, for details)

clients that they have been 'really heard'; simplify complex material; present familiar material in unfamiliar ways; and challenge dysfunctional patterns of thinking and behaving; and throughout all this continue simultaneously to communicate unconditional positive regard for the client.

Professionalism also means that counsellors do not give up on clients. Even when clients are being particularly challenging and difficult to care for, effective counsellors will not abandon or blame their clients and they will do all they can to communicate this dedication to their clients.

Is counselling effective?

In appropriate circumstances, counselling is effective. The summary for the latest relevant Cochrane review (Bower & Rowland, 2006) starts:

Counselling for psychological problems is better than usual general practitioner care. People who receive counselling in primary care from a trained counsellor are more likely to feel better immediately after treatment and be more satisfied than those who receive care from their general practitioner.

STOP THINK Drugs can have the effects they do without individuals knowing that they have been given drugs. That is one way we know that drugs differ from placebos. How might counselling be evaluated in a similar manner to drugs? What implications does your answer have for Jerome Frank's claims about the mechanisms by which all helping relationships work (Box 2)?

Box 2 **Frank's (1961) claimed common factors to *all* helping relationships**

- An emotionally charged, confiding relationship with a helpful person
- A healing setting
- A rationale, conceptual scheme or myth that provides a plausible explanation for the patient's symptoms and prescribes a ritual or procedure for resolving them
- A ritual or procedure that requires the active participation of both patient and therapist and that is believed by both to be the means of restoring the patient's health

(see Duncan, 2002, for details)

People who have received counselling tend to agree. An article in the November 1995 edition of *Consumer Reports* summarized the findings of probably the largest ever consumer satisfaction survey of counselling. Of about 7000 people who completed the relevant part of the survey, about 1200 reported that they had either been 'barely managing to deal with things' or that 'life was usually pretty tough' when they started receiving counselling at some time in the previous 3 years. Approximately 90% of these people reported feeling better by the time of the survey and they attributed this improvement to the counselling they received (Seligman, 1995). Clients who 'shopped around' and chose a counsellor who matched their needs reported better outcomes, as did those who actively engaged in the counselling process. Longer courses of counselling also resulted in greater improvement. No differences in outcome were reported according to the type of counselling that had been received.

Although the *Consumer Reports* respondents showed least satisfaction with counselling from marriage counsellors (relative to other counsellors), approximately three-quarters of people who completed a course of counselling with Relate reported gaining a better understanding of themselves, with more than half also reporting a year after completion that counselling had helped them improve their relationship (McCarthy et al., 1995).

In accordance with such findings, the Department of Health's (2001b) evidence-based clinical practice guideline starts with the following two principal recommendations:

1. Psychological therapy should be routinely considered as an option when assessing mental health problems.
2. Patients who are adjusting to life events, illnesses, disabilities or losses may benefit from brief therapies such as counselling.

Conclusion

Counselling is put to many uses and takes many forms. The role of counselling in promoting the well-being of patients in health care settings has been both empirically demonstrated and acknowledged by government. Key elements of effective counselling can be identified and many of these can be employed to good effect elsewhere, e.g. during doctor–patient interactions (see pp. 96–97).

Case study

Following the birth of his first child, Chris made a series of visits to his GP.

Ali, the GP, became increasingly convinced that Chris was depressed and/or suffering from some form of anxiety disorder. Ali referred Chris to a person-centred counsellor.

The counsellor listened attentively to Chris's account of what was bothering him. Paying particular attention to Chris's non-verbal cues and to areas he seemed anxious to avoid discussing, the counsellor gently helped Chris consider possible links between how he was feeling and the recent birth of his son. As Chris talked, he discovered – somewhat to his surprise – that he was deeply anxious about his ability to fulfil the various responsibilities he felt he had as a father and husband while at the same time pulling his weight at work. Over time and with his counsellor's support, Chris explored these concerns and came to see that he had been unconsciously judging himself by unattainable standards, many of which, on reflection, he rejected. He came to realize that some of the conditions of worth he had attached to his performance in these roles were, without him noticing, based on his father's views, e.g. that men should contribute to family life financially but not domestically. Chris reduced his hours at work to spend more time with his son and did not need to bring these problems back to his GP.

How counselling works

- Most people feel better after it and evaluate it positively.
- Counselling should be routinely considered when people are facing life challenges and mental health problems.
- It is best provided by trained and supervised professionals.
- Counselling benefits from time and a location dedicated to that sole purpose.
- It requires unconditional positive regard plus interventions tailored to individual clients.
- It aims to help clients obtain increased self-sufficiency.
- It requires client motivation.

Adaptation, coping and control

It has frequently been suggested that there is a link between the manner of adaptation to, and coping with, the external environment and physical and mental health. It is, therefore, of considerable importance that we understand the way in which humans respond to external and internal stimuli.

Coping can mean any general adaptive process. It can also mean the mastery or control of major events. The behavioural sciences have developed two complementary ways of describing coping and adaptation – the first concerned with how people manage ordinary everyday things, and the second with the way they deal with major life events. These two approaches have been brought together in what has been called the *stress-coping paradigm*.

The stress-coping paradigm

The stress-coping paradigm was originally developed by Lazarus (1980). Lazarus starts from the position that the social (and biological) worlds are ubiquitously stressful. People have to cope with and adapt to different things, large and small, all the time. The degree to which this produces stress is determined by the extent to which these external stimuli are perceived to exceed the ability of the person to deal with them and, therefore, to endanger well-being. People have to appraise the extent to which the stimuli do this. They will then act or react accordingly.

According to Lazarus, when confronted by a stimulus that is potentially stressful, an individual engages in two processes of appraisal. These are called *primary* and *secondary* appraisal. Primary appraisal is the means whereby people determine whether a stimulus is dangerous or not. If individuals decide it is not dangerous, they may conclude that it is irrelevant to them. Alternatively, they may view it as benign or positive. If the stimulus is appraised as irrelevant, or benign or positive, it is not regarded as a stressor (Fig. 1).

If a stimulus is regarded as stressful, this is because it is perceived to represent harm or loss or threat (anticipated harm or loss). The secondary appraisal process is about mastering the conditions of harm or threat. This can take several forms: seeking out information; taking direct action to confront the stressor; doing nothing and attempting to ignore it; or worrying about it (Fig. 1).

The importance of this model is that it recognizes that stimuli are not in themselves stressful. Stress arises as a consequence of the cognitive or thinking process which people bring to bear on particular stimuli (the appraisal processes) and on the extent to which they can control these stimuli by doing various things. It is when they are not able to control things, because they do not have the resources to do so, that stress arises. It is important to note that researchers have observed that positive feelings can arise even in the most difficult and stressful of experiences. People find meaning and purpose in the difficulties they face, and this helps them deal with the problems they are trying to cope with (Folkman & Moscowitz, 2000, 2004). The observation of positive feelings is a relatively common, if somewhat surprising finding in the case of people coping with illness, especially chronic illness. This stress-coping paradigm emphasizes, therefore, the social context within

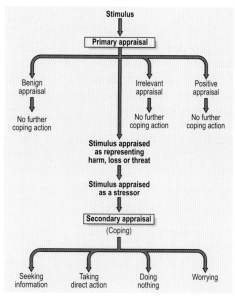

Fig. 1 The stress-coping paradigm (from Kelly & Sullivan, 1992, with permission).

which coping takes place. A very important resource is the social support from others. Social support may come from family members, friends or the caring services. It seems that social support makes coping easier, although in itself social support will not solve all the problems a person has to deal with. Support can come in a variety of forms. It might include practical things like minding children, or providing aids and devices to make life easier around the home. The support might be emotional, in the form of talking and listening. There is no simple recipe, but where support networks are stronger, people seem to be able to withstand difficulties better than those without such support.

Coping and illness

It has been argued that stress, and, by implication, the failure to cope or adapt, is responsible for the development of particular types of illness because certain biological responses in the individual lead to tissue damage (Seyle, 1956). There is a good deal of research that focuses on specific illnesses that seem to follow stressful life events (Holmes & Rahe, 1967; Fisher, 1986; Hemingway & Marmot, 1999).

Although it is undoubtedly the case that exposure to external stimuli that are frightening and threatening may cause physiological changes in the human body, the question of the social environment in which this occurs is important. This is because coping is also related to the resources that people can bring to bear when they have difficult situations to deal with. Support of family and friends (a social network) and financial resources come into this category. These resources can and do have an important mediating effect on difficulties but cannot themselves prevent them. In the absence of social support, other life difficulties can be particularly damaging. A good deal of psychological morbidity can be accounted for in terms of combinations of low self-esteem, lack of financial resources and absence of social support (Brown et al., 1975) (see pp. 114–115).

Strategies of adapting to chronic illness

A number of typical strategies have been observed in the way people cope with, adapt to and try to gain some control over chronic illness. The responses are linked to the amount of threat their illness presents to them, and what they are able to do about the threat.

Normalizing

Here the patient acknowledges the symptoms, for example, of asthma, but redefines them as part of normal experience and hence as nothing to worry about. By defining something abnormal as normal, the patient is neutralizing the threat. This can present particularly difficult clinical management problems, because the more successful patients are in neutralizing the symptoms, the more likely they may be not to comply with treatment (see pp. 94–95).

Denial

Here the patient denies the existence of the illness altogether. This may have profoundly beneficial effects, especially in the early stages of a very worrying or threatening diagnosis. Denial may help the patient draw back, take stock and marshal help. In the longer run, however, denial prevents the patient from confronting the illness, will present particular difficulties for the treating doctor and may have considerable effects on the family or partner of the sufferer.

Avoidance

Patients who practise avoidance do not deny their problem. They set out to avoid those situations that might exacerbate their symptoms or lead to other problems. In this group of behaviours we find the person who suffers from claustrophobia and who therefore never lives or works anywhere where he or she may have to use a lift or get in an airplane. We find the reformed alcoholic who never goes to parties or social gatherings for fear of being tempted by the alcoholic drink. We find the person with epilepsy who never applies for a job where he or she might have to reveal the fact of this illness. While individually each of these strategies is highly adaptive, they also contain within them certain maladaptive or potentially self-destructive elements. The person with claustrophobia or epilepsy may miss out on all sorts of opportunities, while the reformed alcoholic may be cut off from a great deal of social intercourse.

Resignation

In resignation we find individuals who have totally embraced their illness and for whom the most important thing about their life is their illness. Their whole being is consumed by their disease. They resign themselves to their fate. The illness is defined in such a way that instead of being something threatening, it grants certain psychological rewards. At certain times in a serious and grave illness, resignation may be an entirely appropriate way to respond. However, in many less serious conditions, total resignation leads to invalidism. The problem that this type of behaviour presents for physicians is that their best efforts to get patients to attempt to take some control over their own life are resisted as patients work hard to maintain their dependence on others.

Accommodation

Here patients acknowledge and deal with the problems their illness produces – whether this is managing their symptom manifestations like pain, or managing a self-administered drug regime. The everyday work of handling the disease is seen as part of normal living. No attempt is made to build a special status out of the illness. Instead people try to deal with others on the basis of their other characteristics, such as being a keen gardener, a football fan, a member of the church, and so on. They do not make their illness central to their life.

Case study

Childhood diabetes

It is important to avoid defining coping as either good or bad. The manner of people's response to stimuli will vary and in some cases people may draw certain psychological or social rewards from the way they cope, even though others may regard their manner of coping as dangerous or self-destructive. This is sometimes observed in long-term chronic illness.

In childhood-onset diabetes, for example, the family has to cope with illness and the difficulties presented by the symptoms and managing the self-medication and diet. However, it is perfectly possible for the young child to come to enjoy some of the benefits of being a sick person in the family: being spoiled and receiving special privileges, for example. Also the family may come to adapt to the illness in ways that they too find rewarding. Parents may receive psychological rewards from taking on the role of carers. This may work quite well while the child is young, but as the child grows up and tries to free him-/herself from the parents' control, successful earlier coping may become highly maladaptive. The child's attempt to grow and be independent may be seen as a threat by the parents, who may insist on the adolescent remaining in the sick role. The diabetic may respond by taking dietary risks in an effort to cope with parental control. Particular dynamics become established within the family, and these in turn may produce other problems with which the family has to cope.

STOP THINK Although many disorders have been linked directly or indirectly to coping, the precise mechanisms whereby human behaviour in the face of stress produces psychological and biological consequences are very complex, and compared to many branches of medicine, understanding of these mechanisms is limited.

- To what extent are coping and adaptation linked to psychological traits and psychosexual development on the one hand or to social factors, particularly availability of resources, on the other? Is it always going to be the case that what might be seen as maladaptive from a medical point of view would be bad for the patient?

Adaptation, coping and control

- Adaptation and coping refer to behaviours that involve dealing with everyday problems as well as major life events.
- It is the person who deals with these problems who defines them as everyday or major.
- Coping and adaptation are linked to a range of psychological variables and social support and resources.
- Stress results when the ability to deal with events is not equal to the events or stimuli.
- Failure to cope and adapt may have serious health consequences at both a physical and a psychological level.
- Some strategies of coping seem to be inherently unstable or potentially self-destructive.

Cognitive-behavioural therapy

Cognitive-behavioural therapy (CBT) is a set of empirically grounded clinical interventions, applied in a systematic way to help people change their thoughts and behaviours so they can function in a more adaptive and healthy way. The foundational model for CBT was outlined by Aaron Beck (1976; Beck et al., 1979), but as CBT has been applied to new clinical problems there have been significant revisions.

CBT has become an increasingly popular approach for helping people with physical and mental health problems. The National Institute for Clinical Excellence (NICE) recommends CBT as the 'treatment of choice' for most common mental health disorders, including depression, panic disorder, obsessive-compulsive disorder, posttraumatic stress disorder, eating disorder and schizophrenia (Roth & Fonagy, 2004).

The rationale behind CBT

The cognitive model emphasizes that people's emotions and behaviours are influenced by their perceptions of events and the meanings they attach to their experience. It is not simply situations that determine how people feel and behave, but the way in which they *construe* and *appraise* these situations (see pp. 126–127 and pp. 134–135). Depending on their unique development histories and temperaments, people filter incoming information in ways that reflect their particular concerns and beliefs. Consequently, aspects of thinking may become distorted or maladaptive, leading to emotional and behavioural problems. For example, an individual whose parents were excessively preoccupied with the risks associated with illness may develop an unhealthy preoccupation with illness and maladaptive beliefs about illness, e.g. 'Illness is always very harmful', 'Life with illness is unbearable' and 'I should make every possible effort to avoid getting ill'. These beliefs will determine emotional and behavioural responses to possible signs of illness. This individual may be hypervigilant for signs of illness, repeatedly checking his or her body for warning signs so that normal or minor fluctuations in bodily processes may be misinterpreted as evidence of illness. Such people may seek frequent reassurance from doctors and undergo extensive unnecessary medical tests in their search for explanations of symptoms.

CBT emphasizes the dynamic interactions between thoughts, moods and behaviour (see Case study). However, it gives primacy to the role of thinking and cognition in the development and maintenance of emotional disorders. The cognitive model proposes that there are different levels of thinking. At the level closest to conscious awareness are the relatively rapid and involuntary thoughts we have in response to specific current situations. These are called *automatic thoughts*. At a deeper level people develop *core beliefs* about themselves, others and their world. These are deeply felt, but often not easy to access or articulate. Between these two levels sits a group of *intermediate beliefs* that are manifest in the rules, attitudes and assumptions that people live by.

The role of the CBT therapist

The role of the CBT therapist is, firstly, to assist individuals in identifying and clarifying their current patterns of thinking and, secondly, to modify this thinking through a range of strategies that encourage individuals to take on a more rational or evidence-based view of their own experience. CBT is based on the principle of *collaborative empiricism*. Rather than the therapist acting as the expert, the therapist and client work together to resolve problems. Treatment is conducted in a spirit of open-minded enquiry and *guided discovery* to help clients clarify and evaluate their own thoughts and beliefs. An explicit goal of treatment is to teach clients the model of CBT so that they can develop the capacity to be their own therapist (for a list of core CBT competencies, see http://www.ucl.ac.uk/clinical-health-psychology/CORE/CBT_Framework.htm).

The structure of CBT

CBT is a relatively short-term structured therapy. A typical course of CBT may last from 8 to 20 sessions with follow-up sessions to ensure the maintenance of gains. Sessions are approached in a structured fashion and there is a shared plan or agenda for each session that the therapist and client co-construct. Goals are clearly defined in measurable and operationalized terms and progress in therapy is continually monitored.

CBT involves the mutual planning of therapeutic tasks and homework exercises that the client carries out between sessions; what happens between sessions in the client's normal environment is seen as very important. While earlier versions of behavioural therapy approached homework tasks in terms of behavioural rehearsal or exposure to feared situation, contemporary CBT approaches homework tasks as an opportunity for clients to test out existing dysfunctional beliefs and to learn new, more adaptive beliefs (Bennett-Levy et al., 2004). For example, a client with health anxiety who engages in excessive reassurance-seeking might be asked to refrain from seeking medical reassurance for an agreed period to see whether this increases or decreases anxiety.

Some basic techniques

In the early stages of treatment, techniques are focused on eliciting and clarifying underlying negative automatic thoughts and beliefs, and identifying common themes and patterns in these thoughts. Clients are usually asked to keep a record of their thoughts in particular situations. For example, a client with health anxiety may be asked to record automatic thoughts and mood when he or she notices new bodily signs or sensations (Fig. 1).

Clients may be asked to recount specific situations, such as a recent panic attack, in vivid detail to elicit automatic thoughts and appraisals. An effective way of eliciting negative automatic thoughts involves exploring the *worst-consequence scenario*. This usually takes the form of the question: 'What's the worst that could happen if …'? Clients may be asked to engage in certain exposure tasks in order to activate fear and, with it, salient automatic thoughts. Exposure may be to external situations or internal bodily sensations and cues. For example, a client may be asked actively to hyperventilate in order to generate familiar panic symptoms and associated thoughts.

Situation	Thoughts	Mood and rating (0–10)	Behaviour
Got up in the morning and noticed lots of hairs on my pillow	Why is my hair falling out? I've never noticed it before. Could it be the start of alopecia? People with cancer lose their hair.	Worry 7	Checked other pillows to see if there were hairs. Combed hair to see if more hair was falling out. Pulled at hairs on head. Looked up alopecia on internet.

Fig. 1 Thought record showing links between thoughts, mood and behaviour.

In the later stages of treatment, techniques are employed to help clients to modify old beliefs, learn new beliefs and practise new behaviours. The choice of technique is guided by a *case formulation*, which is a working hypothesis about the cognitive and behavioural factors involved in the origins and maintenance of the client's difficulties (Needleman, 1999). Case formulation usually includes several components: (1) formative early experiences, e.g. mother always worried about being ill, repeated early visits to GP; (2) related dysfunctional assumptions and beliefs, e.g. 'If there is pain there must be serious damage'; (3) critical trigger incidents, e.g. recent recurring pain in lower abdomen; and (4) maintenance factors, e.g. excessive use of painkillers, frequent checking for bodily symptoms. The case formulation is openly discussed with the client and it provides a basis for planning subsequent treatment interventions.

Clients are encouraged to question and test out the evidence for their beliefs and to list evidence for and against particular beliefs. They may also be asked to carry out personal experiments to confirm or refute existing beliefs. Clients may be encouraged to identify common cognitive distortions or 'thinking errors', e.g. *black-and-white thinking, personalizing and catastrophizing* (see pp. 132–133). For example, clients may think: 'I should always feel 100% healthy', 'When the doctor coughed it was a sign that he was really worried about me' and 'Life with a chronic illness would not be worth living'. Clients are explicitly helped to develop alternative rational responses to replace less adaptive thoughts.

Applications of CBT to physical health problems

Although CBT was established for the treatment of psychiatric problems, it has also proved effective in the treatment of physical health problems. Chronic medical conditions are frequently associated with psychological problems and the effective treatment of psychological dysfunction is often an important step in enabling patients to cope better with physical illness.

The thought processes relevant to treatment of most physical problems include patients' beliefs about bodily functioning and the causation of physical problems; misinterpretations of bodily symptoms and signs; evaluations of the threat to self and future well-being associated with illness; and changes in behaviour and mood following perceived impairment which may increase emotional distress and the degree of handicap (Salkovskis, 1989). CBT is particularly useful in modifying thoughts and behaviours, which may function to maintain physical problems, even when these originally had a physical cause. For example, excessive avoidance of physical exercise after a viral illness may eventually cause new fatigue symptoms unrelated to the original viral illness.

CBT is demonstrating effectiveness in treatment of a wide range of chronic illnesses and disabilities. For example, there is promising evidence for the use of CBT in treating chronic fatigue syndrome (Deal et al., 1997); rheumatoid arthritis (Sharpe et al., 2003) and chronic pain (Morley et al., 1999). There is also evidence to support the use of CBT to treat somatization (Kroenke & Swindle, 2000) and hypochondriasis (Barsky & Ahern, 2004).

Recent developments in CBT

Recent developments in CBT, including dialectical behaviour therapy, acceptance and commitment therapy and mindfulness-based cognitive therapy, draw on several influences, including eastern philosophy, meditation and yoga. These therapies are less concerned with changing negative thought patterns and more concerned with living in the present moment, acceptance and deepening of emotional experience and the development of a more compassionate response to one's own experience (Hayes et al., 2005). The relationship that clients have with their thoughts is seen as equally significant to the content of their thoughts. The way clients think about their thoughts (e.g. 'If I can't control these thoughts I will go mad') is sometimes called *metacognition* and newer forms of CBT target maladaptive metacognitive processes.

- The next time you feel ill or have unexplained physical symptoms, try to notice your own thought and moods. What beliefs about illness do you have and what experiences in your life might have formed these beliefs?

Case study

A 47-year-old van driver suffered a heart attack 5 months ago while driving home from work. He had stopped the car and flagged down a passing motorist, who took him to hospital. On the day of his heart attack, he had felt unwell and had suffered chest pains when climbing stairs to make deliveries.

He made a full physical recovery and is not thought to be at great risk of another attack, but is now depressed, will not walk uphill or take much exercise at all and thinks it unlikely that he will be able to return to work. Figure 2 gives examples of the likely elements in the cognitive-behavioural cycle.

How would you begin to tackle this man's difficulties? What questions would you ask to enable him to examine his dysfunctional thoughts? Suppose that he agreed to try some gentle exercise, and he did experience chest pain. Are there any possible psychological causes (see pp. 148–149)?

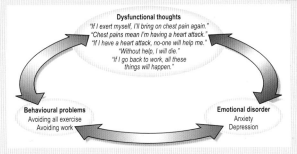

Fig. 2 Dysfunctional thoughts: the vicious circle.

Cognitive-behavioural therapy

- CBT aims to identify, evaluate and test the beliefs and attitudes we hold about ourselves, others and the world around us.
- The aim of CBT is to modify unhelpful and maladaptive beliefs and to generate more flexible, rational and adaptive beliefs.
- CBT emphasizes that the way we think about situations influences our mood and behaviour.
- CBT is a structured therapy that focuses on clearly identified and achievable treatment goals.
- CBT is a widely used treatment for physical and mental health problems, with good evidence for its effectiveness.

Role of carers

Doctors need to be aware of informal carers for two reasons: firstly, because caring for an elderly, chronically sick or disabled relative may affect the health of the carer and, secondly, because community care (see pp. 156–157) relies on families to take on the role of carer.

Caring has been divided into responsibility for the person (as may be the case, for example, when caring for an adult with schizophrenia) or carrying out direct care tasks (as when caring for an elderly parent no longer able to care for him- or herself).

Role of carers

Different models of care give carers different roles. Twigg & Atkin (1991) have suggested four models: (1) carers as a resource; (2) carers as co-workers; (3) carers as co-clients; and (4) when carers are superseded.

Carers as a resource

This is probably the most common view: that it is the natural order for a family to be responsible for the care of its members. The focus of services is on the dependent person and the aim is to maximize the level of informal care. This remains the background against which current British community care policies are set, although increasingly the next model is adopted alongside it.

Carers as co-workers

This model also aims to maintain and increase informal care, but acknowledges that to do so the needs of carers must be recognized – both psychological and physical needs such as domestic help, aids and time away, including holidays. This can be provided through a variety of services, including one-to-one support from health care staff such as nurses or through support offered through services run by charities or voluntary organizations.

Carers as co-clients

Here the carer becomes an indirect client and is thus a legitimate focus for support and services. This may cause confusion in the health service, where the formal status of a patient is clear, but may prove less of a problem for social work, where the definition of 'client' is more accommodating. Thus carers may find it easier to get help and support in the social services than through the NHS unless such services can be seen to have a direct clinical outcome. Family therapy treats all members as 'patients' or 'clients'.

Superseded carers

The last model looks to the future of the dependent person, aiming to make him or her independent and thus not (or less) reliant on the support of the carer. This model may be most appropriate for those dependent on parents. Not only is it better for disabled persons to have greater independence for themselves, but it helps answer the question of who will look after them when their parents are themselves unable to cope.

Impact of caring on the family

The impact on the family has traditionally been referred to as 'burden', although some, particularly those 'cared for', may see it as insulting and stigmatizing to be described as such. Burden is usually described as either objective (that which can be objectively measured and externally validated) or subjective (that which is perceived by the carer). It should be noted that objective burden and subjective burden are not necessarily correlated (Platt, 1985).

Objective burden

Objective burden comprises the things that are externally observable and objectively quantifiable. Financial problems include loss of earnings if the carer has to give up his or her job, as well as additional costs ranging from extra laundry or heating to special aids and trips to hospital. The loss of employment not only affects finances, but also deprives the carer of outside contact and a role other than that of carer.

The disruption of household can be severe, particularly in terms of loss of freedom and privacy, which includes the difficulty couples may have in spending time alone together. Children may be affected through restrictions on their lives, particularly if they become carers for parents.

The tasks vary, depending on the needs of the person being cared for. For elderly dependants care may focus on physical tasks, and the drudgery of the unremitting tasks involved in caring for someone who can do little for him- or herself should not be underestimated. Where the dependent person has a mental illness, care may focus more on supervision and taking responsibility, perhaps for finances or medication. Behaviour that causes most concern to families is usually that which is socially disturbing or embarrassing, or which puts the person at risk.

The effect on the carer's health, both physical and mental, is both an objective burden and the consequence of objective and subjective burdens. Many carers have poor physical or mental health (particularly depression and anxiety) or suffer physical injury, predominantly to their backs, from lifting. Social isolation is a problem both in terms of its own impact on the life of carers and because it contributes to other problems (Social Policy Research Unit, 2004). The majority of carers receive no help from outside sources, and the amount of time spent caring can severely restrict the carers' involvement with the world outside the family.

Subjective burden

Subjective burden is difficult to measure objectively and is, to some extent, how the carer feels about caring. Thus social isolation is not just the absence of outside contacts, but the extent to which the carer feels isolated and withdrawn. Carers may feel their independence is eroded, together with their freedom and their sense of identity.

Stigma is experienced both by people with particular conditions (see pp. 60–61) and by their carers, and reflects society's negative view. It may be a feature of being made to feel that they have contributed to the problem (e.g. a child's mental illness) or it otherwise reflects on them, as the following quotations suggest:

> *How can I tell anyone my husband's schizophrenic? They'll think there must be something wrong with me to have married him in the first place*

(wife).

Sometimes I just want to kill us both. I'm getting on ... can't go on like this much longer ... what's to become of him? If I did it ... we'd both be at peace

(mother)

The emotional impact includes everything from anxiety, depression, despair, hopelessness and helplessness to resentment, frustration and anger. Stress results when the carer is unable to continue coping with the demands being made. This may be exacerbated by guilt and worry that they aren't doing enough or that they have somehow contributed to the problem. Concern about the future is especially important for elderly carers, who worry about what will happen when they die.

Lastly, the role of carer has an impact as it changes the relationship between two people. For a woman, it is often expected and becomes an extension of the role she had been performing all her life, especially if caring for a child who has now grown into an adult. Roles are reversed when caring for parents, and when caring for a spouse the mutual support in the relationship may be lost. The role of carer usually falls on one person in a family, most commonly a woman.

Research has tended to concentrate on the negative aspects of caring and it is easy to ignore that caring for a loved one can bring rewards and pleasure as well as burdens and sorrow (Grant & Nolan, 1993).

Carers' issues

Not being recognized as providers of care is central to other problems such as lack of adequate services, support and lack of information and advice. This may be particularly strong where people feel they had no choice in taking on the caring role. Confidentiality raises a number of issues. Carers may feel they need information about their relative and his/her condition which this person does not want divulged. Although there are guidelines (e.g. Royal College of Psychiatrists, 2004), doctors will still use their judgement in what to share. Thus they may feel more comfortable discussing treatment issues of a person with dementia with that person's spouse than with the mother of a son with schizophrenia. Carers also often need their own support.

Current position

Both social work and the health service now have to take account of carers' views when planning services. The Carers (Recognition and Services) Act 1995 gives carers their place in the provision of care. No new resources, however, have been forthcoming to implement the Act. The National Service Frameworks in both England and Wales and Scotland set out standards for carers. The Clinical Standards Board for Scotland (2001) lays down seven essential criteria for judging services giving information and support to carers of people with schizophrenia (standard 7) (Box 1).

Case study

Mrs McLeod (65) lives alone with her son Alex (34), who has had schizophrenia since he was 19. He has always lived with his parents apart from a few short stays in hospital. Mr McLeod died 8 years ago. They are visited occasionally by Alex's sister, but an older brother has moved away and doesn't want any contact.

Alex hears voices, spends most of the day in bed and is up at night wandering round the house, smoking and playing music loudly. Mrs McLeod asks him to turn the sound down because of complaints from neighbours, but this leads to bitter arguments. At other times Alex gets very anxious and depressed and wakes his mother to talk to her. She gets very little sleep and is constantly tired. Although she had smoke alarms fitted, Mrs McLeod still worries about the risk of fire, as Alex often leaves cigarettes burning. All the furniture has burn marks.

His only trips out of the house are to the clinic for medication and to buy cigarettes. He refuses to attend a day centre.

Mrs McLeod also rarely goes out as she does not like leaving Alex alone, both because she fears what might happen and because she feels guilty when he is alone. Because Alex doesn't like anyone coming into the house and because of his sometimes bizarre behaviour, she has stopped inviting anyone. Her two great worries are whether she did anything that might have made Alex schizophrenic and what is going to happen when she dies.

Box 1 **Information and standards for carers**

1. Carers are given information about schizophrenia and the services available both locally and nationally to support them and the person for whom they are caring
2. Carers are offered the opportunity to meet with the staff supporting the person for whom they are caring, and are actively involved in the discussions about, and planning of, that person's care
3. If a person who has a diagnosis of schizophrenia refuses to give consent for his or her carer to be given information and to be actively involved in discussions about care, then this decision is discussed with the person and with his or her carer, and is recorded in the case notes. A person's decision either to give or refuse consent is reviewed with him/her and with his/her carer on an ongoing basis
4. Carers have access to an independent advocacy service
5. When respite is required, the local social work services are advised of this need
6. Carers have access to information and advice outwith normal working hours
7. Carers are advised of their right to an independent assessment of their need by the local social work services (Clinical Standards Board for Scotland, 2001)

STOP THINK
- As a GP, how does your responsibility to the ill or disabled person (the dependant) conflict with your responsibility to the carer (who may also be your patient)?
- Should relatives have the right to choose whether they care, or to what extent, should they be responsible for a dependent relative? What happens (and who pays) if they choose not to be?

Role of carers

- A relative is the first line of care for most people with chronic illness or disability.
- There are four models of care: carers as resources, co-workers, co-clients and superseded carers.
- Burden can be objective or subjective.
- Major problems are lack of recognition, lack of services and lack of information.

Self-help groups

No doctor or health professional can afford to ignore the rise of the self-help movement in the management of illness, disability and social problems. Self-help ranges from the large national organizations, to small, unique, local groups. All have arisen from people wanting to take more control of their lives and responsibility for the management of their illness/disability. Probably the largest and most famous self-help organization is Alcoholics Anonymous (AA) (see pp. 82–83) with its 12-step programme (Box 1). This is a model followed by others, e.g. Gamblers Anonymous, Narcotics Anonymous and Overeaters Anonymous. The concepts behind the 12-step programme have been incorporated into some professionally run services.

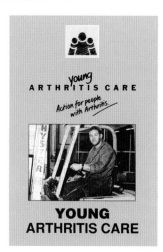

Fig. 1 Booklet produced by the organization Arthritis Care.

Box 1 **Twelve steps of Alcoholics Anonymous**

1. We admitted we were powerless over alcohol, that our lives had become unmanageable.
2. We came to believe that a power greater than ourselves could restore us to sanity.
3. We made a decision to turn our will and our lives over to the care of God as we understood Him.
4. We made a searching and fearless moral inventory of ourselves.
5. We admitted to God, to ourselves and to another human being the exact nature of our wrongs.
6. We were entirely ready to have God remove all these defects of character.
7. We humbly asked Him to remove our shortcomings.
8. We made a list of all persons we had harmed, and became willing to make amends to them all.
9. We made direct amends to such people wherever possible, except when to do so would injure them or others.
10. We continued to take personal inventory and when we were wrong promptly admitted it.
11. We sought through prayer and meditation to improve our conscious contact with God as we understood Him, praying only for knowledge of His will for us and the power to carry that out.
12. Having had a spiritual awakening as the result of these steps, we tried to carry this message to alcoholics and to practise these principles in all our affairs.

Types of self-help groups

Self-help groups divide into two broad categories – those whose aim is to help members and those with a primarily campaigning role, aiming to change public attitudes and policy, although many include both aims.

In the health field, self-help groups exist for practically every condition, whether defined as illness or some 'deviation from the norm'. There are groups for people with lifelong conditions (e.g. Association of Cystic Fibrosis Adults), chronic medical conditions (e.g. Ileostomy Association), mental health problems (e.g. MIND), and people who define themselves as survivors, whether of the system (e.g. Survivors Speak Out) or of abuse (e.g. Incest Survivors Group). Groups exist for relatives (e.g. National Schizophrenia Fellowship, renamed Rethink in 2002). Other groups exist for those experiencing traumatic life events, including bereavement (e.g. Compassionate Friends).

Functions of self-help groups

Support
The emotional support, acceptance and understanding that come from others in a similar position cannot be overestimated and the importance of social support has been discussed elsewhere (see pp. 136–137). For particularly stigmatized or disadvantaged groups their main source of social contact and friendship may come through such groups. However some people may feel more stigmatized by being expected to socialize with such people, or see it as a sign of weakness. Members of the British Council of Organizations of Disabled People (BCODP), which organizes the Rights not Charity demonstrations, are more likely to view themselves as political than those organizations which do not join.

Role models
Those who have overcome or learned to live with the problem provide a powerful model for others in the same position and can offer a hopeful and optimistic view of the future.

Information and advice about coping
Both patients and relatives complain of lack of information; this is collated and disseminated by self-help groups and ranges from public lectures and specially written booklets (Fig. 1) to discussion groups. Information can shade into advice about coping, and even counselling.

Coping strategies
Those with the problem usually have more to offer in the way of practical advice about day-to-day management of the disorder and general strategies for coping than do most professionals.

Ideology
Self-help groups have their own philosophies, with which members identify and which may or may not be in line with current professional thinking. When alternative views are put forward there is likely to be tension, if not hostility, between and within groups. People may seek out groups that support their position and the recognition of shared beliefs is an important part of support.

Mutual aid
In self-help groups, help is reciprocal and the giving as well as receiving of help is fundamental. Giving help has a range of benefits, including: increased meaning and purpose to one's own life; increased feelings of self-worth and confidence; the positive reinforcement, both personal and social, that comes

from helping; and even the rehearsal of coping strategies by advising others. AA is explicit about this reciprocal help: its 12th step requires members to take the message to other alcoholics (Table 1). Carers were explicit about the core value of reciprocity as setting self-help groups apart from those supported by professionals (Munn-Giddings & McVicar, 2007).

Most self-help groups engage in face-to-face contact, although the number of support groups springing up on the internet suggests this is not always necessary (Klemm et al., 1998). The internet offers the opportunity for support outside one's immediate area, anonymity for those who feel stigmatized and important contact for those with mobility problems or in rural areas.

Empowerment

Patients frequently feel powerless in the face of both their illness and the medical profession. Self-help groups foster empowerment in two ways. One is through information, education and advice about the illness and coping, thus giving the individual some sense of mastery and control. Secondly, self-help groups may seek to influence service delivery and policy both nationally and locally, and educate the public with the aim of changing public attitudes. This can be seen as a more consumer-oriented approach to empowerment. Some groups specifically challenge the media portrayal of their disability. Disability rights groups, for example, picket the Children in Need appeal to make people aware of their views and their objection to charity.

Self-help and service provision

Small, local self-help groups that aim to do nothing more than offer support and advice within the group will continue to flourish, although individual groups may wax and wane, dependent largely on the health of those who run them. In the UK as elsewhere, the development of community care (see pp. 156–157) has pushed many self-help groups to become service providers. Groups have gained grants to provide services directly (to client groups rather than just members) and the distinction between self-help groups and voluntary organizations is sometimes not clear. Although this has positive aspects, as services are more likely to be tailored to users' needs and those most involved have a say in the running of services, it can also have some less desirable consequences. Self-help projects usually suffer from insecure short-term funding and can be used to plug gaps in services rather than adequately resourcing statutory agencies. Groups may lose their mutual aid orientation, and the centrality of the user's experience may be diminished as staff are brought in to run the organization and its services. In the chase after money to fund services, some of the campaigning and more political aspects of the group may be lost in an attempt not to offend potential funders, or because the time required is no longer available.

Internet groups

The internet offers a multitude of opportunities for self-help groups to flourish and can be particularly helpful for those with rare conditions or living in rural areas who might otherwise find meeting others difficult. It allows the sharing of experiences linked to evidence-based information (Herxheimer et al., 2000).

The Expert Patients

The self-help approach to management of chronic illness has found official support through *The Expert Patients Programme* introduced by the Department of Health (2006).

Case study

Rethink (formerly the National Schizophrenia Fellowship (NSF))

In its beginning, the NSF was an organization that offered support to carers of people with schizophrenia, and 90% of its membership were carers. Local groups, usually run by a relative, meet regularly to share information, advice, problems, experiences and feelings, and to gain support, acceptance and help with coping. Professionals often give lectures and participate in discussion; although some groups have ongoing professional support to maintain them, the focus is on carer experience and control.

The organization has always had a campaigning role and, although not opposed to the closure of mental hospitals, it campaigned for this not to exceed the rate of replacement community services and also emphasized the need for asylum. The organization developed into a major service provider, changing its name to Rethink. Both locally and nationally Rethink responds to consultation documents and community care plans. It is frequently viewed as the voice of carers of the mentally ill, despite being predominantly white and middle-class. It has always been active educationally, running local and national conferences for members and professionals, and in many areas carers speak to groups of nurses, social workers and doctors in training, giving their perspective on life with schizophrenia, the role of relatives as carers and their response to services.

Rethink is now firmly in the arena of service provision, running community day services, employment projects, cafés, housing projects and respite care. The rapid expansion in service provision can be seen simply by looking at the accounts. In 1988–1989 the turnover was £769 143, but by 1992–1993 this had expanded to £6.1 million and incoming resources for 2006–2007 were £43 847 000.

The NSF spawned similar organizations throughout the world, which meet together as the World Schizophrenia Fellowship. Founded in 1982, its membership includes Australia, Austria, Canada, Colombia, France, Germany, India, Indonesia, Ireland, Israel, Japan, Malaysia, Netherlands, New Zealand, South Africa, UK, Uruguay and USA (www.rethink.org).

- What can professionals gain from being involved with a self-help group?
- Is there a danger that self-help could be seen as a cheap alternative to other services?

- The internet also offers an opportunity to promote non-standard approaches to conditions. There are websites that support anorexia nervosa as a lifestyle choice rather than an illness and offer advice on how to be anorexic. Concern over this has led some servers to deny access to such sites. What do you think about this (see pp. 86–87)?

Self-help groups

- Self-help groups provide an alternative to the traditional approach.
- They value personal experience.
- Self-help groups seek to empower members.
- They have roles as service providers and campaigners as well as offering support.

Palliative care

Development of palliative care

The main pioneer of the hospice (palliative care) movement in the UK was Dame Cicely Saunders, who worked as both a volunteer nurse and a social worker, and later as a doctor, at two of the first London hospices, St Joseph's and St Luke's. This experience made her aware of the need for a place of care that would specialize in pain and symptom control in the terminal stages of disease, but that would also provide an environment that would allow people to adjust emotionally and spiritually to their approaching death (Saunders & Sykes, 1993). Her subsequent foundation of St Christopher's Hospice in London as a centre of excellence in palliative care provided the cornerstone of the modern hospice movement. Its rapid expansion over the past four decades has been accompanied by the recognition of palliative medicine as a medical specialty. It has also become a global movement, with palliative care services available in approximately 100 countries, including the USA, Asia and Africa (Stjernsward & Clark, 2004). These authors estimate that 33 million people currently dying in the world would benefit from a basic palliative-care approach, and this number triples when families and carers are included.

Defining palliative care

In 2002 the World Health Organization redefined palliative care as 'the active care of patients with advanced progressive disease. Management of pain and other symptoms and provision of psychological, social and spiritual support is paramount. The goal of palliative care is achievement of the best quality of life for the patient' (World Health Organization, 2002c). In 1990 it developed guiding principles which stated that palliative care:

- affirms life and regards dying as a normal process
- neither hastens nor postpones death
- provides relief from pain and other distressing symptoms
- integrates the psychological and spiritual aspects of patient care
- offers a support system to help patients live as actively as possible until death
- offers a support system to help the family cope during the patient's illness and their own bereavement.

Although the advent of hospice care has dramatically improved the care of patients, particularly in the area of pain and symptom control, evidence suggests that these goals are still not being met in every setting in which palliative care is provided. There is, therefore, an increasing drive to make hospice standards of care available for all dying patients and not an exception for a small minority. New definitions now distinguish different levels of palliative care according to the setting in which it is provided and the expertise of staff delivering the care, although the number of levels is still being debated. At one level, the palliative-care approach aims to promote both physical and psychosocial well-being as an integral part of all clinical practice, whatever the illness or stage, through a knowledge and practice of palliative care principles (National Council for Hospice and Specialist Palliative Care Services, 1997). At the other end of the spectrum, 'Specialist palliative care is the active total care of patients with progressive far-advanced disease and limited prognosis, and their families, by a multi-professional team who have undergone recognized specialist palliative care training' (National Council for Hospice and Specialist Palliative Care Services, 2000). More recently the definition of palliative care has been expanded to include supportive and end-of-life care as the discipline attempts to encompass the whole disease trajectory (National Council for Hospice and Specialist Palliative Care Services, 2002; NICE, 2004; www.who.int/cancer/palliative/definition/en).

Beyond the hospice

In the past, hospice care has largely been confined to those patients who were dying from cancer, because most were funded by charitable contributions. An important consequence of the expansion of the hospice movement, however, has been the spread of its principles and goals to other places of care. Increasing demands are being made to improve the palliative care of people with other chronic non-malignant conditions and to other sectors of the population, e.g. the elderly and those with learning disabilities (Addington-Hall & Higginson, 2001). Palliative-care services now exist in a wide variety of forms, ranging from autonomous inpatient units and day centres where patients can attend for medical or social care to multidisciplinary hospital support teams that provide specialist palliative care advice to patients in large acute hospitals (www.hospiceinformation.info). Specialist palliative home care teams can also assist GPs in caring for patients at home.

Total pain

The philosophy of the hospice movement is the alleviation of total pain and the affirmation of the remaining quality of life. This means tackling not only physical pain (pp. 148–149), but also any emotional, psychological, social or spiritual problems the patient has that might contribute to the patient's total distress.

Figure 1 shows that the extent of a patient's pain may be affected by a whole range of physical, psychological, social and situational factors that may influence his or her ability to cope with it. Physical effects of disease and treatment (for example,

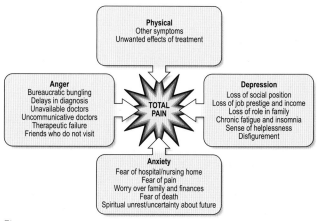

Fig. 1 Composition of total pain, and factors influencing sensitivity (from Twycross, 1994, with permission).

radiotherapy or surgery) may be exacerbated or precipitated by other complications. These may include anger at medical staff over unnecessary delays in diagnosis, lack of communication from them or failure to provide a cure, anxiety about other family members, finances or prognosis, or depression or loss of hope resulting from the loss of job, role or function due to illness. The degree to which individuals are free from total pain will therefore depend on the ability of their professional carers to understand and solve its many causes.

The multidisciplinary team

The need for multidisciplinary teams of health professionals who work together is essential to tackling total pain (Twycross, 1999) and increasingly team-working is seen as an essential to the success of palliative care (NICE, 2004). Core members will include medical and nursing staff, social workers, chaplains, physiotherapists and occupational therapists. However, the individual needs of the patient and his or her family will determine which team member plays a central role. For example, in the case of a patient with persistent nausea it may be the doctor who directs the patient's care. On the other hand, a patient who is facing severe financial difficulties may need most help from the social worker while a patient who has difficulty in coping may benefit from consultations with a psychologist. The team should delegate tasks amongst its members to ensure that its resources are mobilized effectively and care prioritized in order to meet each individual's needs as efficiently as possible. The effectiveness of the team will largely depend on good communication between members, and between itself and other health professionals, as well as with patients and their families.

Measuring palliative care

As with every other medical specialty, practitioners of palliative care are increasingly accountable for the care they provide. Measuring palliative care can enable doctors and researchers to evaluate the care patients receive and allow comparisons of care to be made across settings, between patients with different types of disease and between patients at different stages of the disease process. Standards and guidelines are now being developed to enable palliative-care professionals to deliver and audit the structure, process and outcome of care. Though some people argue that the individual approach to providing palliative care means that it cannot and should not be measured, recognized goals of palliative care such as those of the World Health Organization (Johnston & Abraham, 1995) and concepts such as total pain have allowed the definition of measurable palliative-care outcomes. These include pain and symptom control, communication, psychological well-being, social support and spiritual distress (Higginson, 2004). The importance of quality of life (QoL) in palliative care means that this outcome can also be used to measure and monitor results of care that go beyond the traditional end-points of tumour size, side-effects of treatment and survival (see pp. 40–41). QoL is usually measured by multidimensional instruments that assess the physical, functional, psychosocial and spiritual needs of patients (Kaasa & Loge, 2004). More recently the Gold Standards Framework and the Liverpool Care Pathway have facilitated hospice standards of care being implemented and audited in hospitals, nursing homes and the community by providing guidelines for non-specialist staff to manage palliative and end-of-life care more effectively (Thomas & Noble, 2007; Ellershaw & Wilkinson, 2003).

Case study

Jane was a 49-year-old woman with cancer of the breast and bony metastasis. She was married to Adam, a lawyer, and had two teenage daughters, Sara and Louise. Her prognosis was poor and after receiving a course of palliative radiotherapy, she had come home to spend her remaining time with her family. Neither daughter knew how serious their mother's condition was, though both suspected that it was not good because of the number of health professionals constantly visiting the house. Both Jane and her husband thought that in protecting their daughters from the truth they were shielding them from unnecessary anxiety and grief. As a result, relationships in the family were strained and both girls were doing badly at school. Jane was experiencing uncontrolled pain and nausea, which prevented her from sleeping and eating properly. At this point the GP, after consulting the district nurse, decided to refer Jane to a specialist nurse for advice on pain control and help with improving communications among the family.

As the nurse's visits to the family progressed, Jane and Adam were encouraged to share their knowledge of Jane's prognosis with their daughters. Both learned that instead of protecting their daughters they were in fact alienating them, causing them to feel confused and isolated. Gradually, through open communication, Louise and Sara came to accept that their mother was dying, but that as a family they could still make the most of the time that was left. Jane was also given a different form of pain relief: a syringe driver which administered analgesia continuously while allowing her to remain as mobile and unrestricted as possible. In the end Jane died peacefully and comfortably at home surrounded by Adam and her daughters.

STOP THINK
- Consider the Case study and write down how you think Jane's daughters felt when initially they were not told of the seriousness of her condition.
- Think how you would go about breaking down the barriers to communication between the family. Imagine that you were the GP in this situation, and plan what you would say to Jane and Adam.
- Think how you might negotiate between them and Sara and Louise.

Palliative care

- The provision of palliative care has been revolutionized by the modern hospice movement, particularly in the area of pain control.
- With the growth of the hospice movement has come the recognition of the care of the dying as a medical specialty known as palliative medicine.
- The philosophy of the hospice movement emphasizes the alleviation of total pain, and the patient and his or her carer as a unit of care.
- Palliative care is provided by a multidisciplinary team of health professionals, including doctors and nurses, physiotherapists and occupational therapists, social workers, psychologists, pastoral staff and nurses specifically trained to be advisors in palliative care.
- Quality-of-life measures are now being developed to enable doctors and researchers to measure and evaluate the physical and psychosocial well-being of patients. These conceptualize patients' needs using multidimensional instruments and provide outcomes of care that allow comparisons to be made across settings and between patients with different types of disease and at different stages.

Complementary therapies

'Complementary therapies' is the term used to include complementary and alternative medicine (CAM). The Cochrane Collaboration (www.cochrane.org) defines CAM as 'a broad domain of healing resources that encompasses all health systems, modalities, and practices and their accompanying theories and beliefs, other than those intrinsic to the politically dominant health systems of a particular society or culture in a given historical period'. Complementary therapies are usually, if not invariably, complementary to conventional medical treatment and so the term 'alternative' is less appropriate. They may be described as being in the folk sector of medicine (see pp. 100–101). CAM's popularity has led to suggestions that medical curricula should include awareness of CAM (Cumming, 2007).

The use of complementary therapies

The use of complementary therapies has become very popular in recent years. In a survey of over 1200 British adults, 20% had used CAM in the previous 12 months, of whom 34% had used herbal medicine (Ernst & White, 2000). Sales of CAM-related products in the UK are predicted to rise to over £125 million by 2002 (House of Lords, 2000). A survey of first-year medical students found that 37% had had previous experience of CAM and, of those who used it, 82% said that they had found it helpful (Greenfield et al., 2002).

Patients may ask doctors and other health professionals about the wisdom of trying complementary therapies or may conceal their interest because of a fear of disapproval. They may not perceive CAM as medicine and not report its use. An open discussion of the costs and benefits is essential so that the practitioner is aware of other therapies that the patient may be having. Many have no adverse effect but some may interact with conventional therapy (see Case study). Complementary therapies or remedies may not all be safe and could be toxic (Burton, 2003). There is likely to be increasing government legislation on safety and the 'yellow card' notification system to monitor adverse events is used by professionals (Ross, 2007).

The popularity of CAM is increasing across the westernized world. Increased concern over ecological and environmental issues may have helped to fuel interest in 'natural' healing systems. Astin (1998) identifies key points in society that represent this shift towards alternative medicine, which are linked to holistic beliefs in perceiving the body, mind and spirit in an integrative manner. This is totally different from conventional medicine, where disease is treated by looking specifically at organs or tissue of the body. Other identifiable reasons for this movement are related to patients' rights, a more active role in consumer health, self-care and fitness, and dissatisfaction with conventional medicine (Cassileth, 1998). Many people seek complementary therapy because: they want to use all options in health care; they want a cure without side-effects or pain; they are disappointed with the traditional orthodox consultation; they believe in holistic care; they perceive conventional medicine to be ineffective; or they may be concerned about the side-effects of powerful drugs (Vincent & Furnham, 1997).

Consultations are generally longer and concentrate on a person's overall well-being and own subjective experience. Complementary therapists undoubtedly have well-developed communication skills (see pp. 96–97). It is possible that the efficacy of some complementary therapies may occur because of the placebo effect (see pp. 92–93).

Complementary therapists are often active listeners and are perceived as being 'low-tech' (Fig. 1). In the UK, more GPs are becoming trained in complementary therapies such as homeopathy and hypnotherapy.

Types of complementary therapies

The House of Lords Select Committee on Science and Technology (House of Lords, 2000) published a report on CAM and grouped the different kinds of complementary therapy into three:

- Group 1 included the disciplines of osteopathy, chiropractic, acupuncture, herbal medicine and homeopathy. These are sometimes known as the big five, and acts of parliament regulate osteopathy and chiropractic in their professional activity and education.
- Group 2 includes therapies used to complement conventional medicine and do not claim to diagnose. They include aromatherapy and reflexology.
- Group 3 includes therapies that claim to diagnose as well as treat and generally have a different paradigm of the causes of disease. It includes traditional Chinese medicine, crystal therapy and iridology.

There are many others not mentioned here but conventional medical or health practitioners may encounter the following.

Group 1
Acupuncture
Acupuncture is one of the oldest therapies, originating in China over 2000 years ago. Small needles are inserted into specific points in the body. It is assumed that vital energy 'qi' travels along meridians, and if yin and yang are unbalanced the energy becomes blocked.

Chiropractic
This manipulates the joints and uses massage to treat musculoskeletal complaints, particularly in the back. It assumes that nerves that control posture and movement become irritated, which leads to referred pain.

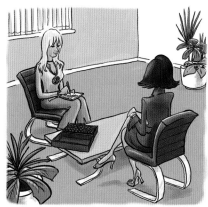

Fig. 1 Listening practitioner.

Herbal medicine or phytotherapy

Remedies derived from plants and plant extracts are used to treat complaints. They are traditional pharmaceuticals, but consist of many chemical constituents and are usually unstandardized.

Homeopathy

Homeopathy is a therapy that treats like with like. Patients are given a small dose of a substance that is thought to produce the same symptoms in a healthy person if given in a higher dose. The remedies are highly diluted so that not even a single molecule may be left in the solution. The patient's constitution is also assessed.

Osteopathy

The therapy involves manipulation of the spine. It assumes that the blood supply is impaired. It may be used together with chiropractic.

Group 2

Aromatherapy

Essential oils extracted from aromatic plants and diluted in vegetable oils are applied to the skin. Small quantities are absorbed through the skin or by inhalation. Essential oils also have mood-altering effects via the limbic olfaction system.

Reflexology

This is massage of the foot, which assumes that there are zones in the body so that each organ has a corresponding location in the foot. It produces feelings of relaxation.

Group 3

Traditional Chinese medicine

If the two types of energy (or 'qi'), yin and yang, are in imbalance, disease may occur. Traditional Chinese medicine restores the balance and may use herbs, massage or acupuncture.

Crystal therapy

Crystals are placed in patterns around the body to adjust the energy field or person's aura.

Iridology

The iris's pigmentation reflects the individual's health status, enabling diagnosis.

The effectiveness of therapies outside the current mainstream of medicine may occur through a variety of methods, which may include conventional biochemical routes, by the effect of the therapeutic interaction, or in ways as yet not understood. Research on the efficacy of these therapies has been difficult to carry out using conventional research designs but there is increasing pressure to evaluate complementary therapies and to provide an evidence base (Lewith et al., 2002).

Case study

St John's wort (*Hypericum perforatum*) (Fig. 2)

Extracts of this herb have long been used in folk medicine. In Germany it is licensed for use in anxiety, depression and sleep disorders. It has been shown to be an effective antidepressant for mild or moderate depression (Williams, 2002; Woelk, 2000). The extracts contain many different chemical classes, so the active agent is a matter of uncertainty. It may be hypericin or hyperforin (Fig. 3) (Kingston, 2001). It may be preferred to conventional antidepressants because of their perceived side-effects. However, there may be herb–drug interactions. St John's wort interacts with oral contraceptives and may lead to reduced blood levels, with a risk of breakthrough bleeding and unplanned pregnancy.

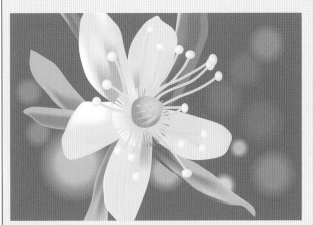

Fig. 2 St John's wort flower.

	R
Hypericin	H
Pseudohypericin	OH

Fig. 3 Diagram of molecules of hypericin and hyperforin (adapted from Mills & Bone, 2000, with permission).

STOP THINK

- Complementary therapies are often considered to be risk-free.
- Why might there be more risks or side-effects with herbal medicine than with homeopathy?
- Balance the costs and benefits of consulting an osteopath to a patient with chronic low-back pain.

Complementary therapies

- Complementary therapies and alternative medicine are growing in popularity.
- Therapies have been grouped on the basis of evidence and regulation.
- The evidence for their efficacy is sparse, but there is a high level of patient satisfaction.
- For further reading, see Cumming et al. (2007).

The management of pain

Pain is defined by the International Association for the Study of Pain as: 'an unpleasant sensory and emotional experience associated with actual or potential tissue damage, or described in terms of such damage'. The experience of pain is subjective and dependent on past experiences of injury. Note that the definition includes the emotional experience, indicating that the pain perception is not just sensory. We often associate pain with an acute injury or event that is assumed to signal harm or damage. This may be an appropriate interpretation where pain has an obvious cause and is of recent onset. However, many people's experience of pain is a more chronic picture. Chronic pain may present in a variety of ways and is estimated to have a prevalence of 10% in the population. Chronic back pain is one of the commonest causes of sickness from work and contributes to escalating figures for disability benefits.

Neurophysiology of pain

Research on the neurophysiology of pain has provided remarkable insights into pain mechanisms. The development of neural plasticity, allows damaged pathways to reconnect. Central sensitization can occur, which causes a 'wind-up' phenomenon of increased firing of nerve pathways. 'Pain memory' is a neural imprint of past pain experiences. These developments have built on the earlier concepts of a gate-control mechanism described by Melzack & Wall (1999). This model clarified that the experience of pain is also modulated by downward neural pathways, i.e. from the brain, facilitating psychological regulation of pain.

The way forward – a biopsychosocial approach

It is no longer appropriate to dismiss pain as being 'all in the mind' if investigations show no to the cause. The neurophysiology of pain allows a much more complex understanding. Management of pain is also complex. Psychological and social factors contribute significantly to the way in which pain is perceived and managed.

Why psychosocial factors are important

Continuing pain can lead to losses, such as an inability to work, medical retirement, financial restrictions and an inability to continue with normal activities – all of which may in turn lead to relationship difficulties and reduced quality of life. This may result in the development of depression, hopelessness and reduced sense of control. Constant pain may make it difficult to sleep, reduce ability to concentrate and, subsequently, increase irritability. Sexual activity may be reduced and thoughts of suicide are not uncommon.

Health beliefs and misconceptions

Health beliefs can powerfully influence people's response to their symptoms and expectations of treatment (see pp. 38–39). If individuals with chronic pain believe that their pain is a signal of harm and damage, then they are likely to avoid doing things that will bring on pain. This usually leads to a gradual reduction in physical mobility and can result in secondary problems, such as postural changes, stiffness in joints or the lack of use of an affected limb. Individuals may be fearful of exercise and less compliant with advice. This kind of health belief can lead to anxiety and significant unhelpful behavioural changes.

Cognitive-behavioural approaches

There are three linked components to the management of pain: dealing with unhelpful patterns of thinking, which can then lead to changes in behaviour and subsequent improvement in mood (see pp. 136–137). These psychological principles can be applied by all clinicians who have contact with pain patients. A more integrated and intensive approach is commonly used in pain management programmes.

Changes in cognitions

- Identify and help to reshape misconceptions about pain (Box 1), to ensure that the patient has a good understanding of the principles of pain mechanisms early on.
- People are often fearful of exercise and activity in case this causes pain to flare up, which will then be attributed to having caused harm and damage. Fear avoidance can lead to a decrease in mobility and to lower levels of fitness.
- Help patients to recognize and reframe unhelpful patterns of negative thoughts, e.g. 'I used to be able to decorate my house in no time – now I'm useless – there's no point in trying' could be changed to: 'If I get some help with the heavy bits, I could do this decorating in chunks of half an hour. It may take me longer but it means I will have done it without having to rely on others'.

Box 1 **Common misconceptions about pain**

- 'I've been told my X-rays show wear and tear. This must mean that my bones are wearing away. I had better not do too much in case I wear things away even further.'
- 'If you have pain it means that you have damaged and harmed something. I had better not do anything that gives me pain in case I harm myself.'
- 'It's best to avoid getting dependent on medication, so I'll go as long as possible without taking anything.'

Changes in behaviour

Pain often leads to behaviour that is shaped by operant conditioning (see pp. 22–23):

- 'Good days' often lead to doing too much and trying to catch up. This usually results in 'bad days', when little can be done while waiting for the pain to settle. Mood is then often low, and frustration and anxiety are high (Fig. 1).
- This cycle can be broken by setting behavioural goals where a level of activity is found that does not cause pain to flare up. The level is then gradually increased, which reduces the 'wind-up' effect of pain and helps improve mood and confidence. This can apply to exercise as well as other activities such as housework, gardening, sports, concentration tasks, social activity and hobbies (Fig. 2).
- Setting levels of activity as goals that are achievable helps to increase the likelihood of positive results, which in turn helps to increase a sense of control and positive thinking.

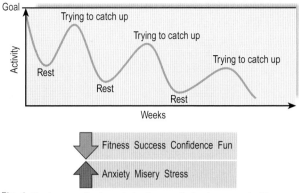

Fig. 1 The impact of pain on behaviour and behaviour on pain. The overactivity–rest cycle.

■ Learning relaxation techniques can greatly improve a sense of being in control of pain. With regular relaxation practice, it is possible to alter the vicious cycle where pain causes increasing frustration and irritability, raised adrenaline levels and increased spasm, all of which lead to changes in pain threshold. Relaxation skills can also help improve sleep.

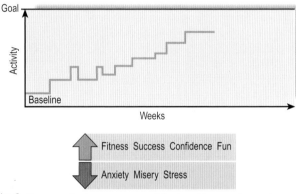

Fig. 2 Elements of pain management. Behavioural intervention: pacing, activity scheduling and goal-setting.

Changes in mood and sense of control or self-efficacy

■ As people accumulate skills and strategies to build up activity, and so regain some of what was lost. This reduces frustration and improves mood.
■ Correcting misconceptions and helping people to reframe negative patterns of thinking improves perceived control and mood.

What is the evidence?

Waddell (1998) has synthesized the evidence on treatment of back pain and concluded that most medical specialist services are inappropriate and may be harmful for patients with simple backache. These patients need a biopsychosocial approach to early mobilization and to address misconceptions and psychological distress. A systematic review of pain treatments by McQuay et al. (1997) found large and sustainable improvements in outcomes using a psychological approach. A meta-analysis and systematic review of randomized controlled trials for cognitive-behavioural therapy for chronic pain by Morley et al. (1999) found that cognitive-behavioural treatments were associated

with significant effects on pain experience, measures of coping and behavioural expression of pain.

A comprehensive account of an interdisciplinary approach to chronic pain is found in Main & Spanswick (2000).

 STOP THINK ■ Why is bed rest no longer recommended for people with back pain?

The management of pain

■ Lack of findings on investigation does not mean that pain is not genuine.
■ The mind/body split (i.e. all physical or all psychological) is in not a helpful way to conceptualize pain.
■ Injuries from accidents can lead to posttraumatic stress disorder or similar symptoms, which are frequently missed and contribute to the maintenance of pain and disability.
■ A cognitive-behavioural approach is effective in managing pain.
■ Identify and correct patients' misconceptions.
■ Help patients to reframe negative thinking.
■ Help patients set achievable goals.
■ Affirm patients' progress and improvements in their sense of control and self-efficacy of progress.

Case study

John has had back and neck pain for 4 years, following a road accident in which he suffered minor whiplash. An MRI scan shows some degenerative changes, but no indications for surgery. John was medically retired 1 year ago and reports disturbed sleep and poor concentration. His wife works full time and he feels guilty about not working. He tends to push himself and then has to recover for the rest of the week. He has given up golf, is gaining weight, rarely sees friends, and is increasingly angry. Recently John was assessed in a multi-disciplinary pain clinic and given explanations about chronic pain and its effect on physical and psychological state. He began a pain-management programme and initially found it difficult to shift from his pattern of overactivity. However, with regular setting of activity and exercise goals he was able to gradually increase what he could do, and felt les anxious about harm, which lead to increasing confidence. He initially found relaxation difficult, but gradually built up skills, resulting in less irritability and he is now able to enjoy things with his family. He began some voluntary work and feels less guilty about not working.

Organizing and funding health care

The organization and funding of health care affect patients as well as health care providers. Doctors, as health care providers, may be restricted in their actions owing to the existing organization of health care, or they may feel that their patients' access to certain expensive tests or interventions is restricted.

Health care systems all over the world seem to be facing a funding crisis. The main issue is the allocation of scarce resources. This is not simply a question of money but also of political decision-making and priorities. In order to understand the current organization and funding of health care, we have to look at historical developments and the underlying political decision-making process.

We concentrate on three countries, the UK (with a predominantly state-run welfare system), the USA (with a predominantly free-market system), and Germany (with a mixed-health economy), representing the major ways health care is organized and funded (Table 1). Total expenditure per capita on health (including private and public health expenditure) in these three countries differs considerably, as does the proportion of the gross national product spent on health care.

UK

All citizens of the UK are included in the NHS. The NHS is a universal, tax-funded health care system. Doctors, nurses and hospitals are paid by the state. The NHS requires some additional payments from patients, for example, for prescriptions and dental check-ups, but the overwhelming majority of care provision is free of charge. Treatment is decided on (mostly) by doctors. GPs are gate-keepers in this system, selecting patients and referring patients to the appropriate specialist. Medical care is available to all, and is therefore without stigma or significant financial cost to the poor. However, there is a problem of waiting lists in certain areas (see pp. 154–155). This has stimulated an increase in the small but growing private health care sector. In the UK this includes sales of over-the-counter medicines and private payments for alternative therapies and hospital treatment. The latter is often provided by the same doctors in the same hospitals as the standard NHS care.

USA

The system in the USA is predominantly commercial insurance-based. Most people take out their own private health insurance, or are insured through their employer. These insurance companies reimburse doctors, hospitals and others for care provided. Most people have the freedom to go to the medical professional or hospital of their choice. A limited number of people are covered by state-organized schemes, such as Medicaid, which provides health care for the poor, but eligibility is incomplete and coverage usually excludes dental services and prescribed drugs, and Medicare, for all people over 65, which provides limited coverage. Over 45 million people are not insured or are seriously underinsured.

Germany

Of the German population, most are insured by one of 250 sick funds, which are funded by income-related contributions and are self-governing non-profit institutions. The average contribution rate is approximately 15% of an employee's gross income. Just under half of the contributions are paid by the employers and the other half by the employees. Self-employed persons and employees earning over a certain ceiling (47 700 Euros in 2007) are allowed to opt out of the statutory insurance scheme and join one of the 50 or so private health insurance companies. As in the UK, family doctors are gate-keepers, selecting and referring patients to the appropriate specialist. Patients receive comprehensive coverage, which entitles them to primary and hospital care, but patients pay a small fee for the first doctor or dentist visit each quarter and for prescriptions. The sick funds reimburse the doctors, hospitals and pharmacists for delivery of their services. Privately insured people pay the doctor or pharmacist and their insurance company reimburses the patient. Legal restrictions and government regulations limit the freedom of the sick funds to control cost, prices and the quantities and range of provisions.

What are the advantages of each system?

The German national insurance-funded and the British tax-funded systems have many similarities as predominantly universal and comprehensive systems. The two are more similar to each other than either is to the US system. Therefore the European collective system will be compared with the private system in the USA.

Box 1 lists some of the main advantages and disadvantages of collective health care systems. Some of the listed issues are political, others more clearly medical. For example, the first advantage is obviously political: it expresses ideals of shared citizenship and enhances social cohesiveness in society. The issue that 'free care encourages trivial complaints' has a direct impact on the doctor. If care is free for the patients we might

Table 1 **Three different ways of funding and organizing health care provision**		
UK	**USA**	**Germany**
■ State-run national health service mainly funded through taxation	■ Mainly private health insurance system with market-based health care provision	■ National health insurance-based system with a market-based health care system
■ Every citizen covered, but small fees paid on prescriptions	■ 10% of the population not covered	■ Every citizen covered, but small fees paid on use
■ Per capita spending on health US$2428	■ Per capita spending on health US$5711	■ Per capita spending on health US$3204
■ 8.0% of gross national product (GNP) spent on health services	■ 15.2% of GNP spent on health services	■ 11.1% of GNP spent on health services

Box 1 Collective systems of health care: advantages and disadvantages

Advantages

- Social citizenship/cohesion
- Combats the inverse-care law
- No fee results in less over-doctoring
- More scope for coordinated planning
- Bargaining-power economies of scale
- Tax revenue is cheap to collect
- Easier to meet emergencies, e.g. AIDS, war

Disadvantages

- Reduces individual responsibility
- Increases deference towards the doctor
- Free care encourages trivial complaints
- Impedes search for market solutions
- Vote-catching discourages quality
- Higher public spending
- Makes health a political football

*The inverse-care law argues that the provision of health care in a market economy is inversely related to the need for it; in other words poor facilities are to be found in depressed areas characterized by high morbidity, and better facilities in affluent areas characterized by low morbidity (Tudor Hart, 1971: 405).

Box 2 Advantages and disadvantages of private systems of health care

Advantages

- Liberal citizenship/choice
- Market: best mechanism for regulating any distribution
- Similar-quality care for low price; better care for higher price
- Direct service and short waiting lists
- Improvements stimulated by market
- Patients = consumers, i.e. know their rights

Disadvantages

- Choice only for those who can pay
- Health insurance market does not equate health care market
- Many cannot afford the higher price
- Inverse-care law: services concentrated
- Improvement stimulated by profit, not need
- Patients still depend on doctors' opinion

expect that more people will come forward with relatively minor complaints.

Box 2 shows some of the main advantages and disadvantages of private health care. For example, in the first advantage, 'liberal citizenship/choice', Americans have the freedom to shop around for their health care; they can decide to have an all-inclusive insurance or only insure for hospital treatment. They are not told by the state what they must do; this is a very political argument. The first disadvantage, 'choice only for those who can pay', refers to the fact that many Americans do not have access to proper health care, and therefore no choice at all. In the USA, only people with enough money or a good health insurance scheme can buy the best available medical care. Consequently, people who have a good medical insurance cover have little incentive to seek lower prices for health care. This is one of the reasons why the system is so expensive. Finally, an issue concerning doctors directly is the extent to which patients have a choice. For example, someone with lower back pain can opt for

physiotherapy, chiropractic or drug treatment. However, this is not a completely free choice, since most patients are unable to judge the quality and the usefulness of the services on offer (see pp. 88–89). Furthermore, the increase in patients' complaints and litigation indicates that patients are dissatisfied with the services provided. However, this is not completely a problem of private medicine, since the number of complaints and court cases in the UK is also on the increase.

Paying the doctor

These are observations of imperfections in the different ways of organizing health care, not judgements about these systems. Similarly, there is no right way of fixing the doctor's payment. Every method has significant disadvantages: a fee-for-service payment may have the effect of encouraging some doctors to advise more treatment than is really necessary, whereas payment on a capitation basis, i.e. number of patients on the roll, may mean that doctors are in too much of a hurry to give adequate individual attention to each patient.

Convergence

There appears to be a tendency for the different models of health care provision to converge. In the 1990s the Clinton administration pushed for reforms in the health care system that would increase the role of the state, while in countries with a national health care system (e.g. the UK) or national health insurance system (e.g. Germany), governments are trying to increase the role of the market (see Case study).

Case study

In 2000 the UK Secretary of State for Health signed an official concordat with the private health care sector. The arrangement meant that regional health authorities/boards were, for the first time, able to make local contracts with the private health care sector. In this way NHS patients could benefit from spare capacity in the private sector (see pp. 154–155).

- In what ways is the government of your country involved in the provision of health care?

- What are the main differences in the way health care is organized in the USA, Germany and the UK?

Organizing and funding health care

- The organization of a nation's health care system is closely related to the way it is funded.
- Both public and private health care and health-funding systems have specific advantages and disadvantages
- It seems as if the different health care systems are converging (http://devdata.worldbank.org/wdi2006/contents/index2.htm).

Assessing needs

The health services are constantly in a state of flux due to alterations at the supply side of care, for example, the appearance of new drugs, the introduction of new medical technology and attempts to make services more efficient and effective. Health services are also changing through alterations in demand, for example, the changing composition of the population, as people live longer (see pp. 16–17), migration flows change (see pp. 48–49) or new diseases appear (HIV/AIDS in the late 20th century) and preferences and expectations among consumers change for certain kinds of treatment. Somewhere in this pool of potentially conflicting interests we have to establish the needs of individuals, communities and populations whilst ensuring that each receives maximum benefit within the limits of available resources, such as staff, buildings and funding (Powell, 2006).

Different kinds of need

The first distinction to make is the difference between the need for health and the need for health care. The former refers to the World Health Organization (1946) definition of health as 'all aspects of physical and mental well-being'. The latter refers to the ability to benefit from health care or prevention services. It is therefore more specific and, as such, will depend on the health care and preventive services (potentially) available.

The need for needs assessment

Why does a service provider, a policy-maker, a doctor or a hospital manager set about identifying the needs of people? Providers of health care need to know: (1) what users need in the way of health care; and (2) what is needed in a particular area, in order to achieve an improvement in the health of the population. These two objectives are not the same. What potential or actual service users feel they need (Fig. 1) might only partially overlap with what policy-makers consider to be the best possible range of services in an area that can improve the health of the people there (normative needs). Both types have to be distinguished from

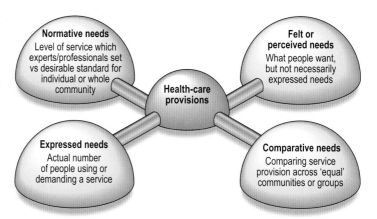

Fig. 1 Types of needs in health care provision (from Bradshaw, 1972, with permission).

expressed needs, the actual use or demand for a service, and *comparative needs*, which compare services across similar communities or client groups; for example, comparing the services available to people with HIV and those with cancer, or comparing services available in New York with those in Washington DC. Thus need is not a unified concept.

Needs assessment

It is difficult to assess all needs at the same time, since needs assessment exercises require funding and can be time-consuming, like any other piece of research. Consequently, needs assessments usually focus on a specific illness and a limited area of care, thus assessing the needs of a particular group of (potential) patients in order to determine how their need might be met. When we consider the needs of the population in a given area we also have to ask questions such as: 'Whose needs do we take into consideration?' and 'Are we looking at the present needs of people currently ill or the potential future needs of the total population?' The assessment of the needs of the local population should also be performed on a regular basis, since a population changes over time, and their actual or perceived needs might change. Planning health care provision takes time, whether it be training of doctors and nurses or building hospitals. Changing funding from one type of health service to another, such as the transformation from hospital care to community-based services, is also time-consuming.

Thus one of the main issues is: 'How do we firstly define, and secondly

measure, need?' The next main questions are: 'Who should perform a needs assessment?' and 'Whose definition of 'needs' is it to be based on: (1) lay people; (2) professionals; (3) researchers; (4) politicians; (5) managers; or (6) a combination of groups?'

One main issue in needs assessment exercises is the way one measures health needs. We can focus on all people (healthy or unhealthy), or only on those with the specific disease or illness. The former is the most equal way of assessing the overall need in a population, whereas the latter ensures that those who know what it is to have a particular illness help to establish an overview of the needs of its sufferers. Both approaches also have drawbacks. Asking a sample of all people to identify needs will result in highlighting the need for provisions related to more common illnesses and related health services, and will underrepresent specific needs for people with rarer or less acceptable conditions (Hopton & Dlugolecka, 1995). Conducting a needs assessment among people with specific conditions will highlight needs that might be specific to them only, but not to the general population or to people with other conditions. Thus, although previous users are likely to have a bias towards existing services, non-users are likely to lack experience and knowledge of the topic and will generally opt for provision for more common conditions.

How a needs assessment is conducted can have an influence on its outcome. An uncritical social marketing approach may lead to more service for the general population, at the expense of specific services for those most in distress.

The case study shows that all the needs assessed by different people have a role to play in the provision of health services.

It is important to remember that a prediction of more pregnancies in a certain area does not automatically mean that more hospital beds and doctors are needed to cope with the increase in deliveries. Different illnesses require different approaches to service provision, and the needs assessment itself might vary according to the illness in question. It is likely that service users have less input in a needs assessment of hospital-based orthopaedic surgery than in one of community-based mental health care.

Unmet and unlimited needs

There is a potential problem of unmet needs, as well as unlimited needs. The former issue refers to missing out people in assessing needs, whilst the latter refers to whether we will be able to fulfil the needs we identify in a needs assessment exercise. Asking people about their health problems in order to identify unmet needs might raise expectations about the service they expect to receive, but which we cannot provide.

In Figure 2 three circles represent needs, demand and supply. Demand in this figure can be seen as the expressed needs mentioned above. Figure 1 indicates that there might be needs that are not recognized as such by those who have them. This implies that people other than the users have conducted the needs assessment.

The realization that health needs are far more than demands from patients presented to the medical profession gave rise to the idea of a clinical iceberg or iceberg of disease. From a social science perspective the concept of an iceberg of disease is an indication that different perceived needs in different groups of people can lead to different reactions; some will result in seeking medical help while others will lead to self-medication or are simply ignored.

STOP THINK
- Can lay people assess their own health care needs?

STOP THINK
Considering the case study on the organization of maternity care, what do you think will be the main needs identified by the following groups?
- GPs in the community
- Obstetricians in the regional hospital
- Regional health administrators
- Local politicians
- Community midwives
- Pregnant women
- Women of child-bearing age but not currently pregnant

Remember to have another look at the spread on pp. 4–5.

Needs assessment and users

Needs assessment cannot be left completely to users: for example, recreational drug users might not feel that they have a drugs problem, so a needs assessment exercise conducted among this group would indicate that there is no need for a problem drug service. However, a small proportion of these recreational drug users will develop problems in the near future, leading to a need for specific drug services. Furthermore, needs assessment has to be linked to the provision of services. If needs assessments are conducted in different health and social services areas, we (society as a whole, i.e. our politicians) have to decide which of those needs have priority over others.

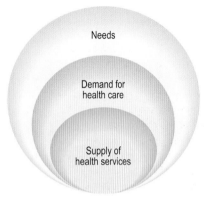

Fig. 2 The relationship between needs, demand and supply.

Case study

The organization of maternity care
Epidemiologists and policy-makers can establish the likely number of healthy babies that will be born in a city, region or any other area. This estimate will be based on: (1) the number of women of child-bearing age in the area; and (2) the birth rate for that area, subtracting the likely number of mothers and babies needing specialist obstetric care before, during or after the delivery.

This information in itself will not be sufficient to predict the need for maternity services in the area. We need to ask women and their partners how and where they want the maternity services to provide health care. Do women want a predominantly midwife-led care, or do they want GP maternity care, or do they want shared care between doctors and midwives, or shared care between obstetricians and GPs? A further set of questions is: Where should these maternity services be delivered – at home, in a GP maternity unit, in a midwifery unit, or in a specialist obstetric hospital?

Assessing needs
- There is a difference between the need for health and the need for health services.
- There are four ways of defining need: normative need, felt need, expressed need and comparative need.
- Needs assessment should include the views of different stakeholders, including service users (i.e. patients), as well as lay public, professionals, managers, politicians and researchers.
- Needs assessment runs the risk of raising people's expectations and of not having the resources to meet them.

Setting priorities and rationing

The medical profession often has to prioritize treatment and ration services at a patient level. Any practising doctor can tell a personal story of having to choose between patients because resources are limited – whether staff, money, theatres or organ donors.

Rationing of health care has always taken place, however wealthy the country, but until recently it was done implicitly and was often invisible and inequitable (see pp. 150–151). As spending on health services has increased in most countries, discussion about priorities and rationing has become more explicit. Thus, the question is not, 'Will we have rationing?', but 'How will we organize rationing?' (Box 1).

(see pp. 150–151)

Box 1

1. A BBC survey suggests that a quarter of local health groups in England are asking patients to wait longer for hospital care to bring down NHS deficits.
2. Family doctors have been told they cannot send patients to hospital for a long list of treatments for non-urgent conditions for the last 3 months of the financial year. These include in vitro fertilization (IVF), vasectomies, varicose vein treatment, wisdom teeth and other minor operations.

This story from the BBC (9 February 2007) illustrates two typical ways of rationing in the UK: (1) increased waiting time for funded treatments; and (2) not funding selected treatments.

Setting priorities

Setting priorities implies choosing a limited number of options from a wider range and ranking these in order of importance. Following on from priority-setting is a process of rationing. Rationing is often defined as allocating scarce resources by some criteria other than the price mechanism. This does not mean that the price is not an important consideration, but that the price (or cost, which may not be the same as price) of a service, say a hip replacement, is not the only factor in the decision whether or not a patient who is in need of such surgery will receive treatment. Priority-setting is a dynamic process, and in every budget cycle new technologies and information on health outcomes are taken into consideration in setting new priorities.

Forms of rationing

Rationing is a trade-off between providing all services to a limited number of people and providing a limited number of services to all people. Rationing often involves a limitation of both the range and the volume of service provision (Box 2). Decisions regarding rationing also have to be made at different levels: at an individual, local/regional and national level.

A variety of rationing mechanisms have been identified (Klein et al., 1996):

- Denial: for example, refusing to treat people over 70 years of age for certain conditions
- Deterrence: putting up social, economic or psychological barriers

---

Box 2

Neonatal care may become too expensive: Doctors at Sheffield's main maternity unit have been told that if demand for neonatal services continues to rise an 'arbitrary ban' may have to be introduced according to Panorama, a British television documentary programme. This could mean that babies born more than 15 weeks prematurely could be refused treatment.

This cutting from the *British Medical Journal* (1994; 309: 282) highlights limited availability of resources and the ever-growing demand for medical services.

- Dilution: prescribing cheaper non-brand-name drugs, or reducing length of stay in hospital
- Delay: hospital waiting lists
- Deflection: having GPs as gate-keepers, or referring an elderly person for local authority services rather than keeping him/her in hospital.

Free-market provision of care is often not regarded as a form of rationing. Everybody who has enough money can buy any treatment, e.g. expensive operations, privately. However, many will not have the money either to buy the service directly or to take out comprehensive private insurance. Hence, practically, the effect is similar to rationing.

Rationing: underlying principles

We now consider some of the principles that underpin rationing. The key principle is generally considered to be equity but a number of other principles are also important (Harrison & Hunter, 1994):

- Equity: ideally everyone should have a fair opportunity to attain their full health potential and, more pragmatically, no one should be disadvantaged from achieving their potential if it can be avoided. Equity could refer to access to health care, but also to healthy living conditions or equity of autonomy.
- Needs: the NHS was introduced on the principle that people should receive health services on the basis of their health and medical need rather than their ability to pay, but need is not a simple, clear concept (see pp. 152–153).
- Equality: all individuals have an equal access to health care. Should a 70-year-old smoker and heavy drinker have the same chance of getting the next available donor kidney as a 21-year-old non-smoker and non-drinker?
- Effectiveness: the ability of an intervention to achieve its intended effect in those to whom it is offered (i.e. does it work?).
- Cost-effectiveness (efficiency): the effectiveness of an intervention in relation to the resources used (e.g. time, labour, equipment and materials).
- Quality-adjusted life years (QALYs): a technique for estimating the extra years of life gained from particular interventions, adjusted for the quality of the extra years. They are often combined with costs to give a cost per additional QALY, but there are many assumptions built into their calculation (see pp. 40–41).

(see pp. 152–153). ... (see pp. 40–41).

Medical consideration

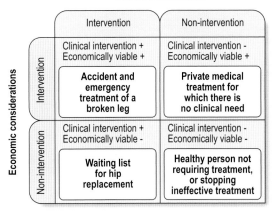

Fig. 1 Overview of medical and economic considerations in decision-making.

Decision-making

In a democracy we have to establish who should set priorities and ration services. Should it be doctors, administrators, politicians, service users, pressure groups, courts or some sort of consensus group?

Commissioning is one of the growing fields in health care, where decisions have to be made by the purchasers of health care regarding the range, quantity and quality of health services bought for a specific population at a specific time. Local NHS health care trusts and health authorities are effectively taking decisions on the rationing of services. This is a case where decision-making about priority-setting and rationing lies predominantly with the health care managers and, to a lesser extent, the medical profession, but certainly not the services users.

The National Institute for Clinical Excellence (NICE) assesses the effectiveness of drugs, treatment and medical technology in the UK. NICE is trying to balance clinical effectiveness and cost-effectiveness (www.nice.org.uk).

STOP THINK
- What principles should guide a decision to spend more money on either clinical psychology services for people with depression or hip replacement surgery, both of which have 6-month waiting lists? What information would you need to help you make a decision between them?
- What effect would using different principles have on the decision?

Consultation of users

The appeal of the Oregon experiment (see Case study 2) lies partly in its explicit approach to rationing and partly in community participation in priority-setting. It is interesting to note that prevention comes high on the priority list.

Figure 1 shows the main different forms of rationing, whereby medical and economic considerations are taken into account. The bottom left-hand corner is the situation often found in the UK, whereas the top right-hand corner is a serious possibility in countries with private medicine working for profit.

Case study 2

The Oregon experiment
The US state of Oregon pioneered a system for prioritizing health care in an attempt to address the widespread problem of the growing number of people who are without private health insurance and who are not eligible for federal assistance programmes. Most controversial of the reforms is the use by the legislature of a priority list of health services to determine benefit levels for the insurance programmes. In addition, Oregon aimed to bring cover for the rationed services to everyone in the population. Priorities were set by a Health Services Commission, initially on the basis of a technical methodology similar to 'cost per QALY', and, subsequently, on broad-based consensus through public consultation. The Commission came up with the following priorities:
- Acute, fatal conditions where treatment prevents death and leads to full recovery
- Maternity care
- Acute, fatal conditions where treatment prevents death, but does not lead to full recovery
- Preventive care for children
- Chronic, fatal conditions where treatment prolongs life and improves quality of care
- Comfort or palliative care.

The next step was for the politicians to determine how much could be funded from existing and additional sources. This clearly brought the provision of health care to the centre of the political arena, since an increase in the health budget meant an increase in taxation or a decrease in the provision of other state provisions, for example, in education. Thus the Oregon experiment introduced a rational plan for expanding services to the entire population of the state, while acknowledging the limitations of funding resources (based on Kitzhaber, 1993).

Setting priorities and rationing

- All health care systems have some inbuilt form of rationing.
- Rationing takes different forms.
- The key principles of rationing care are equity, equality, effectiveness and cost-effectiveness. Needs and value are also important but difficult to operationalize.
- Much rationing and setting of priorities takes place implicitly. Explicit rationing forces people to make difficult choices. Who makes these choices and decisions is another key issue.

Case study 1

During World War II penicillin was scarce on the battlefields. Doctors had to make decisions on which soldiers would be treated and which not. The recovery rate of getting the soldiers back to the front was considerably higher among those with a sexually transmitted infection (STI) than those with serious shot and shrapnel wounds. However, medical considerations (i.e. the highest recovery rate) were overruled by political (what people at home might think) and ethical considerations, such as 'soldiers with an STI are less deserving than those with bullet wounds'.

Community care

For 20 years, community care has been a cornerstone in the development of health services, and many doctors who previously spent their lives in hospitals are increasingly based in community settings. Community care is a concept embraced by people of all professions and political persuasions.

At its broadest, community care involves service delivery, economic policy, political rhetoric and philosophical ideology. It can be seen as a way of delivering services, of enhancing quality of life or of reducing spending by an out-of-control welfare state. It has come from the New Right in both the UK and the USA, and from a Marxist background in Italy. The development of community care throughout developed countries has come about through a variety of clinical, social and political influences (Fig. 1).

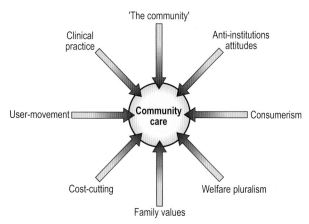

Fig. 1 Influences on community care.

The most numerous group within community care is the elderly, but it also covers people with mental health problems, and people with learning, physical or sensory disabilities. Some of the problems in discussing community care come from translating what is a generic policy to services appropriate for different patient and client groups. Guiding users through a variety of different agencies and organizations, all of which should cooperate and interrelate (Fig. 2), adds to the problem.

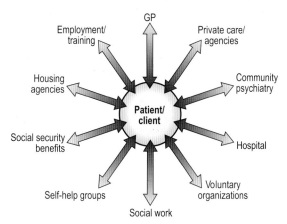

Fig. 2 Agencies with whom the patient/client may be involved.

Influences on community care

The community

There are two powerful beliefs at work here. The first is that there is a community that cares and that will accept its old, its ill and its disabled people and treat them as equal and valued members of that community. The second is that living in the community is, by definition, better than living in an institution. For those who receive good care and support, have appropriate housing and a good social network, living in the community empowers them to make choices over their lives, freed from the restrictions of institutions. For those who are ignored by their neighbours, with a very low income from benefits and little support from services, living in the community can be a nightmare existence of loneliness and poverty. Recent political emphasis on social inclusion influences the provision of services within the mainstream as far as possible.

Anti-institutions

Institutions are clearly expensive and can be dehumanizing and lead to loss of abilities, apathy and dependence (Goffman, 1968b). As the population of long-stay psychiatric patients diminished, their place was taken by the growing number of elderly people with dementia. The true meaning of asylum as sanctuary has been forgotten and, as the number of beds are cut, it can be difficult to admit patients in acute crisis.

Consumerism

The political right supports the view that market forces should dictate, services are thus needs-led not service-led. Consumers (formerly patients) are to be consulted about service delivery. The left supports consumerism more from a position of advocacy and empowerment.

Welfare pluralism

There is a move from the welfare state (in the UK, for example) towards a mixed economy of care, in which services are provided by statutory agencies, voluntary organizations and the private sector. This can incorporate means testing for certain kinds of care.

Cost-cutting

The growing elderly population means that the cost of residential care is escalating for welfare-state countries. Community care is a way of capping this cost by restricting residential care and moving costs to families. This has also involved trying to make the divide between health care and social care more distinct. In continuing care of elderly people in England and Wales, distinctions are made between medical care, which requires hospitalization, and nursing care, which can take place in nursing homes and thus is not part of free health care. In Scotland this distinction has been removed and personal care for the elderly is funded.

Family values

A return to traditional family values has been a major political theme for conservative governments in both the UK and North America for the last decade. The family is promoted as the front line of care, and services are directed at helping families care rather than replacing that care with state or private facilities (see pp. 140–141).

User movement

Although this can be linked to consumerism, it has more to do with advocacy, the promotion of patients' rights and often an antimedical, antipsychiatry model of mental health problems (see pp. 142–143).

Clinical practice

From the 1950s onwards new advances in treatment, including the introduction of phenothiazines, behaviour therapy, rehabilitation and psychosocial therapies, meant that custodial care for groups such as those with mental health problems became less relevant.

Recovery

These changes have contributed to a change in emphasis on the types of services and outcomes. In mental health services in particular there is an emphasis on recovery and the 'recovery movement'. The focus is less on the illness, but on developing a positive approach to tackling the adverse impact of having a mental health problem, with individuals seeing themselves as being able to have a positive life and being involved in their own recovery, rather then simply being passive recipients of services (Repper & Perkins, 2003).

Underlying problems

Coherence of vision

Community care requires multidisciplinary cooperation at all levels: staff and policy in housing, social work, benefits, medicine, nursing, occupational and physiotherapy, psychology and employment are all involved. Current policy requires joint planning and working between health and social services to provide seamless services to community care clients. Different professional views and priorities can cause practical problems. In mental illness, for example, the biomedical versus the social–environmental view requires radically different approaches to clients and services. A biopsychosocial approach brings these together and is advocated by many. The reality of service delivery, however, can be difficult as many agencies that have to cooperate have different views and priorities.

The role of women

By and large women relatives and friends are expected to fill the gaps left by the shortage of public service resources and provide informal care at home (see pp. 140–141). Community services tend to be staffed by low-paid, predominantly female workers with poor conditions and terms of employment.

'Them' and 'us'

The well-known NIMBY (not in my back yard) syndrome means that the community is often not willing to accept people with problems. Plans to develop hostels or sheltered housing are frequently met with local opposition.

Community care in the UK

Community care in the UK has been both defined and limited by the NHS and Community Care Act 1990, which came into operation on 1 April 1993.

Whereas previously patients were fitted into established services, now patients are to be assessed as to their needs, with services being designed and provided to meet these needs (see pp. 152–153). This ties in with who provides services. Health boards and social work departments now buy in services from the mixed economy rather than provide them themselves. Many residential establishments for the elderly, or sheltered housing for those with mental health problems, are expected to be provided by private companies or voluntary organizations rather than social work departments.

The impact of this for patients is that there is no longer free-at-point-of-delivery care by the NHS, but means-tested care through social work. Services are targeted to 'concentrate on those with greatest needs'; they should 'allow for a range of options', 'respond flexibly and sensitively to the needs of individuals and carers', and, above all, 'intervene no more than is necessary to foster independence'. Key objectives for service delivery include:

- to promote the development of domiciliary, day and respite services to enable people to live in their own homes wherever feasible and sensible
- to ensure that service providers make practical support for carers a high priority
- to make proper assessment of need and good case management the cornerstones of high-quality care
- to promote the development of a flourishing independent sector alongside good-quality public services
- to clarify the responsibilities of agencies and so make it easier to hold them to account for their performance
- to secure better value for tax-payers' money by introducing a new funding structure for social care.

STOP THINK
- Is the community willing and able to accept everyone with a problem?
- Is there a role for institutions/asylums?

Case study

Tom was born with cerebral palsy and until he was 25 was cared for by his mother. As her health deteriorated both realized that other provisions would have to be put in place. Tom took this opportunity to assert his independence; he had not done so earlier, fearing hurting his mother's feelings.

An advocate from a local advocacy service worked with him to develop and achieve his plans. Tom wanted to try living independently but was worried about being lonely. He was housed in a specially adapted flat in mainstream accommodation through a supported housing project, which provides carers to help with personal care and daily living tasks and a support worker to facilitate a social and personal life. Tom attends an employment support project where he is learning computing skills, which both aids his communication and he hopes will gain him employment. A volunteer befriender goes out with him socially, e.g. to the cinema and pub, and although he has experienced some negative behaviour and insults he is taking that in his stride. He has made many friends through the internet and enjoys the freedom the internet gives. He has a girlfriend he met through his computer classes. He looks to the future when he might get married but for the moment says he is too young to settle down.

Community care

- Community care is a generic policy.
- It is both inter- and multidisciplinary.
- It is a needs-led service.
- Community care relies on care by families.
- It places care outside institutions.

Health: a global perspective

The world has become a much smaller place as more people travel. Hence diseases spread much faster across national boundaries, as travellers are accompanied by bugs, bacteria and viruses. There were nearly 200 million international migrants (3% of the world's population) in 2006. Health scares about bird flu and severe acute respiratory syndrome (SARS) have highlighted this global mobility. Patterns in the prevalence of diseases vary by geographical location, for example, the prevalence of HIV is significantly higher in sub-Saharan Africa than in most other regions of the world.

Some use the term 'international health' others 'global health'. The word 'international' is defined in terms of crossing national borders, whereas the word 'global' encompasses the entire world. We can study different patterns of disease, but also ways of providing health care (see pp. 150–151), and health policy-making. Therefore, it is not just health *problems* that cross borders or are common to countries around the world; *solutions* can also cross borders, countries can both learn from each other and also share their own experiences and information.

We group countries into three categories using health, education and economic indicators (also known as human development index). The common practice is to group Japan, Canada, the USA, Australia, New Zealand and western Europe as 'developed' or industrialized regions, or 'first world'. All countries in South and Middle America, Africa and most in Asia are grouped together as 'developing' countries or 'third world', whilst Russia and the Eastern European countries (or 'second world') are somewhere in between. The 'developing' countries are subdivided into the 'least developed' (or 'fourth world'). The World Bank classifies countries into three categories on the basis of gross national income (GNI) per capita per year: low-income ($905 or less); middle-income ($906–$11 115); and high-income (more than $11 116).

A *developing country* tends to have the following features:
1. Agriculture is more important than manufacturing.
2. There is limited specialization and exchange.
3. There are not enough savings to finance investment.
4. The population is expanding too rapidly for available resources.
5. There is a low standard of living.

The use of terms such as 'third world', or 'low-income' or 'developed' country can create the illusion that nations are homogeneous with similar social, political and/or cultural circumstances and problems. Developing countries are not equally poor, neither is the population in even the poorest country equally poor. Moreover, terms like 'developing country', 'third world' or even 'Africa' may carry a notion of inferiority, poverty, disease, corruption and failure.

The level of development in countries has a direct effect on its population. For example, one of the characteristics of developing countries is their relatively young population; in Europe 20% is under the age of 15, in North America 22%, in Asia 34% and in Africa 45%. They represent the next generation to become sexually active (see pp. 30–31), and will affect the birth rate and population growth.

Current international health issues

There are different patterns of disease between developing and developed countries (Table 1). In high-income countries two-thirds of people live beyond the age of 70 and the main causes of mortality are chronic and non-infectious diseases. In low-income countries less than a quarter of people reach 70 and, although the causes of mortality included coronary heart disease, infectious diseases (e.g. HIV) and complications of pregnancy and childbirth continue to be major causes of death. Governments will need to prioritize (see pp. 154–155) differently to provide the health services needed to combat these different causes of death.

Box 1 suggests that malnutrition (largely due to poverty) is the single most important cause of death. The average person in a developed country will probably attribute this to famine and disasters as these get media attention (see pp. 52–53). However, for many in the third world poverty comes in a form of chronic malnutrition. This type of hunger does not make world news, but it is estimated that it takes many more lives than the better-publicised famines.

HIV relates to the second risk factor – unsafe sex. An estimated 40 million people are living with HIV. There were 4.3 million new infections in 2006, with 2.8 million (65%) of these occurring in sub-Saharan Africa. In 2006, 2.9 million people died of AIDS-related illnesses, and some 14 000 are infected each day. The AIDS epidemic has an impact on households, education, workplaces and economies, not just health and health care.

Inequality

While global health improves, inequalities in health remain and in many instances are increasing. This is the case within many countries, but also between countries, so whilst life expectancy has been improving worldwide, in sub-Saharan Africa this improvement has been halted by HIV.

The poorest 20% of people in the world are 10 times more likely to die before the age of 14 than the richest 20% (DFID, 2000). Women in the poorest countries are 500 times more likely to die in childbirth than in developed countries. Developing countries account for 84% of the world

Table 1	**Leading causes of death by broad income group (2002)**		
	Disease	**Deaths (millions)**	**% of all deaths**
High-income countries	Coronary heart disease	1.34	17.1
	Stroke and other cerebrovascular diseases	0.77	9.8
	Trachea, bronchus, lung cancers	0.46	5.8
	Lower respiratory infections	0.34	4.3
	Chronic obstructive pulmonary disease	0.3	3.9
Middle-income countries	Stroke and other cerebrovascular diseases	3.02	14.6
	Coronary heart disease	2.77	13.4
	Chronic obstructive pulmonary disease	1.57	7.6
	Lower respiratory infection	0.69	3.3
	HIV/AIDS	0.62	3
Low-income countries	Coronary heart disease	3.1	10.8
	Lower respiratory infections	2.86	10
	HIV/AIDS	2.14	7.5
	Perinatal conditions	1.83	6.4
	Stroke and other cerebrovascular diseases	1.72	6

Adapted from World Health Organization (2007).

population and 93% of the worldwide burden of disease. However, they account for only 18% of global income and 11% of global health spending.

The same inequality can be found in research, as less than 10% of global spending on health research is devoted to diseases or conditions which account for 90% of the global disease burden – this is referred to as the 10/90 gap. Poverty is the single biggest cause of preventable death in the world. It underscores lack of education, access to food, resources, medical services and adequate housing.

Globalization

Globalization refers to integration across the globe. It means that human interaction has become more intense in a range of fields including economics, health, politics, knowledge and technology transfer (Lee, 2003). It has had both positive and negative impacts on the health of poor people. New technologies and the development of health systems have resulted in a 50% reduction in child mortality in the last 20 years (DFID, 2000).

The globalization of pharmaceutical markets has increased the availability of drugs through both public and private sectors in some of the remotest areas of the world. However, pharmaceutical companies are nearly all large multinational companies which exist to make profits, but profits are much higher in countries where people have money. Therefore, these companies develop drugs for minor lifestyle issues in middle-class consumers rather than drugs for life-threatening diseases in poor populations without spending power. Moreover, the pharmaceutical industry spends millions of dollars to convince doctors to prescribe their products. Commercial information provided by sales representatives of pharmaceutical companies has greater influence than scientific sources on GPs' prescribing behaviour in developing countries.

The tobacco industry (also large multinationals) has been able to shift its focus from western countries to developing country markets, with major implications for health (see pp. 84–85).

Health care staff migration

There is a migration of trained health workers, mainly from developing to developed countries. Poor wages, economic instability, poorly funded health care systems, the burden and risks of HIV and safety concerns are other factors that 'push' nurses to leave developing countries. Additional factors 'pull' health workers to developed countries, including higher wages, better living and working conditions and opportunities for advancing their education and expertise. Some countries, despite their own domestic health care needs, cannot offer enough jobs for all health professionals

they train, thus motivating them to emigrate. However, the loss of skilled personnel (the so-called *brain drain*) is a major concern for many developing countries (Fig. 1).

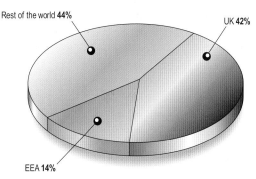

Fig. 1 New full registration of doctors in the UK by place of training (2002). EEA, European economic area.

War, terror, natural disasters and disease epidemics can all have an effect on large groups of people, either directly through disaster or war or indirectly because of displacement of people. According to the International Red Cross (IRC) over 3 million people lost their lives due to conflict and disasters over the last decade and 242 million are affected by disasters and conflicts every year. Developing countries account for three-quarter of global deaths reported due to conflicts and disasters.

STOP THINK
■ What can you give to developing countries and what can (or do) you take from developing countries?

Millennium Development Goals

The MDGs are eight goals to be achieved by 2015 that respond to the world's main development challenges. It is agreed to by all the world's countries and their leading development institutions. Three goals relate directly to health. Health is also an important contributor to several other goals (Box 2).

Although the MDGs are unlikely to be reached the last century has seen a greater improvement in health than at any time in the last three millennia.

Health: a global perspective

■ Globalization and especially air travel have made the world a smaller place, where diseases spread easier over greater distances.

■ Disease prevalence varies between high-, middle- and low-income countries.

■ Major health inequalities exist between countries, which are often made worse by factors such as health worker migration, the way pharmaceutical companies operate and/or lack of health research funding for problems specific to developing countries.

Health: a rural perspective

There are advantages, in terms of health, of living and working in rural areas, but providing appropriate health care in sparsely populated and remote areas brings its own particular challenges as well as additional costs for members of the public and health care providers alike.

Health and health care needs

There are common characteristics relating to health and health care in remote and rural areas; however it is important to remember that not all rural communities are the same. Although by definition remote and rural areas are geographically distant from urban centres and are often sparsely populated, different rural areas will have distinct demographic, geographic and socioeconomic profiles. For example, a small fishing community in Shetland will have a very different population from that of a deprived village in Wales where the main source of employment was a coalmine which closed down 15 years ago. This in turn will determine health priorities and challenges.

Although the particular health needs will vary, rural communities in developed countries often have a relatively high ageing population. Social care needs and support services then become a priority. Injuries relating to certain occupations such as farming, fishing, game-keeping or forestry are also more common in rural areas. Rural communities in many industrial countries are also becoming increasingly dependent on tourism which brings seasonal variations in health care need. This may be in the form of people with chronic conditions, accidental injury resulting from increasingly popular adventure sports or greater numbers of road traffic accidents. Research comparing the health of rural and urban populations in the UK is inconclusive and varies with type of condition. Canada and Australia, with many more remote and rural communities and generally greater travelling distance, have invested more in rural health research.

Access to health care is also complex. Rural communities may benefit from improved access to primary care compared to urban populations but

are disadvantaged in terms of access to secondary and specialized care. There is consistent evidence to suggest that people in rural areas have lower levels of health service use and that they present later with medical problems. Later presentation and diagnosis of diseases can have an impact on prognosis and morbidity and mortality.

STOP THINK
- How do you think it would be different as a doctor in a small rural town compared to a big city?

Rural communities

Service provision is often less comprehensive in rural areas compared to many urban ones, not just with regard to health care, but also education, libraries, financial services or entertainment. Service provision is poorer because of distance to (health) services, poorer public transport and the fact that transport is at the mercy of the weather. Moreover, over the past decades we have seen the decline of services in many rural areas in the UK with the closure of small schools, garages, pharmacies, pubs, post offices and the discontinuation of local bus services. Local GP surgeries and community hospitals have suffered the same fate. For example, in England the number of maternity units fell by 17.3% in an 8-year period from 341 in 1996 to 282 in 2004 (Community Health Statistics, 2006). Many of these units were located in rural parts of the country. Although it is generally accepted that it is impossible to have a full-scale academic hospital or an opera house in every village and hamlet of the country (see pp. 154–155) for reasons of economies of scale, the decline in service provision may be less acceptable to local communities.

Rural patients do expect to have to travel; they need to do so for some of their food shopping, to get to certain indoor sport facilities, schooling, library, pub or police station. Although car ownership in rural areas of the UK is higher than in the cities, there are people who have no access to a car and rely on the poorer public transport. Rural poverty is not always recognized.

This means that services are even more difficult to access for vulnerable groups in society, often those most in need. People with young children, adolescents (especially those too young to drive), elderly people without their own transport (see pp. 16–17), the disabled and the poor (see pp. 44–45) may find it hard to attend clinics and hospital appointments.

Health care in rural communities

People in small communities are more likely to know each other and each others' business. This may make it, for example, more difficult for a young person in a rural area to obtain condoms in the local chemist or to make an appointment with the local doctor to discuss drug misuse. Anonymity and confidentiality are harder to maintain, and stigma (see pp. 60–61) is harder to avoid. People in rural areas may choose to travel to a more anonymous clinic in an urban area to receive screening, testing or treatment related to, for example, mental illness, domestic violence or sexually transmitted infections.

The closeness of communities also has advantages for health. It is possible to achieve greater continuity with health care professionals and establish better relationships (Farmer et al., 2006). GPs are more familiar with the wider context of their patients' lives, families and relationships, which can lead to a better understanding and the prescription of more effective psychosocial and medical interventions. However, recent changes in the provision of out-of-hour services in the UK may have an impact on continuity of care as out-of-hours duties will not necessarily be carried out by local GPs known to the community. This will have implications for patients and health care professionals.

Providing health services is more expensive in rural areas due to fewer patient consultations per health care worker (higher staff–patient ratios) and more staff time spent on travelling. Doctors and nurses having to travel greater distances not only brings with it higher transport expenditure, but also more time wasted on sitting in cars. Training and staff development costs are also higher in rural areas for similar reasons. Health care is also more expensive to patients compared to their urban counterparts. Travel costs are higher and people are likely to have to take more time off work to attend hospital appointments, perhaps with overnight stays the day before in a hotel.

Community-level initiatives such as voluntary hospital car services are often established to help those who need it to access hospital care but this is then a cost borne by the individual and community rather than the health service. Centralization of services may result in greater efficiency for the health service but may result in an increase in indirect costs such as travel.

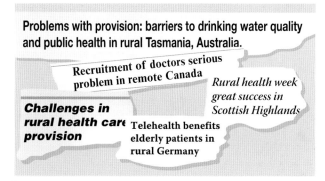

Fig. 1 Problems with rural health provision often hit the headlines.

Staffing problems

Recruitment and retention of health care staff in rural areas are problems throughout the world. Extra incentives in terms of a remote and rural allowance or relocation package can be offered to ensure key posts are filled. There is some evidence that medical students who do (part of) their training in rural areas are more likely to settle there as doctors. It is harder to keep up certain skills in rural areas, especially around rarer health care problems. For example, if recommendations are that GPs need to attend at least 12 normal deliveries a year, or do 25 minor surgical procedures, GPs in rural areas simply might not get enough practice as there are not enough patients in their catchment area needing these interventions.

One possible solution to help community-based practitioners to keep up their skills is to rotate them in a central hospital for a week or fortnight a year. This solution has the disadvantage that the rural practitioner is away from the rural community where locum cover is more difficult to organize. Some posts have been specially created for rural roaming practitioners who regularly alternate between rural practices to allow permanent GPs to maintain training, and rural fellowships offer additional training to GPs (Siderfin, 2005).

One way of providing services to dispersed populations in rural areas is using mobile services, e.g. for dentistry or breast cancer screening, more care at home, or doctors (GPs or specialists) may offer branch surgeries one morning a week or month. These services can be subject to disruption, especially during winter months when the weather is bad. Maintaining skills is a fundamental requirement but there have been suggestions of professional snobbery among hospital-based specialist staff against their rural more generalist colleagues

Centralization of health services

Even with a highly centralized service we need to consider what we need to offer in rural areas in case of an emergency. For example, over the past three decades maternity services have been more and more centralized in the UK. Many community maternity units run by midwives and/or GPs have been closed, especially in rural areas. This means more women and/or their babies have to travel greater distances when something goes wrong. Moreover, they need to travel earlier to avoid travelling in labour and as a consequence may end up waiting in the central obstetric units until labour starts. Women and their babies may be kept in hospital slightly longer after the delivery because of the long distance between where women live and their health care facility.

Similarly, services once provided by cottage hospitals such as dealing with minor injuries have now been centralized to urban hospitals. As travel is not always possible due to adverse weather conditions (e.g. in gales and bad mist helicopters cannot fly to some of the islands off the UK coast), we still need to have some kind of provision to deal with emergencies in rural areas. The UK sometimes uses flying squads, where hospital specialists come out by ambulance or air ambulance to provide emergency cover in case of, for example, road traffic accidents or obstetric emergencies. Other countries, like Australia, with its vast rural areas and low population density, have developed a flying-doctor service.

Tele-health

One possible solution for remote and rural communities has been the use of internal and computer-based technology. For example, a rural GP examining a patient with skin problems in her local practice could have a video link with a dermatologist in a teaching hospital 500 miles away. Or a woman coming in for her antenatal care check-up with a local midwife in rural Cornwall can be linked with a consultant obstetrician using tele-ultrasound. This would allow the obstetrician to help the midwife in her diagnosis and act as back-up in emergency or unexpected or unusual situations.

Rural practitioners can also use computer technology to update their skills, knowledge and competencies on a regular basis. Distance learning, whereby rural practitioners update their skills using video and internet links with trainers in central hospitals, has been promoted as a way forward. This has been helped by the extension of broadband services into remote areas.

Health: a rural perspective

- Health care needs, expectations and facilities in rural areas can differ greatly from those in urban areas.
- Working as a rural doctor brings all the advantages and disadvantages of living in a rural community.
- Anonymity and confidentiality are harder to maintain for patients and health care providers alike.
- In many high-income countries health care facilities have been centralized over the past few decades, leaving people in rural areas with fewer services, lower-quality services and/or larger travel distances and time.
- Some solutions, such as the introduction of tele-medicine, have the potential to improve rural health care.

Medical students' experience

Wherever you train to be a doctor, there are some experiences common to all medical students. These set you apart from the rest of the undergraduate population. Thinking about how you solve problems during this time should enable you to see how you might tackle challenges in the future. It will also facilitate an understanding of how other people (including patients) deal with their own difficulties.

Research into students' experience of UK medical education began in the early 1980s (Firth-Cozens, 1986; Firth, 2001) and continued into the early 1990s (Miller, 1994; Guthrie et al., 1998; McManus et al., 1999), but this impetus has not been sustained through the years of major UK curriculum reform following the publication of *Tomorrow's Doctors* (General Medical Council, 1993), and the overall research-based picture has developed only slightly over the last 10 years.

What is different about medicine?

Many of the pressures on medical students are not qualitatively different from those on other students: they worry about coursework, exams, money and relationships, but the workload is heavier and the length of the course potentially increases the burden of financial debt (Ross et al., 2006). The new developments of problem-based, self-directed learning and earlier clinical contact have been positively received by students and supervisors (Jones et al., 2002), although they require some adjustment and the time spent in preparation is not substantially less than the time spent rote-learning.

Family background may add to the pressure, since parents may have high expectations of medical student offspring. There is evidence that where this is the case, it adds to the stress experienced throughout the medical career (Brewin & Firth-Cozens, 1997; Firth-Cozens, 1998). This may operate by setting up specific personal beliefs about the need for high achievement. These then influence both feelings and behaviour, and in some individuals can lead to excessive self-criticism, which has been found to be a strong predictor of subsequent stress and depression (Firth-Cozens, 2001).

Personality influences a student's reactions to the medical course. One factor is the student's ability to tolerate ambiguity and uncertainty. Medical students are all excellent at science, but people, including patients, are often seemingly irrational and unpredictable. The realization of this fact can cause distress in students, and there is evidence that this influences career choice. Those most intolerant of ambiguity tend to choose specialties such as pathology, anaesthesiology, radiology and surgery: those with greater tolerance go into general practice and psychiatry, where they have closer contact with people.

Adjustment to university and medical school takes time. The first term seems to be stressful, as it is for many other students. Miller (1994) surveyed a complete class cohort of first-year students at Edinburgh medical school. He found that in the first term, half the class (50.3%) scored above the threshold on a screening device (the General Health Questionnaire (GHQ)) for psychological distress. By the summer term, only one-third showed these levels of distress (Fig. 1). Learning to balance social relationships and activities with heavy academic commitments was particularly stressful.

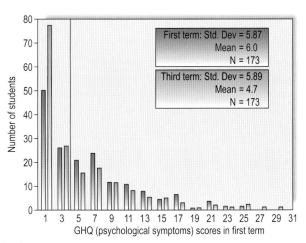

Fig. 1 Proportion of students above the General Health Questionnaire threshold in first and third term. Vertical line indicates threshold for significant psychological symptoms. (Data reproduced by permission of P Miller.)

In contrast, Moffat et al. (2004) reported that only a quarter (24.9%) of first-year Glasgow undergraduates (following a new problem-based learning curriculum) reported psychological distress (also using the GHQ-12). However, this was reversed for term 3 of year 1, when 52.4% of Glasgow medical students reported raised GHQ-12 scores. Uncertainty about individual study behaviour, progress and aptitude when coming close to exam time was the main stressor.

In the more traditional courses, the sources of stress change with clinical experience. Firth-Cozens (1986) found the item most commonly reported as 'particularly stressful' in fourth-year students in the UK was 'relationships with consultants'. A common complaint is that some senior staff teach by humiliation rather than encouragement (Moss & McManus, 1992; Allen, 1994), and some students can become so anxious that they fail to attend ward rounds. Any objective assessment of teaching would recognize this as not only grossly inappropriate and unfair, but a very poor teaching method. Reporting such incidents through a formal feedback mechanism, anonymously if necessary, would help to stop it. Discussing them with others could reduce distress. It is to be hoped that earlier introduction to clinical experience, better educational training of clinical teachers and more community-based clinical teaching have reduced these complaints but there is, as yet, no research evidence to support such a belief. Indeed, Radcliff & Lester (2003) found that it was still a major concern amongst fourth-year students, though things improved in the fifth year, when they reported being more appreciated by senior clinical staff, particularly if they were made to feel part of a team.

Coping strategies

There are some well-known maladaptive responses. One is avoidance, for example, by putting off work that is difficult. Similarly, denial and dismissal of a negative event have been found to be coping strategies that increase stress levels, not reduce them. Alcohol abuse is another poor coping strategy. Alcohol consumption amongst university students has been rising, and consumption by medical students has followed this trend (Newbury-Birch et al., 2000). This study reported that 49% of men and 43% of women were drinking above the 'low-risk' level of alcohol (respectively < 21 units/week and < 14 units/week). Alcohol use was also strongly correlated with cannabis use. In a related study, Newbury-Birch et al. (2001) report that, contrary to expectation, mean alcohol consumption, and drinking above the recommended safe limits, had increased in a cohort of medical students as they progressed from second year to final year and into their preregistration year. Although there was a negative relationship between alcohol use and anxiety levels at all 3 years, and no association between alcohol use and depression, qualified doctors have a higher than average risk of developing alcohol problems, and these student studies suggest that the habit may be established early in their medical careers.

Tackling stress can be done on all levels (see pp. 126–127). Try to deal with the source of the stress:

- Manage the workload. Prioritize what you are doing, then delegate, delay or drop things that are not urgent.
- Seek support. Talk to others. If you are worried, listen to someone else's point of view.
- Look at your thinking style. If you think that you may set unrealistic standards for yourself, try to challenge this (see pp. 136–137). Ask yourself what you would say to a friend in a similar situation, then take your own advice.
- Relax. Trying to work all the time leads to tiredness and inefficiency. Set aside time to switch off by doing something else: sport, yoga, music or seeing friends.

In the competitive environment of a medical school, students can sometimes feel inadequate. Classmates may enjoy demonstrating their knowledge and skills. Remember that the requirements for being a good doctor are diverse and not necessarily based on being the first to display textbook knowledge. For example, giving an immediate diagnosis on the basis of the initial information given by a patient can be faulty. Research on students has shown that many of them start off with a wide-ranging interview style (being unsure of possible diagnoses). They explore all possibilities. Over the course of medical school, however, they gradually use increased medical knowledge to home in early on a diagnosis. They may fail to investigate the other possibilities. In this situation, a more open-minded approach would be more appropriate.

In the early experience of clinical work, remember that you are still a student. Set realistic standards for yourself. If you have persistent thoughts about leaving medicine, it is important to talk this over with someone. You may feel great pressure from your family or a medical member of staff. It may be helpful to talk to an outsider. Most universities have counsellors or those who can offer careers guidance. It is important that the decision is yours and not dominated by feelings of duty or consideration of how much you have already invested. Remember that there are many branches of medicine that you may not have considered: the choice is not limited to general practice versus hospital medicine.

Satisfaction

Despite the demanding conditions of medical training, there are many rewards in the practice of medicine. Students and young doctors can have experience of different specialties and are likely to settle eventually in one that suits their personality and abilities. Those who derive most interest from the science can move towards laboratory research and those who enjoy the 'art' of medicine will go into specialties that include closer contact with patients. Although very

different, both types of career can bring enormous personal satisfaction.

Case study

Ian, a third-year medical student, appeared before a faculty committee appealing to stay on, despite having twice failed an exam in paediatrics. He said that he had fallen behind in studying, but assured the committee that he would not do so again.

When asked whether there were any relevant circumstances, he described a catalogue of misfortune. During his third year he had been off for several weeks with abdominal pain that eventually proved to be appendicitis and resulted in an appendectomy. Just before Christmas, his parents separated, and he kept going home at weekends to help his depressed mother. In the spring, his landlord evicted him because a drunken flatmate had smashed furniture. By the summer term, he was camping out in friends' flats, trying to study and missing many days on clinical attachments. He was extremely anxious and unable to sleep or concentrate. Having failed the exam, he attempted to revise over the summer, but had to earn money by working in a bar and made little progress.

The committee took a sympathetic view of his circumstances, but criticized him for not discussing his difficulties with a tutor and arranging to have time off officially, especially when he was ill. He was permitted to repeat his third year, but strongly advised to make contact with the accommodation service, the counselling service and his tutor. He did this and scraped through his repeated year. In subsequent years, he maintained reasonable passes and graduated successfully.

STOP THINK There is evidence that levels of anxiety and depression in students are, to some extent, predetermined by personality, but it has also been shown that teaching stress management to medical students enables them to control the symptoms of stress. Another view is that some experience of anxiety and depression may not be a bad thing anyway, since doctors who score more highly on these symptoms are more empathetic and approachable.

Given these various findings, and that lack of support from senior staff is a common complaint, should more be done for students – stress management courses, regular meetings with members of staff or support groups across years? Or is it the case that 'If you can't stand the stress, you should get out of the medical school?'

Medical students' experience

- Medical students' experience of stress is different from that of other students: at first in terms of the amount of work, then later in terms of clinical contact.
- Adaptation to medical school is influenced by family background and personality: these factors also influence career choice.
- Relationships with senior medical staff are often stressful in the clinical years.
- Students' use of alcohol to relieve stress may establish a habit that puts them at risk of becoming doctors with alcohol problems.
- If you have doubts about medicine as a career, talk it over with someone and make your own decision.

Life as a trainee doctor

Introduction

From the UK to Australia, postgraduate medical training is undergoing considerable reform (Grant, 2007, van Der Weyden, 2007; www.mmc.nhs.uk/). Consequently, some of what is written here will have changed by the time you read this. What is certain is that you will be working fewer hours than previous generations of young doctors. What has not changed is the steep learning curve required at the beginning of your first post. However, shadowing the previous trainee, a good induction and support from senior medical and nursing colleagues will all help to make this particular transition easier than it might otherwise be. This is the time when you really start to put all the theory you have learned as a medical student into practice.

Foundation programmes

In the UK, final-year medical students may apply for a place on a 2-year foundation programme via a national electronic application system (www.foundationprogramme.nhs.uk/pages/home). Most foundation programmes consist of 4 months in six different posts. The programme aims to help medical graduates to build upon what they have learned at medical school and to increase their confidence and competence as doctors. There is a national curriculum and attendance at formal teaching is compulsory throughout the 2 years. Successful completion of the first year, together with a minimum of 4 months spent in general medicine and 4 months in general surgery, is required to gain full General Medical Council registration.

The emphasis of foundation training is on acquiring generic rather than specialty-specific knowledge and skills, and time spent in a specialty is not a prerequisite for acceptance into training in that specialty. However, some trainees are convinced that they might be disadvantaged at interview by lack of experience in their chosen specialty (French et al., 2007), and it is generally held that it is important to do over and above the minimum assessment requirements if an applicant wishes to stand out when it comes to competitive entry to specialty training.

 ■ How do you think you will react to your first job? Can you predict what will give you satisfaction, and what you will find most difficult? Although medical students may be aware that the first postgraduate year can be difficult, many of them seem surprised by the demands of the early years.

Specialty training

During their second year, foundation doctors may apply for entry to specialty training. In 2007, a national electronic recruitment system was introduced, the Medical Training Application System (MTAS: www.mtas.nhs.uk/). There were considerable problems in its first year and these received wide publicity. The government set up an independent inquiry, led by Professor Sir John Tooke. The inquiry reported in January 2008 (www.mmcinquiry.org.uk/index.htm) and made 47 recommendations. One of these was to separate the first and second foundation years and to make the second year into the first year of core specialty training. However, at the time of writing, no definite decision has been made.

European working-time directive

One of the main reasons for the changes in postgraduate medical training has been the implementation of the European working-time directive. All training-grade doctors now work considerably fewer hours than they did in the past, which is a considerable improvement for doctors' health and well-being. New grades of staff such as phlebotomists and ward assistants have been employed to do some of the routine tasks that used to be done by junior doctors. Some specialties are busier than others so working some antisocial hours can still be a regular occurrence in some posts. Most foundation doctors still do out-of-hours work, although in some hospitals it has been decided to restrict this to F2 doctors only. Many foundation doctors think that this would be a mistake because the experiences they get whilst working at night can be extremely valuable. New ways of working are being introduced so that Hospital-at-Night teams (spearheaded by the Hospital-at-Night nurse practitioner) are the first port of call for ward staff rather than the foundation doctor. Foundation doctors have reported that Hospital-at-Night teams provide valuable support, allowing them to concentrate on the more difficult aspects of patient care at night (French et al., 2007).

Reduced working hours have meant that trainee doctors have less time for on-the-job learning than in the past. To compensate there is more emphasis on formal teaching away from the hospital ward and maximizing learning opportunities during working hours. There is also greater emphasis on assessment of acquired competencies. For example, foundation doctors are assessed on their practical skills and their interpersonal skills and professionalism. With advances in technology, new methods of training are becoming available all the time, which will help to make up for the reduction in working hours – for example, clinical skills laboratories.

 ■ How good are you at using your time effectively? Are you good at prioritizing your workload and seeking out learning opportunities?

Making mistakes

In medicine, it is inevitable that doctors will sometimes make mistakes, whatever their grade. The majority of serious mistakes made by young doctors are made through ignorance or inexperience; less common are mistakes through lack of information or poor communication, and tiredness. The most common mistakes are misdiagnosis (including 'deliberately' picking the least severe scenario because it is the least scary) and procedural errors. The fear of making mistakes is an important source of stress for young doctors and this is exacerbated by the fear of litigation, which is becoming increasingly common.

Senior staff will understand that you are learning so where there is doubt about clinical management, it is always wise to get another opinion. It is also important not to be overconfident as this too can result in mistakes. In general, senior staff would prefer that you asked for help rather than make a mistake, no matter how irritable or unapproachable they may appear. Senior doctors are also under pressure and they may not be around as much as they would like. If you are anxious about asking for help, overcoming your anxiety is likely to be easier than accepting that you have made a mistake.

Apart from any legal worries associated with making mistakes, there are always emotional effects. Junior doctors, in particular, experience feelings of remorse and guilt, even when they were not responsible. In good teams, the incident will be discussed so that feelings of remorse can be shared, put into perspective and lessons learned. Often junior doctors have a distorted perception of the incident, believing themselves to be wholly to blame when, in fact, they were only partly, or not at all, responsible. In most cases, the prevention of similar incidents in the future lies in good organizational practice, teamwork and support, rather than in the hands of the individual doctor. Significant-event analysis is a core part of the foundation curriculum. This will give you a valuable opportunity to look at what went wrong and why and how it can be prevented in the future. Following incidents involving a death there may have to be a discussion with the procurator fiscal or police as the death may be classified as a sudden death.

Case study

Debbie was in her first job in a teaching hospital, intending to go into paediatrics. Her boyfriend, Peter, was training in surgery 350 miles away. On one of their rare weekends together, Peter was very bitter and depressed, and expressed doubts about medicine as a career. Debbie returned after the weekend and was herself then very low. She had a difficult week during which she contracted tonsillitis. One night she admitted an elderly man but did not realize the severity of his unstable angina. He was not treated and died in the early hours of the morning. Although a more senior member of staff said that this was likely to have happened even with appropriate treatment, her consultant implied that she was negligent in front of nursing staff. She was devastated and decided to give up hospital medicine and go into general practice, where she would be away from hospitals and able to be nearer Peter. On telephoning him, she learned that he had decided to leave surgery. Being now less concerned about her consultant's reference, she took time off to recover from tonsillitis. She then went to stay with Peter for the weekend and told him what had happened. He was sympathetic and helped put the incident in perspective.

A year later, Debbie was in another teaching hospital in paediatrics, and despite regularly working extra hours, was enjoying good clinical supervision and had resumed her original career plans. Peter was in medical publishing and only 60 miles away.

Several factors had helped her to get through her crisis: the temporary relief of knowing that she could leave hospital medicine if she wanted to; taking time off to recover from illness; catching up on sleep; and talking about her misery. Her next job was one with better senior support, she was nearer to Peter and this was enough to sustain her in working towards her career in paediatrics.

How can you prepare to cope?

You can approach this stressful situation in the same way as other difficulties (see pp. 126–127). Looking at three different aspects may help you: these are cognitions, feelings and behaviour.

Cognitions

- Put the situation in perspective: you are still learning and your confidence and competence will steadily improve.
- Focus on what you have achieved on a day-to-day basis. Junior doctors are highly skilled and play a vital part in the clinical team.
- Some mistakes are inevitable: what is important is to learn from them and to assess them objectively. It will help to discuss them with other people, either your peers or senior colleagues.
- Think about what you want from your career. Do you want to: be an eminent specialist, have a good work–life balance, work in the community or get involved in teaching? You may want to be in a specific geographical location for a variety of reasons and this may require some compromises regarding specialty choice. Make choices that fit in with your own needs.

Feelings

- Discuss feelings with others in a similar situation, whether these are feelings of pleasure, fatigue, disillusionment, guilt, incompetence, pride or anger.
- Discuss feelings with friends, partner or family. They may not know what it is like, but they can still empathize with you and it may help them to understand your situation.

Behaviour

- Look after your health. Try to rest when you can and to eat properly whenever possible. If you are ill, despite the culture of working through illness, take time off and see a doctor if necessary.
- Find good ways to unwind: going away, going out, taking exercise, reading, watching television, socializing. Do whatever works for you.
- Seek support from others: junior medical staff at work, friends and family at home.

 STOP THINK

- Remember that you are still learning and may be unsure of what to do. Will you be willing to ask for help from more senior members of medical or nursing staff? Why might this be difficult?

Life as a trainee doctor

- Long hours have been shown to affect young doctors' cognitive performance, mood, general health and functioning.
- Stressful factors reported by young doctors are having too much responsibility, the effects of work on their personal life and concern about making mistakes.
- Mistakes happen most often through ignorance and inexperience. It is important to seek help, however uncomfortable this may be.
- Most junior doctors feel useful and are satisfied with their choice of medicine as a career.
- Stress management techniques can be helpful: focus on cognitions, feelings and behaviour.

The profession of medicine

Being a medical student means learning about the discipline of medicine. However, more is learnt that is not part of the official medical curriculum. Implicit in medical training is showing students how to behave and act as doctors. Your medical education is a socialization into medicine. Socialization refers to a new recruit being exposed to the predominant norms (expected ways of behaving) and values of an occupation, and gradually absorbing these ideas until they become 'natural'. Students, for example, learn to take decisions, to deal or cope with cutting up bodies in pathology practicals, but also to adhere to a dress code on the wards, or to talk to patients and staff in a certain way. In other words, one learns to become a medical professional as much as a medical doctor.

The nature of professions

Professions are an important element in the organization of medical care and the structure of society. The former refers to the position that the medical profession has in the health services; the latter refers to the way professions are regarded as special occupations in society. We could ask: 'What do professionals such as doctors, clergy and lawyers have in common?' or 'What is the difference between doctors and rubbish collectors, two occupations we cannot really do without?' (Fig. 1).

There are two main perspectives on the origin and nature of professions. Professions, in the older of the two perspectives, represent the institutionalization of altruistic values, since the professions are seen as committed to providing services for the common good. Thus, stockbrokers and company directors differ from teachers, lawyers and doctors in that the former occupations consist of people working for an immediate personal gain, be it money, prestige or promotion. The latter occupations consist of people who are motivated not only by personal interest or by financial gains. Those engaged in a profession are often said to have a vocation, or a calling. Sociologists who studied professions in the 1950s drew up lists of characteristics of professions as opposed to other occupations. Greenwood (1957) developed one such list:

1. Systematic theory
2. Authority recognized by its clientele
3. Broader community sanction
4. Code of ethics
5. Professional culture sustained by formal sanctions.

The medical profession incorporates all the above features:

1. It has a theoretical basis.
2. Patients come to doctors for advice/help, and also governments come to the medical profession for advice/help.
3. No one is allowed to practise medicine without a licence.
4. The Hippocratic oath and the Declaration of Geneva are its code of ethics.
5. It has strong professional organizations that guard the quality of the work done by its members, leaving it relatively free of lay evaluation or legal contracts.

Continuous professional development, the doctor's obligation to keep up to date in both skills and knowledge, is part of this professional culture.

Professions and competition

More recent thinking approaches professions from the notion of *autonomy*, which is based on the profession being able to exercise power and control over, for example, other occupations, policy-makers and clients (Turner, 1995). Such approaches emphasize competition between different occupations. For example, the crucial feature of the division of labour in health care is the control that doctors exercise over their own work and that of allied occupations. The original function of nursing, for example, was to serve the doctor. Today nursing has developed to a more autonomous profession with its own education (with professors of nursing in many universities), field of knowledge, control over its members and some power to exclude other occupations from its area of expertise. The maintenance of the medical profession requires the continuing exercise of dominance over allied and competing occupations. As a result the medical profession can be seen to possess an officially approved monopoly of the right to define health and illness, and to treat illness. For example, in many countries it is illegal to practise medicine without a licence.

Depending on which approach one takes, a profession is defined as either an altruistic occupation serving the common good or a particularly successful competitor in the occupational arena. Perhaps we can see elements of both approaches at different times or in different types of doctors.

In many countries doctors belong to the best-paid categories of professionals. One way of being able to guarantee jobs for medical graduates is to limit the intake of students. Matching the supply of and demand for doctors maintains a sense of exclusiveness and enables the medical profession to claim a high remuneration.

Professions can be seen as occupations that somehow reduce risk and uncertainty in our lives. The priest, the lawyer and the doctor look after our soul, our well-being and/or our body. Some have argued that this factor gives these occupations a higher status in society.

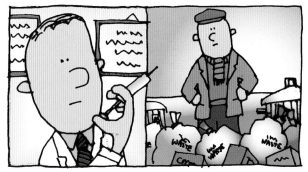

Fig. 1 Which is more important for public health?

STOP THINK ■ What makes medicine a profession rather than just an occupation?

The organization of the medical profession

Doctors in nearly every country have a strong professional organization, which acts both as an advisory body to governments and the public and as a trade union. The medical view is often aired in prestigious medical journals, which are in themselves part of the organization of the profession. More significantly, such medical journals are regarded as important by the general population and government officials, which makes them highly influential. The importance and influence of professions are not so much based on their claims as on society's reaction to these claims. Aromatherapists, clinical psychologists, kinesiologists and faith healers make claims that are often not dissimilar to those made by doctors, but most people in industrialized societies put their faith most of the time in the medical profession and not in the other healers.

Challenges to medical autonomy

The medical profession is self-regulating in many countries, and in the UK it is regulated by the General Medical Council. Doctors often argue that the only person who can evaluate the work of a doctor is a fellow doctor. However, medical autonomy has been increasingly challenged and eroded in recent years:

- The state has varying degrees of control over professionals, such as regulating their income, training or the right to practise.
- Hospital administrators/managers and health insurance companies have a certain amount of control over doctors. Managers can direct funding from one medical specialty to another, or from hospital- to community-based practitioners, while insurance companies can influence the kind and amount of medical interventions conducted.
- Challenges have also come from the professionalization of other paramedical occupations, particularly nursing.
- Within medicine, there have been attempts to change the hierarchical structure of the profession and to embrace complementary therapies such as homeopathy and acupuncture.
- Consumers (and patients) have begun to question the kind of services they receive. In the UK the introduction of the Patient Charter has changed the balance towards the lay public. Moreover, the internet has given patients easier access to medical information, guidelines, government reports and policy documents.
- The effectiveness of medical treatments has been challenged and the number of complaints against doctors has increased, and the number of court cases against doctors, especially in the USA, has made indemnity insurance very costly. The consequence of all these societal factors is that doctors have increasingly limited autonomy over medical issues.
- Negative media publicity has also led to calls for more control over the medical profession (see pp. 52–53).

 STOP THINK ■ How altruistic is medicine as a profession?

 STOP THINK ■ What does it mean to be a professional?

Box 1 **The World Medical Association Declaration of Geneva: physician's oath**

At the time of being admitted as a member of the medical profession:

I solemnly pledge to consecrate my life to the service of humanity;

I will give to my teachers the respect and gratitude which they are due;

I will practise my profession with conscience and dignity; the health of my patients will be my first consideration;

I will maintain by all means of power the honour and the noble traditions of the medical profession; my colleagues will be my brothers;

I will not permit considerations of religion, nationality, race, party politics or social standing to intervene between my duty and my patient;

I will maintain the utmost respect of human life from the time of conception, even under threat; I will not use my medical knowledge contrary to the laws of humanity;

I make these promises solemnly, freely and upon my honour.

Case study

The development of the medical profession in the UK

It was only as the 19th century progressed that doctors became the dominant group in treating illness. The British Medical Association was founded in 1832, and one of its roles was to transform the status of medicine into a profession ranking with other learned professions.

After 15 unsuccessful attempts to convince parliament that doctors could be trusted with monopoly powers, the 1858 Medical Act unified the profession, combining surgeons, physicians and apothecaries, and created the General Medical Council, which was empowered to keep a register of qualified practitioners. As a result, employment positions were increasingly open only to registered doctors, particularly those posts controlled by the state's Poor Law hospitals and by the mutual Friendly Societies that provided insurance protection and medical care to working-class patients, often through trade unions. In 1911, again after successful political lobbying, the National Insurance Act brought the control of these Friendly Societies under local health committees with strong medical representation, thereby reducing the degree of external and lay control over these doctors' activities.

The profession of medicine

- Professionals are said to work towards professional standards, which are higher than the standards to which other occupations work.
- Professional standards combine an element of altruism with a well-developed system of quality control.
- Students are socialized into the profession.
- The state is the most limiting factor on professional freedom.
- The rise in importance of managers, other health practitioners and patients has eroded the professional power of doctors.

References

Abraham HD, Aldridge AM 1993 Adverse consequences of lysergic-acid diethylamide. Addiction 88: 1327–1334

Abraham C, Sheeran P 2003 Acting on intentions: the role of anticipated regret. British Journal of Social Psychology 42: 495–511

Abraham C, Sheeran P 2005 Health belief model. In: Conner M, Norman P (eds) Predicting health behaviour: research and practice with social cognition models, 2nd edn. Open University Press, Buckingham, UK

Acheson D 1998 Independent inquiry into inequalities in health. The Stationery Office, London

Addington-Hall JM, Higginson IJ 2001 Palliative care for non-cancer patients. Oxford University Press, Oxford

Ahmedzai S 1982 Dying in hospital: the residents viewpoint. BMJ 285: 712-714

Ainsworth MDS, Blehar MC, Waters E et al. 1978 Patterns of attachment. Erlbaum, Hillsdale, NJ

Ajzen I 1991 The theory of planned behavior. Organisational Behaviour and Human Decision Processes 50: 179–211

Albrecht GL, Devlieger PJ 1999 The disability paradox: high quality of life against all odds. Social Science and Medicine 48: 977–988

Alder EM 2002 How to assess quality of life: problems and methodology. In: Schneider HPG (ed.) Hormone replacement therapy and quality of life. Parthenon Publishing, Lancaster

Allbutt H, Amos A, Cunningham-Burley S 1995 The social image of smoking among young people in Scotland. Health Education Research 10: 443–454

Allen I 1994 Doctors and their careers: a new generation. Policy Studies Institute, London

Alonzo AA, Reynolds NR 1995 Stigma, HIV, and AIDS: an exploration and elaboration of a stigma trajectory. Social Science and Medicine 41: 303–335

American Psychiatric Association 2000 Diagnostic and statistical manual of mental disorders IV – text revision (DSM-IV-TR). American Psychiatric Association, Washington

Andersen BL, Cacioppo JT, Roberts DC 1995 Delay in seeking a cancer diagnosis: delay stages and psychophysiological comparison processes. British Journal of Social Psychology 34: 33–52

Anderson P 2007 A safe, sensible and social AHRSE: New Labour and alcohol policy. Addiction 102: 1515–1521

Anderson P, Baumberg B 2006 Alcohol in Europe: a public health perspective. Brussels: European Commission. http://ec.europa. eu/health-eu/news_alcoholineurope_en.htm, accessed 15/5/07

Anionwu EN 1993 Sickle cell and thalassaemia: community experiences and official response. In: Ahmad W (ed.) 'Race' and health in contemporary Britain. Open University Press, Buckingham

Armitage CJ, Conner M 2001 Efficacy of the theory of planned behaviour: a meta-analytic review. British Journal of Social Psychology 40: 471–495

Armstrong D 1994 An outline of sociology as applied to medicine. Butterworth/ Heinemann, London

ASH 2006a Smoking statistics: illness and death – fact sheet 2. ASH, London

ASH 2006b Secondhand smoke – fact sheet 8. ASH, London

ASH 2006c The economics of tobacco – fact sheet 16. ASH, London

ASH 2007 Smoking statistics: who smokes and how much – fact sheet 1. ASH, London

Astin J 1998 Why patients use alternative medicine: results of a national study. Journal of the American Medical Association 279: 1548–1553

Astley-Pepper M 2005 Social erosion or isolation in palliative care. In: Nyatanga B, Astley-Pepper M (eds) Hidden aspects of palliative care. Quay Books, London, pp.74–86

Audit Commission 1993 What seems to be the matter: communication between hospitals and patients. HMSO, London

Aveyard P, West R 2007 Managing smoking cessation. British Medical Journal 335: 37–41

Azoulay E, Pochard F, Kentish-Barnes N et al. 2005 Risk of post-traumatic stress symptoms in family members of intensive care unit patients. American Journal of Respiratory and Critical Care Medicine 171: 987–994

BACP 2007 Ethical framework for good practice in counselling and psychotherapy. British Association for Counselling and Psychotherapy. Available online at: http:// www.bacp.co.uk/ethical_framework/

Bajekal M, Primatesh P, Prior G 2001 Health survey for England: disability. HMSO, Norwich, UK

Bandura A 1997 Self-efficacy: the exercise of control. Freeman, New York

Barry CA, Bradley CP, Britten N et al. 2000 Patients' unvoiced agendas in general practice consultations: qualitative study. British Medical Journal 320: 1246–1250

Barsky AJ, Ahern DK 2004 Cognitive behaviour therapy for hypochondriasis: a randomised controlled trial. Journal of the American Medical Association 291: 1464–1470

Barsky AJ, Saintfort R, Rogers MP et al. 2002 Nonspecific medication side effects and the nocebo phenomenon. Journal of the American Medical Association 287: 622–627

Bartholomew LK, Parcel GS, Kok G et al. 2006 Planning health promotion programs. An intervention mapping approach. Jossey-Bass, San Francisco, CA

Bartley M 2004 Health inequality. Polity Press, Cambridge

Bartley M, Blane D, Davey Smith G 1998 The sociology of health inequalities. Blackwell, Oxford

Batchelor S, Kitzinger J 1999 Teenage sexuality in the media. Health Education Board for Scotland, Edinburgh

Bates I 2001 The supply and consumption of over-the-counter drugs. In: Taylor K, Harding G (eds) Pharmacy practice. Taylor and Francis, London

Beale N, Nethercott S 1985 The health of industrial employees four years after compulsory redundancy. Journal of the Royal College of General Practitioners 37: 390–394

Beck AT 1976 Cognitive therapy of the emotional disorders. New American Library, New York

Beck JS 1995 Cognitive therapy: basics and beyond. Guildford Press, London

Beck AT, Rush AJ, Shaw BF et al. 1979 Cognitive therapy of depression. Guilford Press, New York

Becker HM, Heafner DP, Kasl SV et al. 1977 Selected psychosocial models and correlates of individual health-related behaviours. Medical Care 15 (suppl.): 27–46

Bennett-Levy JB, Butler G, Fennell M et al. 2004 Oxford guide to behavioural experiments in cognitive therapy. Oxford University Press, Oxford

Bergh C, Soderston P 1996 Anorexia nervosa, self-starvation and the reward of stress. Nature Medicine 2: 21–22

Berkman LF, Breslow L 1983 Health and ways of living: the Alameda County Study. Oxford University Press, Oxford

Bibace R, Walsh ME 1980 Development of children's concepts of illness. Pediatrics 66: 912–917

Biener L, Harris JE, Hamilton W 2000 Impact of the Massachusetts tobacco control programme: population based trend analysis. British Medical Journal 321: 351–354

Biggs S 1999 The mature imagination: dynamics of identity in midlife and beyond. Open University Press, Buckingham

Bissell P, May CT, Noyce PR 2004 From compliance to concordance: barriers to accomplishing a re-framed model of health care interactions. Social Science and Medicine 58: 851–862

Bisson JI, Ehlers A, Matthews R et al. 2007 Psychological treatments for chronic post-traumatic stress disorder. Systematic review and meta-analysis. British Journal of Psychiatry 190: 97–104

Blaxter M 1987 Self reported health. In: Cox BD (ed.) The health and life style survey. Health Promotion Trust, London

Blaxter M 1990 Health and lifestyles. Tavistock Routledge, London

Blaxter M, Paterson E 1982 Mothers and daughters: a three-generation study of health attitudes and behaviour. Heinemann, London

Bloor M, McKeganey NP, Finlay A et al. 1992 The inappropriateness of psycho-social models of risk behaviour for understanding HIV-related risk practices among Glasgow male prostitutes. Aids Care 4: 131–137

Booth-Kewley S, Vickers RR Jr 1994 Associations between major domains of personality and health behavior. Journal of Personality 62: 281–298

Bosley CM, Fosbury JA, Cochrane GM 1995 The psychological factors associated with poor compliance with treatment in asthma. European Respiratory Journal 8: 899–904

Bower P, Rowland N 2006 Effectiveness and cost effectiveness of counselling in primary care. Cochrane Database of Systematic Reviews, 2. Article no. CD001025. 10.1002/14651858. CD001025.pub2

Bowlby J 1969 Attachment and loss. vol. 1. Attachment. Hogarth Press, London

Bowlby J 1998 Attachment and loss, vol. 3. Loss, sadness and depression. Pimlico, London

Bowling A 1995a Measuring disease: A review of disease-specific quality of life measurement scales. Open University Press, Buckingham

Bowling A 1997 Measuring health: a review of quality of life measurement scales. Open University Press, Buckingham

Bowling A 2007 Quality of life assessment. In: Ayers S, Baum A, McManus C et al. (eds) Cambridge handbook of psychology, health and medicine, 2nd edn. Cambridge University, Cambridge, UK

Boyce T 2007 Health, risk and news: the MMR vaccine and the media. Peter Lang, Oxford

Bradshaw J 1972 A taxonomy of social need. In: McLachlan G (ed.) Problems and progress in medical care, 7th series. Oxford University Press, Oxford

Bramley G, Doogan K, Leather P et al. (eds) 1987 Homelessness and the London housing market. School for Advanced Urban Studies, Bristol

Brandstater J, Greive W 1994 The ageing self: stabilising and protective processes. Developmental Review 14: 52–80

Brewin CR 2001 A cognitive neuroscience account of posttraumatic stress disorder and its treatment. Behaviour Research and Therapy 39: 373–393

Brewin CR 2003 Post-traumatic stress disorder: malady or myth? Yale University Press, New Haven

Brewin CR, Firth-Cozens J 1997 Dependency and self-criticism as predicting depression in junior doctors. Journal of Occupational Health 2: 242–246

Brown G, Davison S 1978 Social class, psychiatric disorder of mother and accidents to children. Lancet 1: 368–380

Brown GW, Harris T 1978 Social origins of depression. Tavistock Publications, London

Brown GW, Moran PM 1997 Single mothers, poverty and depression. Psychological Medicine 27: 21–33

Brown G, Brolchain M, Harris T 1975 Social class and psychiatric disturbance among women in an urban population. Sociology 9: 225–254

Buckman R 1994 How to break bad news. Pan Macmillan, London

Bunton R, Burrows R 1995 Consumption and health in the 'epidemiological' clinic of late modern medicine. In: Bunton R, Nettleton S, Burrows R (eds) The sociology of health promotion. Routledge, London

Burgess C, O'Donohoe A, Gill M 2000 Agony and ecstasy: a review of MDMA effects and toxicity. European Psychiatry 15: 287–294

Burish TG, Jenkins RA 1992 Effectiveness of biofeedback and relaxation training in reducing the side effects of cancer chemotherapy. Health Psychology 11: 17–23

Burton B 2003 Complementary medicines industry in crisis after recall of 1546 products. British Medical Journal 326: 1001

Bytheway B 1995 Ageism. Open University Press, Buckingham

Cabinet Office 2007 Early intervention. Prof. David Olds of the USA shares experiences and ideas with English audience. Available online at: www.cabinetoffice.gov.uk/social_exclusion_task_force/news/2007/070515_olds.aspx

Calman KC 1984 Quality of life in cancer patients – an hypothesis. Journal of Medical Ethics 10: 124–127

Calnan M 1987 Health and illness: the lay perspective. Tavistock, London

Campbell DA, Yellowlees PM, McLennan G et al. 1995 Psychiatric and medical features of near fatal asthma. Thorax 50: 254–259

Cannon WB 1931 Again the James–Lange and the thalamic theories of emotion. Psychological Review 38: 281–295

Carey MP, Burish TG 1988 Etiology and treatment of the psychological side effects associated with cancer chemotherapy: a critical review and discussion. Psychological Bulletin 104: 307–325

Carpenter PA, Just MA, Shell P 1990 What one intelligence test measures: a theoretical account of the processing in the Raven Progressive Matrices Test. Psychological Bulletin 97: 404–431

Carpenter M, Nagell K, Tomasello M et al. 1998 Social cognition, joint attention, and communicative competence from 9 to 15 months of age. Monographs of the Society for Research in Child Development 63(4)

Carson AJ, Ringbauer B, MacKenzie L et al. 2000 Neurological disease, emotional disorder, and disability: they are related: a study of 300 consecutive new referrals to a neurology outpatient department. Journal of Neurology, Neurosurgery and Psychiatry 68: 202–206

Carver CS, Pozo C, Harris SD et al. 1993 How coping mediates the effect of optimism on distress: a study of women with early stage breast cancer. Journal of Personality and Social Psychology 65: 375–390

Cassileth B 1998 The social implications of questionable cancer therapies. Cancer 63: 1247–1250

Cattell RB 1971 Abilities: their structure, growth and action. Houghton Mifflin, Boston

Chadwick DJ, Gillat DA, Gingell JC 1991 Medical or surgical orchidectomy: the patients' choice. British Medical Journal 302: 572

Chaiken S 1980 Heuristic versus systematic information processing and the use of source versus message cues in persuasion. Journal of Personality and Social Psychology 37: 1397

Champion VL 1994 Strategies to increase mammography utilization. Medical Care 32: 118–129

Chandola T, Bartley M, Sacker A 2003 Health selection in the Whitehall II study, UK. Social Science and Medicine 56: 2059–2072

Clark D, Seymour J 1999 Reflections on palliative care. Open University Press, Buckingham

Clark M, Hampson SE, Avery L et al. 2004 Effects of a tailored lifestyle self-management intervention in patients with type 2 diabetes. British Journal of Health Psychology 9: 365–379

Clarke A 1995 Population screening for genetic susceptibility to disease. British Medical Journal 311: 35–38

Clarke V, Lovegrove H, Williams A et al. 2000 Unrealistic optimism and the health belief model. Journal of Behavioral Medicine 23: 367–376

Clement S 1995 Diabetes self-management education. Diabetes Care 18: 1204–1214

Clinical Standards Board for Scotland 2001 Schizophrenia. CSBS, Edinburgh

Cohen S, Herbert TB 1996 Health psychology: psychological factors and physical disease from the perspective of psychoneuroimmunology. Annual Review of Psychology 47: 113–142

Coker N (ed.) 2002 Understanding race and racism in medicine. An agenda for change. King's Fund Publishing, London

Coleman J, Hendry L 1999 The nature of adolescence, 3rd edn. Routledge, London

Coleman P, Bond J, Peace S 1993 Ageing in the twentieth century. In: Bond J, Coleman P, Peace S (eds) Ageing in society: an introduction to social gerontology, 2nd edn. Sage, London

Collison D, Dey C, Hannah G et al. 2007 Income inequality and child mortality in wealthy nations. Journal of Public Health 29: 114–117

Colom R, Lluis-Font JM, Andrés-Pueyo A 2005 The generational intelligence gains are caused by decreasing variance in the lower half of the distribution: supporting evidence for the nutrition hypothesis. Intelligence 33: 83–91

Colom R, Garcia-Lopez O 2003 Secular gains in fluid intelligence: evidence from the culture fair intelligence test. Journal of Biosocial Science 35: 33–39

Committee on Health Promotion 1996 Women and coronary heart disease. Guidelines for health promotion no. 45. Faculty of Public Health Medicine, London

Community Health Statistics 2006 NHS maternity statistics, England. Available online at: www.ic.nhs.uk/webfiles/publications/maternityeng2005/NHSMaternityStatistics260506_PDF.pdf

Conrad P 1985 The meaning of medications: another look at compliance. Social Science and Medicine 20: 29–37

Copeland L 2003 An exploration of the problems faced by young women living in disadvantaged circumstances if they want to give up smoking: can more be done at general practice level? Family Practice 20: 393–400

Cornwell J 1984 Hard-earned lives: accounts of health and illness from East London. Tavistock, London

Coulthard M, Chow YH, Dattati N et al. 2004 Focus on social inequalities. Office of National Statistics, London, Chapter 6

Coupland N, Coupland J, Giles H 1991 Language, society and the elderly. Blackwell, Oxford

Cox T, Griffiths A, Barlowe C et al. 2000 Organisational interventions for work stress: a risk management approach. HMSO, Norwich

Crawford R 1987 Cultural influences on prevention and emergence of a new health consciousness. In: Weinstein N (ed.) Taking care: understanding and encouraging self-protective behaviour. Cambridge University Press, Cambridge

Cromarty I 1996 What do patients think about during their consultations? A qualitative study. British Journal of General Practice 46: 525–528

Cumming AD 2007 Learning about CAM: reasons, recommendations and strategies. In: Cumming AD, Simpson K, Brown D (eds) Complementary and alternative medicine: an illustrated colour text. Elsevier Churchill Livingstone, Edinburgh

Cumming AD, Simpson K, Brown D (eds) (2007) Complementary and alternative medicine: an illustrated colour text. Elsevier Churchill Livingstone, Edinburgh

Cunningham-Burley S, Boulton M 2000 The social context of the new genetics. In: Albrecht G, Fitzpatrick R, Scrimshaw C (eds) Handbook of social studies in health and medicine. Sage, London

Cunningham-Burley S, Irvine S 1987 'And have you done anything so far?' An examination of lay treatment of children's symptoms. British Medical Journal 295: 700–702

Cunningham-Burley S, Maclean U 1987 The role of the chemist in primary health care for children with minor complaints. Social Science and Medicine 24: 371–377

Cunningham-Burley S, Maclean U 1991 Dealing with children's illness: mothers' dilemmas. In: Wyke S, Hewison J (eds) Child health matters. Open University Press, Milton Keynes

DAFNE Study Group 2002 Training in flexible, intensive insulin management to enable dietary freedom in people with type 1 diabetes: dose adjustment for normal eating (DAFNE) randomized controlled trial. British Medical Journal 325: 746–752

Danaei G, Vander Hoorn S, Lopez AD et al. 2005 Causes of cancer in the world: comparative risk assessment of nine behavioural and environmental factors. Lancet 366: 1784–1793

Danner DD, Snowdon DA, Friesen WV 2001 Positive emotions in early life and longevity: findings from the nun study. Journal of Personality and Social Psychology 80: 804–813

Davey Smith G, Hart C, Blane D et al. 1997 Lifetime socioeconomic position and mortality: prospective observational study. British Medical Journal 314: 547–552

Davey Smith G, Shaw M, Mitchell R et al. 2000 Inequalities in health continue to grow despite government's pledges. British Medical Journal 320: 582

Davies R, Wakefield M, Amos A et al. 2007 The hitchhiker's guide to tobacco control: a global assessment of harms, remedies, and controversies. Annual Review of Public Health 28: 171–194

Davis MS 1968 Physiologic, psychological and demographic factors in patient compliance with doctor's orders. Medical Care 5: 115–122

Davison G, Neale JM 2001 Abnormal psychology, 8th edn. Wiley & Sons, London

Davison C, Davey Smith G, Frankel S 1991 Lay epidemiology and the prevention paradox: the implications of coronary candidacy for health education. Sociology of Health and Illness 13: 1–19

DCCT Research Group 1993 The effect of intensive treatment of diabetes on the development and progression of long-term complications in insulin-dependent diabetes mellitus. New England Journal of Medicine 329: 977–986

Deal A, Chalder T, Marks I et al. 1997 Cognitive behaviour therapy for chronic fatigue syndrome: a randomised controlled trial. American Journal of Psychiatry 154: 408–414

de Beauvoir S 1960 The second sex. Four Square Books, London

Dennis M, Barbor TF, Roebuck MC et al. 2002 Changing the focus: the case for recognizing the treatment of cannabis use disorders. Addiction 97 (suppl. 1): 4–15

Department of Economic and Social Affairs, Population Division 2006 World Mortality Report 2005, New York: United Nations

Department of Health 1991 Drug misuse and dependence: guidelines on clinical management. HMSO, London

Department of Health 2001a Valuing people: a new strategy for learning disability for the 21st century. Cm 5086. The Stationery Office, London

Department of Health 2001b Treatment choice in psychological therapies and counselling: evidence based clinical practice guide. Department of Health, London

Department of Health 2005 Self care – real choice, self care support – a real option. Department of Health, London

Department of Health, Chief Medical Officer 2006 The expert patients programme. Department of Health, London

Department of Health 2007 Self care support: the evidence pack. Department of Health, London

DFID 2000 Better health for poor people. Department for International Development, UK

Di Blasi Z, Harkness E, Ernst E et al. 2000 Influence of context effects on health outcomes: a systematic review. Lancet 357: 757–762

Diego MA Field T, Hernandez-Reif M 2005 Prepartum, postpartum and chronic depression effects on neonatal behaviour. Infant Behavior and Development 28: 155–164

Dieppe PA 2004 Relationship between symptoms and structural changes in osteoarthritis. What are the important targets for osteoarthritis therapy? Journal of Rheumatology 31 (suppl. 70): 50–53

Dingemans AE, Bruna MJ, van Furth EF 2002 Binge-eating disorder: a review. International Journal of Obesity 26: 299–307

DiPietro JA, Hilton SC, Hawkins M et al. 2002 Maternal stress and affect influence fetal neurobehavioral development. Developmental Psychology 38: 659–668

Ditton J, Hammersley R 1996 A very greedy drug: cocaine in context. Harwood, Reading

Doka KJ (ed.) 2002 Disenfranchised grief. New directions, challenges and strategies in practice. Research Press, Illinois

Doll R, Peto R 1981 The causes of cancer. Oxford Medical Publications, Oxford University Press, Oxford

Donaldson M 1978 Children's minds. Fontana, London

Donaldson ML, Elliot AS 1990 Children's explanations. In: Grieve R, Hughes M (eds) Understanding children. Blackwell, Oxford

Donovan JL, Blake DR 1992 Patient non-compliance: deviance or reasoned decision-making. Social Science and Medicine 34: 507–513

Drever F, Whitehead M (eds) 1997 Health inequalities: decennial supplement, DS 11. HMSO, London

Duncan B 2002 The founder of common factors: a conversation with Paul Rosenzweig. Journal of Psychotherapy Integration 12: 10–31

Dunn C, Deroo L, Rivara FP 2001 The use of brief interventions adapted from motivational interviewing across behavioral domains: a systematic review. Addiction 96: 1725–1742

Eaker ED, Pinsky J, Castelli WP 1992 Myocardial infarction and coronary death among women: psychosocial predictors from a 20-year follow-up of women in the Framingham Study. American Journal of Epidemiology 135: 854–864

Eaton WW 2002 Epidemiologic evidence on the comorbidity of depression and diabetes. Journal of Psychosomatic Research 53: 903–906

Edwards G 2000 Alcohol: the ambiguous molecule. Penguin, London

Egbert LD, Battit GE, Welch CE et al. 1964 Reduction of post-operative pain by encouragement and instruction of patients. New England Journal of Medicine 270: 825–827

Eiser C, Havermans T, Casas R 1993 Healthy children's understanding of their blood: implications for explaining leukaemia to children. British Journal of Educational Psychology 63: 528–537

Ekman P 1993 Facial expression and emotion. American Psychology 48: 384–392

Ellershaw J, Ward C 2003 Care of the dying patient: the last hours or days of life. British Medical Journal 326: 30–34

Ellershaw J, Wilkinson S (eds) 2003 Care of the dying. A pathway to excellence. Oxford University Press. Oxford

Elliott R, Greenberg LS, Lietaer G 2003 Research on experiential psychotherapy. In: Lambert MJ, Bergin AE (eds) Garfield's handbook of psychotherapy and behavior change, 5th edn. Wiley, New York, pp. 493–539

Engelhard IM, van den Hout MA, Arntz A 2001 Posttraumatic stress disorder after pregnancy loss. General Hospital Psychiatry 23: 62–66

Epstein LH 1984 The direct effects of compliance on health outcome. Health Psychology 3: 385–393

Erikson EH 1968 Identity: youth and crisis. Norton, New York

Ernst E, White A 2000 The BBC survey of complementary medicine use in the UK. Complementary Therapies in Medicine 8: 32–36

Eysenck HJ 1967 The biological basis of personality. Charles Thomas, Springfield, IL

Eysenck M 1996 Simply psychology. Psychology Press, Hove, pp. 115–131

Fallowfield L 1990 The quality of life. The missing measurement in health care. Souvenir Press, London

Fallowfield L, Jenkins V 2004 Communicating sad, bad and difficult news in medicine. Lancet 363: 312–319

Farmer J, Iverson L, Campbell NC et al. 2006 Rural/urban differences in accounts of patients' initial decisions to consult primary care. Health and Place 12: 210–221

Farrell M, Boys A, Bebbington P et al. 2002 Psychosis and drug dependence: results from a national survey of prisoners. British Journal of Psychiatry 181: 393–398

Faulkner A 1995 Working with bereaved people. Churchill Livingstone, Edinburgh

Faulkner A, Maguire P, Regnard C et al. 1994 Breaking bad news – a flow diagram. Palliative Medicine 8: 145–151

Faull C, Woof R 2002 Palliative care. Oxford University Press, Oxford

Ferrie JE, Matikainen P, Shipley MJ et al. 2001 Employment status and health after privatization in white collar civil servants: prospective cohort study. British Medical Journal 322: 647

Festinger L 1957 A theory of cognitive dissonance. Row Peterson, Evanston, Illinois

File SE, Fluck E, Leahy A 2001 Nicotine has calming effects on stress-induced mood changes in females, but enhances aggressive mood in males. International Journal of Neuropsychopharmacology 4: 371–376

Fiore MC, Bailey WC, Cohen SJ et al. 1996 Smoking cessation. Clinical practice guideline no. 18, publication no. 96–0692. Agency for Health Care Policy and Research, US Department of Health and Human Services, Rockville, MD

Firth S 2001 Wider horizons. Care of the dying in a multicultural society. National Council for Hospice and Specialist Palliative Care Services, London

Firth-Cozens J 1986 Levels and sources of stress in medical students. British Medical Journal 292: 1177–1180

Firth-Cozens J 1998 Individual and organisational predictors of depression in general practitioners. British Journal of General Practice 48: 1647–1651

Firth-Cozens J 2001 Interventions to improve physicians' well-being and patient care. Social Science and Medicine 52: 215–222

Fisher S 1986 Stress and strategy. Lawrence Erlbaum, London

Fisher JD, Fisher WA 1992 Changing AIDS-risk behavior. Psychological Bulletin 111: 455–471

Fisher K, Johnston M 1996 Experimental manipulation of perceived control and its effect on disability. Psychology and Health 11: 657–669

Fitzmaurice DA 2001 Written information for treating minor illness. British Medical Journal 322: 1193–1194

Flynn JR 1987 Massive IQ gains in 14 nations: what IQ tests really measure. Psychological Bulletin 101: 171–191

Folkman S, Moskowitz JT 2000 Positive affect and the other side of coping. American Psychologist 55: 647–654

Folkman S, Moskowitz JT 2004 Coping: pitfalls and promise. Annual Review of Psychology 55: 745–774

Folkman S, Lazarus RS, Dunkel-Schetter C et al. 1986 The dynamics of a stressful encounter. Journal of Personality and Social Psychology 50: 992–1003

Foster GD, Sarwer DB, Wadeen TA 1997 Psychological effects of weight-cycling in obese persons: a review and research agenda. Obesity Research 5: 474–488

Foster J, Newburn T, Sauhami A 2005 Assessing the impact of the Stephen Lawrence inquiry. Home Office Research, Development and Statistics Directorate

Foxwell M, Alder E 1993 More information equals less anxiety. Anxiety and screening: an intervention by nurses. Professional Nurse 9: 322–336

Frank JD 1961 Persuasion and healing: a comparative study of psychotherapy. Wiley, New York

Frasure-Smith N, Lesperance F, Talajic M 1993 Depression following myocardial infarction. Impact on 6-month survival. Journal of the American Medical Association 270: 1819–1825

Frasure-Smith N, Lesperance F, Talajic M 1995 Coronary heart disease/myocardial infarction: depression and 18-month prognosis after myocardial infarction. Circulation 91: 999–1005

Freeman GK, Horder JP, Howie JGR et al. 2002 Evolving general practice consultations in Britain: issues of length and context. British Medical Journal 324: 880–882

Freidson E 1975 Profession of medicine – a study of the sociology of applied knowledge. University of Chicago Press, London

French F, Wakeling J, Rooke C et al. 2007 What do foundation doctors, consultants and nurses think about the new foundation programmes? Oral presentation. Association for Medical Education in Europe Annual Conference, August

Friedman M, Rosenman RH 1974 Type A and your heart. New York, Knopf

Friedman HS, Tucker JS, Tomlinson-Keasay C 1993 Does childhood personality predict longevity? Journal of Personality and Social Psychology 65: 176–185

Gamble JA, Creedy D 2001 Women's preference for a caesarean section: incidence and associated factors. Birth 28: 101–110

Gannon L 2000 Psychological well-being in aging women. In: Usher JM (ed.) Women's health. Contemporary international perspectives. BPS Books, Leicester, pp. 476–484

Gardner H 2001 Intelligence reframed: multiple intelligences for the 21st century. Basic Books, New York

Gaston CM, Mitchell G 2005 Information giving and decision-making in patients with advanced cancer: a systematic review. Social Science and Medicine 61: 2252–2264

Geddes J 2003 Efficacy and safety of electroconvulsive therapy in depressive disorders: a systematic review and meta-analysis. Lancet 361: 799–808

General Medical Council 1993 Tomorrow's doctors. GMC, London

General Medical Council 2002a http://www.gmc-uk.org/med_ed/tomdoc.htm

General Medical Council 2002b Withholding and withdrawing life-prolonging treatments. Good practice in decision making. GMC, London

General Medical Council 2006 Good medical practice. Available online at: http://www.gmc-uk.org/guidance/good_medical_practice/

General Registers Office for Scotland. Scottish index of multiple deprivation. Available online at: www.isdscotland.org/isd/3067.html

George J, Kong DCM, Thoman R et al. 2005 Factors associated with medication non-adherence in patients with COPD. Chest 128: 3198–3204

Ghosh S, Shand A, Ferguson A 2000 Ulcerative colitis. British Medical Journal 320: 1119–1123

Glanz K, Rimer BK, Lewis FM 2002 Health behavior and health education: theory, research, and practice. Jossey-Bass, San Francisco

Glasgow RE, La Chance P, Toobert DJ et al. 1997 Long term effects and costs of brief behavioural dietary intervention delivered in the medical office. Patient Education and Counseling 32: 175–184

Glasziou P, Alexander J, Beller E et al. 2007 Which health-related quality of life score? A comparison of alternative utility measures in patients with type 2 diabetes in the ADVANCE trial. Health and Quality of Life Outcomes 5: 21

Goffman E 1968a Stigma. Penguin, London

Goffman E 1968b Asylums. Penguin, Harmondsworth

Gollwitzer PM 1999 Implementation intentions: strong effects of simple plans. American Psychologist 54: 493–503

Gollwitzer PM, Sheeran P 2006 Implementation intentions and goal achievement: a meta-analysis of effects and processes. Advances in Experimental Social Psychology 38: 249–268

Graham H 1984 Women, health and the family. Harvester Wheatsheaf, Hemel Hempstead

Graham H (ed.) 2000 Understanding health inequalities. Open University Press, Milton Keynes

Grant L 1998 Remind me who I am, again. Granta Books, London

Grant JR 2007 Changing postgraduate medical education: a commentary from the United Kingdom. Medical Journal of Australia 186 (Suppl): S9–S13

Grant G, Nolan M 1993 Informal carers: sources and concomitants of satisfaction. Health and Social Care in the Community 1: 147–159

Greenfield S 2000 Brain story. BBC Worldwide, London

Greenfield SM, Innes MA, Allan TF et al. 2002 First year medical student's perceptions and use of complementary and alternative medicines. Complementary Therapies in Medicine 10: 27–32

Greenwood E 1957 Attributes of a profession. Social Work 2: 45–55

Greer S, Morris TE, Pettingale KW 1979 Psychological responses to breast cancer: effect on outcome. Lancet ii: 785–787

Gross JJ 1998 The emerging field of emotion regulation: an integrative review. Review of General Psychology 2: 271–299

Guilford JP 1967 The nature of human intelligence. McGraw-Hill, New York

Guthrie D, Black H, Bagalkote C et al. 1998 Psychological stress and burnout in medical students: a five-year prospective longitudinal study. Journal of the Royal Society of Medicine 91: 237–243

Hallowell N 2000 Doing the right thing: genetic risk and responsibility. In: Conrad P, Gabe J (eds) Sociological perspectives on the new genetics. Blackwell, Oxford

Hammen C 1997 Depression. Psychology Press, Hove

Hammen C, Watkins E 2007 Depression. Psychology Press, Hove

Hammersley R, Ditton J 2005 Binge or bout? Quantity and rate of drinking by young people in licensed premises. Drugs, Education, Prevention and Policy 12: 493–500

Hammersley R, Reid M 2002 Why the pervasive addiction myth is still believed. Addiction Research and Theory 10: 7–30

Hannay D 1979 The symptom iceberg – a study of community health. Routledge and Kegan Paul, London

Haran J, Kitzinger J, McNeil M et al 2007 Human cloning in the media: from science fiction to science practice. Routledge, London

Harding S, Brown J, Rosato M et al 1999 Office for National Statistics. The Stationery Office, London

Harrison S, Hunter DJ 1994 Rationing health care. Institute for Public Policy Research, London

Harrison JA, Mullen PD, Green LW 1992 A meta-analysis of studies of the health belief model with adults. Health Education Research 7: 107–116

Hassell K, Rodgers A, Noyce P et al. 1998 Advice provided in British community pharmacies: what people want and what they get. Journal of Health Services Research and Policy 3: 219–225

Hassell K, Rodgers A, Noyce P 2000 Community pharmacy as a primary health and self-care resource: a framework for understanding pharmacy utilization. Health and Social Care in the Community 8: 40–49

Hayes SC, Follette VM, Linehan M (eds) 2005 Mindfulness and acceptance: expanding the cognitive-behavioural traditions. Guilford Press, New York

Haynes RB, McKibbon KA, Kanani R 1996 Systematic review of randomized trials of interventions to assist patients to follow prescriptions for medications. Lancet 348: 383–386

Health and Safety Executive 2000a Revitalising health and safety. HSE, Suffolk

Health and Safety Executive 2000b Securing health together. HSE, Suffolk

Health and Safety Executive 2008 HSE statistics – key figures for 2006/7. Available online at: http://www.hse.gov.uk/statistics/index.htm

Health Scotland/ASH Scotland 2004 Cessation guidelines for Scotland updated. Health Scotland, Edinburgh

Heather N, Robinson I 1983 Controlled drinking. Routledge, London

Heather N, Robinson I 1996 Let's drink to your health! Routledge, Oxford

Hemingway H, Marmot M 1999 Evidence based cardiology: psychosocial factors in the aetiology and prognosis of coronary heart disease: systematic review of prospective cohort studies. British Medical Journal 318: 1460–1467

Henderson L 2007 Social issues in television fiction. Edinburgh University Press, Edinburgh

Henderson L, Kitzinger J 1999 The human drama of genetics: 'hard' and 'soft' media representations of inherited breast cancer. Sociology of Health and Illness 21: 560–578

Henderson L, Kitzinger J, Green J 2000 Representing infant feeding: content analysis of British media portrayals of bottle feeding and breastfeeding. British Medical Journal 321: 1196–1198

Hepworth M 1995 Images of old age. In: Nussbaum JF, Coupland J (eds) Handbook of communication and ageing research. Lawrence Erlbaum, Mahwah, NJ

Herbert JD, Lilienfeld SO, Lohr JM et al. 2000 Science and pseudoscience in the development of eye movement desensitisation and reprocessing: implications for clinical psychology. Clinical Psychology Review 20: 945–971

Herxheimer A, McPherson A, Miller R et al. 2000 Database of patients' experience (DIPEx): a multi-media approach to sharing experiences and information. Lancet 355: 1540–1543

Higginson IJ 2004 Clinical and organizational audit. In: Doyle D, Hanks G, Cherny N et al. (eds) Oxford textbook of palliative medicine, 3rd edn. Oxford University Press, Oxford, pp. 184–196

Hilton S, Sibbald B, Anderson HR et al. 1986 Controlled evaluations of the effects of patient education on asthma morbidity in general practice. Lancet 1: 26–29

Hilts PJ 1995 Memory's ghost. Simon & Schuster, New York

Hing E, Cherry DK, Woodwell DA 2006 National ambulatory medical care survey: 2004 summary. Available online at: http://www.cdc.gov/nchs/data/ad/ad374.pdf

Hlatky MA, Boothroyd D, Vittinghoff E et al. 2002 Quality-of-life and depressive symptoms in postmenopausal women after receiving hormone therapy. Journal of the American Medical Association 287: 591–597

Holm JE, Holroyd KA 1992 The Daily Hassles scale (revised): does it measure stress or symptoms? Behavioral Assessment 14: 465–482

Holman H, Lorig K 2000 Patients as partners in managing chronic disease. British Medical Journal 320: 526–527

Holmes TH, Rahe RH 1967 The social readjustment scale. Journal of Psychosomatic Research 11: 213–218

Home Office 2005/06 British crime survey. Available online at: http://www.homeoffice. gov.uk/rds/bcs1.html

Hope T, Savulescu J, Hendrick J 2003 Medical ethics and law 2003. The core curriculum. Churchhill Livingstone, Edinburgh

Hopton JL, Dlugolecka M 1995 Patients' perceptions of need for primary health care services: useful for priority setting? British Medical Journal 310: 1237–1240

Horne R, James D, Petrie K et al. 2000 Patients' interpretation of symptoms as a cause of delay in reaching hospital during myocardial infarction. Heart 83: 388–393

Hospers HJ, Jansen A 2005 Why homosexuality is a risk factor for eating disorders in males. Journal of Social and Clinical Psychology 24: 1188–1201

House of Lords 2000 Select committee on science and technology, Sixth report. Stationery Office, London

Howie JGR, Hopton JL, Heaney DJ et al. 1992 Attitudes to medical care, the organisation of work, and stress among general practitioners. British Journal of General Practice 42: 181–185

Howie JGR, Heaney D, Maxwell M et al. 1998 A comparison of a patient enablement instrument (PEI) against two established patient satisfaction scales as an outcome measure of primary care consultations. Family Practice 15: 165–171

Hunt S 1997 Housing-related disorders. In: Charlton J, Murphy M (eds) The health of adult Britain 1841–1994, vol. 1. Office for National Statistics. Decennial supplement no. 12. Stationery Office, London, pp. 156–170

Innes NJ, Reid A, Halstead J et al. 1998 Psychosocial risk factors in near-fatal asthma and in asthma deaths. Journal of the Royal College of Physicians London 32: 430–434

Jackson C 2006 Shut up and listen: a brief guide to clinical communication skills. Dundee University Press, Dundee

Jackson PR, Wall TD, Martin R et al. 1993 New measures of job control, cognitive demand and production responsibility. Journal of Applied Psychology 78: 753–762

James W 1884 What is an emotion? Mind 9: 188–205

Janis LL 1958 Psychological stress. Wiley, New York

Janssen I, Hanssen M, Bak M et al. 2003 Discrimination and delusional ideation. British Journal of Psychiatry 182: 71–76

Janz NK, Becker HM 1984 The health belief model: a decade later. Health Education Quarterly 11: 1–47

Jenkins V, Fallowfield L, Saul J 2001 Information needs of patients with cancer: results from a large study in UK cancer centres. British Journal of Cancer 84: 48–51

Jerrome D 1992 Good company: an anthropological study of old people in groups. Edinburgh University Press, Edinburgh

Johnson M 2003 Ethnic diversity in social context. In: Kai J (ed.) Ethnicity, health and primary care. Oxford University Press, Oxford

Johnson SR 2004 The epidemiology of premenstrual syndrome. Primary Psychiatry 11: 27–32

Johnston M 1980 Anxiety in surgical patients. Psychological Medicine 10: 145–152

Johnston G, Abraham C 1995 The WHO objectives for palliative care: to what extent are we achieving them? Palliative Medicine 9: 123–137

Johnston G, Abraham C 2000 Managing awareness: negotiating and coping with a terminal prognosis. International Journal of Palliative Nursing 6: 485–494

Johnston M, Vögele C 1993 Benefits of psychological preparation for surgery: a meta-analysis. Annals of Behavioural Medicine 15: 245–256

Johnston M, Wright S, Weinman J 1995 Measures in health psychology: a user's portfolio. NFER-Nelson, Windsor

Johnston M, Pollard B, Morrison V et al. 2005 Functional limitations and survival following stroke: psychological and clinical predictors of 3-year outcome. International Journal of Behavioral Medicine 11: 187–196

Jones A, McArdle PJ, O'Neill PA 2002 Perceptions of how well graduates are prepared for the role of pre-registration house officer: a comparison of outcomes from a traditional and an integrated PBL curriculum. Medical Education 36: 16–25

Judge K, Paterson J 2001 Poverty, income, inequality and health. Treasury working paper 01/29. The Treasury, Wellington

Kaasa S, Loge JH 2004 Quality of life. In Doyle D, Hanks G, Cherny N et al. (eds) Oxford textbook of palliative medicine, 3rd edn. Oxford University Press, Oxford, pp. 196–210

Kai J 1996 Parents' difficulties and information needs in coping with acute illness in preschool children: a qualitative study. British Medical Journal 313: 987–990

Kai J, Bhopal R 2003 Ethnic diversity in health and disease. In: Kai J (ed.) Ethnicity, health and primary care. Oxford University Press, Oxford

Kaplan SH, Greenfield S, Ware JE 1989 Assessing the effects of physician–patient interaction on the outcomes of chronic disease. Med Care 27: s110–s127

Karasek RA 1979 Job demands, job decisions latitude and mental strain: implications for job design. Administrative Science Quarterly 24: 285–308

Katz AH, Bender EI (eds) 1976 The strength in us: self-help groups in the modern world. Franklin Watts, New York

Kaye P 1996 Breaking bad news (pocket book). EPL Publications, Northampton

Kaye WH, Klump KL, Frank GKW, et al. 2000 Anorexia and bulimia nervosa. Annual Review of Medicine 51: 299–313

Kelleher D 1994 Self-help groups and their relationship to medicine. In: Gabe J, Kelleher D, Williams G (eds) Changing medicine. Routledge, London, pp. 104–117

Keller MB, McCullough JP, Klein DN et al. 2000 A comparison of nefazodone, the cognitive behavioral-analysis system of psychotherapy, and their combination for the treatment of chronic depression. New England Journal of Medicine 342: 1462–1470

Kelly M 1991 Coping with an ileostomy. Social Science and Medicine 33: 115–125

Kelly M 1992 Colitis. Routledge, London

Kelly MP, Sullivan F 1992 The productive use of threat in primary care: behavioural responses to health promotion. Family Practice 9: 476–480

Kerse NM, Flicker L, Jolley D et al. 1999 Improving the health behaviours of elderly people: randomised controlled trial of a general practice education programme. British Medical Journal 319: 683–687

Kessler RC, Berglund P, Demler O et al. 2005 Lifetime prevalence and age-of-onset distributions of DSM-IV disorders in the National Comorbidity Survey Replication. Archives of General Psychiatry 62: 593–602

Kiecolt-Glaser JK, Newton TL 2001 Marriage and health: his and hers. Psychological Bulletin 127: 472–503

Kiecolt-Glaser JK, Garner W, Speicher CE et al. 1994 Psychosocial modifiers of immunocompetence in medical students. Psychosomatic Medicine 46: 7–14

Kiecolt-Glaser JK, Marucha PT, Marlakey WB et al. 1995 Slowing of wound healing by psychological stress. Lancet 346: 1194–1196

Kiecolt-Glaser JK, McGuire L, Robles TF et al. 2002 Psychoneuroimmunology. Psychological influences on immune function and health. Journal of Consulting and Clinical Psychology 70: 537–547

King JB 1982 The impact of patients' perceptions of high blood pressure on attendance at screening. An extension of the health belief model. Social Science and Medicine 16: 1079–1091

Kingston R 2001 It's only natural. Chemistry in Britain January: 18–21

Kinmonth A, Woodcock A, Griffin S et al. 1998 Randomised controlled trial of patient centred care of diabetes in general practice: impact on current well-being and future disease risk. British Medical Journal 317: 1202–1208

Kinnersley P, Stott N, Peters T et al. 1999 The patient-centredness of consultations and outcome in primary care. British Journal of General Practice 49: 711–716

Kister MC, Patterson CJ 1980 Children's conceptions of the causes of illness: understanding of contagion and use of imminent justice. Child Development 51: 839–846

Kitwood T 1997 Dementia reconsidered: the person comes first. Open University Press, Buckingham

Kitzhaber JA 1993 Prioritising health services in an era of limits: the Oregon experience. British Medical Journal 307: 373–376

Kitzinger J 1995 The face of AIDS. In: Markova I, Farr R (eds) Representations of health and illness. Harwood Academic Publishers, Newark

Kitzinger J 2001 Transformations of public and private knowledge: audience reception, feminism and the experience of childhood sexual abuse. Feminist Media Studies 1: 91–104

Klass D, Silverman PR, Nickman S (eds) 1996 Continuing bonds. New understandings of grief. Taylor and Francis, London

Klee H, Morris J 1997 Amphetamine misuse: the effects of social context on injection related risk behaviour. Addiction Research 4: 329–342

Klein R, Day P, Redmayne S 1996 Managing scarcity. Open University Press, Buckingham

Kleinman A 1985 Indigenous systems of healing: questions for professional, popular and folk care. In: Salmon J (ed.) Alternative medicines: popular and policy perspectives. Tavistock, London

Kleinman A 1986 Social origins of distress and disease. Yale University Press, New Haven

Klemm P, Repperty K, Lori V 1998 A non-traditional cancer support group: the internet. Computers in Nursing 16: 31–36

Korsch BM, Gozzi EK, Francis V 1968 Gaps in doctor–patient communication: 1. Doctor–patient interaction and patient satisfaction. Pediatrics 42: 855–871

Kroenke K, Swindle R 2000 Cognitive-behavioural therapy for somatization and symptom syndromes: a critical review of controlled clinical trials. Psychotherapy and Psychomatics 69: 205–215

Krohne HW, Slangen KE 2005 The influence of social support on adaptation to surgery. Health Psychology 24: 101–105

Kübler-Ross E 1969 On death and dying. Collier Macmillan, London

Kubler-Ross E 1970 On death and dying. Tavistock Publications, London

Kulik JA, Mahler HI, Moore PJ 1996 Social comparison and afiliation under threat: effects on recovery from major surgery. Journal of Personality and Social Psychology 71: 967–979

Kurtz S, Silverman J, Draper J 2004 Teaching and learning communication skills in medicine, 2nd edn. Radcliffe Publishing, Oxford

Kury SP, Rodrigue JR 1995 Concepts of illness causality in a pediatric sample. Clinical Pediatrics 34: 178–182

Lader D, Meltzer H 2001 Drinking: adults' behaviour and knowledge in 2000. Office for National Statistics, London

Lazarus R 1980 Stress and coping paradigm. In: Bond L, Rosen J (eds) Competence and coping during adulthood. University Press of New England, Hanover, NH

Lee K 2003 Globalisation and health, an introduction. Palgrave Macmillan, London

Leeson J, Gray L 1978 Women and health. Tavistock, London

Lemert E 1951 Social pathology. McGraw Hill, New York

Leon D, McCambridge J 2006 Liver cirrhosis mortality rates in Britain from 1950 to 2002: an analysis of routine data. Lancet 367: 52–56

Levine JD, Gordon NC, Fields HL 1978 The mechanisms of placebo analgesia. Lancet 2: 654–657

Levinson DJ, Darrow DN, Klein EB et al. 1978 The seasons of a man's life. Knopf, New York

Lewis G, Sloggett A 1998 Suicide, deprivation and unemployment: record linkage study. British Medical Journal 317: 1283–1286

Lewith G, Jones WB, Wlach H 2002 Clinical research in complementary therapies. Churchill Livingstone, Edinburgh

Ley P 1997 Communicating with patients; improving communication, satisfaction and compliance. Stanley Thornes Publishers, Cheltenham

Ley P, Whitworth MA, Woodward R et al. 1976 Improving doctor–patient communication in general practice. Journal of the Royal College of General Practitioners 26: 720–724

Little P, Everitt H, Williamson I et al. 2001 Preferences of patients for patient centred approach to consultation in primary care: observational study. British Medical Journal 322: 468–472

Little AC, Jones BC, Burriss RP 2007 Preferences for masculinity in male bodies change across the menstrual cycle. Hormones and Behavior 51: 633–639

Lok IH, Neugebauer R 2007 Psychological morbidity following miscarriage. Best Practice and Research in Clinical Obstetrics and Gynaecology 21: 229–247

Love RR, Leventhal H, Easterling DV et al. 1989 Side effects and emotional distress during cancer chemotherapy. Cancer 63: 604–612

Low JTS, Payne S 1996 The good and bad death perceptions of health professionals in palliative care. European Journal of Cancer Care 5: 237–241

Luck M, Bamford M, Williamson P 2000 Men's health: perspectives, diversity and paradox. Blackwell Science, Oxford

Luria AR 1969 The mind of a mnemonist: a little book about a vast memory. Cape, London

Lustman PJ, Clouse RE 2002 Treatment of depression in diabetes: impact on mood and medical outcome. Journal of Psychosomatic Research 53: 917–924

Luty SE, Carter JD, McKenzie JM et al. 2007 Randomised controlled trial of interpersonal psychotherapy and cognitive-behavioural therapy for depression. British Journal of Psychiatry 190: 496–502

Lydeard S, Jones R 1989 Factors affecting the decision to consult with dyspepsia: comparison of consulters and non-consulters. Journal of the Royal College of General Practitioners 39: 495–498

Mackay J, Eriksen M, Shafey O 2006 The tobacco atlas, 2nd edn. WHO, Geneva

Maguire EA, Burgess N, Donnett JG et al. 1998 Knowing where and getting there: a human navigation network. Science 280: 921–924

Main C J, Spanswick C C 2000 Pain management: an interdisciplinary approach. Churchill Livingstone, Edinburgh

Malecka-Tendera E, Mazur A 2006 Childhood obesity: a pandemic of the twenty-first century. International Journal of Obesity 30 (Suppl. 2): S1–S3

Manuck SB, Kaplan JR, Clarkson TB 1983 Social instability and coronary artery atherosclerosis in cynomolgus monkeys. Neuroscience and Behavioural Reviews 7: 485–491

Marmot M 1989 Socioeconomic determinants of CHD mortality. International Journal of Epidemiology 18: 196–202

Marmot M, Adelstein AM, Bulusu L et al. 1984 Immigrant mortality in England and Wales 1970–78. OPCS studies on population and medical subjects no. 47. HMSO, London

Marmot MG, Davey Smith G, Stanfeld SA et al. 1991 Health inequalities among British civil servants: the Whitehall II study. Lancet 337: 1387–1393

Marteau T, Anionwu E 1996 Evaluating carrier testing: objectives and outcomes. In: Marteau T, Richards M (eds) The troubled helix. Cambridge University Press, Cambridge

Matthews KA 1988 Coronary heart disease and type A behaviours: update on and alternative to the Booth-Kewley and Friedman (1987) quantitative review. Psychological Bulletin 104: 373–380

Mathews A, Ridgeway V 1984 Psychological preparation for surgery. In: Steptoe A, Mathews A (eds) Health care and human behaviour. Academic Press, London

Maunder R, Hunter J, Vincent L et al. 2003 The immediate psychological and occupational impact of the 2003 SARS outbreak in a teaching hospital. Canadian Medical Association Journal 168: 1245–1251

Mayer JD, Gaschke YN 1988 The experience and meta-experience of mood. Journal of Personality and Social Psychology 55: 101–111

Mayou R, Farmer A 2002 Trauma. British Medical Journal 325: 426–429

McCarthy P, Walker J, Kain JW 1995 Telling it as it is: the client experience of Relate counselling. Newcastle Centre for Family Studies, Newcastle

McCrae RR, Costa PT 1987 Validation of the five-factor model of personality across instruments and observers. Journal of Personality and Social Psychology 54: 81–90

McDonald IG, Daly J, Jelinek VM et al. 1996 Opening Pandora's box: the unpredictability of reassurance by a normal test result. British Medical Journal 313: 329–332

McGuffin P, Katz R, Watkins S et al. 1996 A hospital-based twin register of the heritability of DSM-IV unipolar depression. Archives of General Psychiatry 53: 129–136

McKeown T 1979 The role of medicine: dream, mirage or nemesis? Blackwell, Oxford

McKinlay JB 1973 Social networks, lay consultation and help seeking behaviour. Social Forces 51: 279–292

McKinnis KJ 2000 Exercise and obesity. Coronary Artery Disease 11: 111–116

McLauchlan CAJ 1990 Handling distressed relatives and breaking bad news. British Medical Journal 301: 1145–1149

McManus IC, Richards P, Winder BC 1999 Intercalated degrees, learning styles, and career preferences: prospective longitudinal study of UK medical students. British Medical Journal 319: 542–546

McQuay HJ, Moore RA, Eccleston C et al. 1997 Systematic review of outpatient services for chronic pain control. Health Technology Assessment 1: i–iv, 1–135

Mead N, Bower P, Hann M 2002 The impact of general practitioners' patient-centredness on patients' post-consultation satisfaction and enablement. Social Science and Medicine 55: 283–299

Measham F 2006 The new policy mix: alcohol, harm minimisation, and determined drunkenness in contemporary society. International Journal of Drug Policy 17: 258–268

Mehler PS 2001 Diagnosis and care of patients with anorexia nervosa in primary care settings. Annals of Internal Medicine 134: 1048–1059

Melzack R, Wall PD 1999 The textbook of pain, 4th edn. Churchill Livingstone, Edinburgh

Menzies D, Nair A, Williamson PA et al. 2006 Respiratory symptoms, pulmonary function, and markers of inflammation among bar workers before and after a legislative ban on smoking in public places. Journal of the American Medical Association 296: 1742–1748

Meredith C, Symonds, P, Webster L et al. 1996 Information needs of cancer patients in west Scotland: cross sectional survey of patients' views. British Medical Journal 313: 724–726

Merskey H, Bogduk N (eds) 1994 Classification of chronic pain. Descriptions of chronic pain syndromes and definitions of pain terms, 2nd edn. International Association for the Study of Pain, Seattle

Miles A 1991 Women, health and medicine. Open University Press, Buckingham

Milgram S 1963 Behavioural study of obedience. Journal of Abnormal and Social Psychology 67: 371–378

Miller PMcC 1994 The first year at medical school: some findings and student perceptions. Medical Education 28: 5–7

Miller MA, Rahe RH 1997 Life changes scaling for the 1990s. Journal of Psychosomatic Research 43: 279–292

Miller WR, Rollnick S 1991 Motivational interviewing: preparing people to change addictive behaviour. Guilford Press, London

Miller WR, Sanchez-Craig M 1996 How to have a high success rate in alcohol treatment. Addiction 91: 779–785

Miller TQ, Smith TW, Turner CW et al. 1996 A meta-analytic review of research on hostility and physical health. Psychological Bulletin 119: 322–348

Miller D, Kitzinger J, Eilliams K et al. 1998 The circuit of mass communication: media strategies, representation and audience reception in the AIDS crisis. Sage, London

Mills S, Bone K 2000 Principles and practice of phytotherapy. Modern herbal medicine. Churchill Livingstone, Edinburgh, p. 544

Moffat KJ, McConnachie A, Ross S et al. 2004 First year medical student stress and coping in a problem-based learning medical curriculum. Medical Education 38: 482–491

Molfino NA, Nannini LJ, Rebuck AS et al. 1992 The fatality-prone asthmatic patient. Follow-up study after near-fatal attacks. Chest 101: 621–623

Montoya P, Pauli P, Batra A et al. 2005 Altered processing of pain-related information in patients with fibromyalgia. European Journal of Pain 9: 293–303

Moore TH, Zammit S, Lingford-Hughes A et al. 2007 Cannabis use and risk of psychotic or affective mental health outcomes: a systematic review. Lancet 370: 3129–3328

Morisky DE, Green LW, Levine DM 1986 Concurrent and predictive validity of a self-report measure of medication adherence. Medical Care 24: 67–74

Morley S, Greer S, Bliss J et al. 1999 Systematic review and meta analysis of randomised controlled trials of cognitive behaviour therapy and behaviour therapy for chronic pain in adults, excluding headaches. Pain 80: 1–13

Morris JK, Cook DG, Shaper AG 1994 Loss of employment and mortality. British Medical Journal 308: 1135–1139

Morris CJ, Cantrill JA, Weiss MC 2003 Minor ailment consultations: a mismatch of perceptions between patients and GPs. Primary Health Care Research and Development 4: 365–370

Moser KA, Fox AJ, Jones DR 1984 Unemployment and mortality in the OPCS longitudinal study. Lancet ii: 1324–1329

Moss F, McManus C 1992 The anxieties of new clinical students. Medical Education 26: 17–20

Muldoon MF, Barger S, Flory JD et al. 1998 What are quality of life measurements measuring? British Medical Journal 16: 542–545

Mullen P D 1997 Compliance becomes concordance. British Medical Journal 314: 691–692

Muller T 2007 Breaking the cycle of children's exposure to tobacco smoke. British Medical Association, London.

Munn-Giddings C, McVicar A 2007 Self-help groups as mutual support: what do carers value? Health and Social Care in the Community 15: 26–34

Murray L, Cooper PJ 1997 Postpartum depression and child development. Psychological Medicine 27: 253–260

Murray L, Fiori-Cowley A, Hooper R et al. 1996 The impact of postnatal depression and associated adversity on early mother infant interactions and later infant outcome. Child Development 67: 2512–2516

Myant KA, Williams JM 2005 Children's concepts of health and illness: understanding of contagious illnesses, non-contagious illnesses and injuries. Journal of Health Psychology 10: 805–819

Myers LB, Midence K 1998 Concepts and issues in adherence. In: Myers LB, Midence K (eds) Adherence to treatment in medical conditions. Harwood Academic Publishers, Amsterdam, pp. 1–24

Myrtek M 2001 Meta analysis of prospective studies on coronary heart disease, type A personality and hostility. International Journal of Cardiology 79: 245–251

Narayanasamy A, White E 2005 A review of transcultural nursing. Nurse Education Today 25: 102–111

National Alcohol Strategy 2007 Safe, sensible, social. The next steps in the National Alcohol Strategy. Available online at: http://www.dh.gov.uk/en/Publicationsandstatistics/Publications/PublicationsPolicyAndGuidance/DH_075218

National Council for Hospice and Specialist Palliative Care Services 1997 Making palliative care better. Quality improvement, multiprofessional audit and standards. Occasional paper, 12 March 1997. NCHSPCS, London

National Council for Hospice and Specialist Palliative Care Services 2000 Specialist palliative care. Palliative care 2000. Commissioning through partnership. NCHSPCS, London

National Council for Hospice and Specialist Palliative Care Services 2002 Definitions of supportive and palliative care. Briefing paper 11. NCHSPCS, London

Nazroo JY 2003 The structuring of ethnic inequalities in health: economic position, racial discrimination, and racism. American Journal of Public Health 93: 277–284

Neale J 2002 Drug users in society. Palgrave, London

Needleman LD 1999 Cognitive case conceptualisation: a guidebook for practitioners. Lawrence Erlbaum, London

Neisser U, Boodoo G, Bouchard TJ et al. 1996 Intelligence: knowns and unknowns. American Psychologist 51: 77–101

Nerenz DR, Leventhal H, Love RR 1982 Factors contributing to emotional distress during chemotherapy. Cancer 50: 1020–1027

Newbury-Birch D, White M, Kamali F 2000 Factors influencing alcohol and illicit drug use amongst medical students. Drug and Alcohol Dependence 59: 125–130

Newbury-Birch D, Walshaw D, Kamali F 2001 Drink and drugs: from medical students to doctors. Drug and Alcohol Dependence 64: 265–270

Newcomb MD 1995 Identifying high-risk youth: prevalence and patterns of adolescent drug abuse. In: Rahdert E, Czechowicz D (eds) Adolescent drug abuse: clinical assessment and therapeutic interventions. NIDA research monograph 156. National Institute on Drug Abuse, Rockville, MD

New Zealand National Health Committee Available online at: http://www.acc.co.nz/for-providers/operational-guidelines/WCM2_020215?ref=2#pcguidelines

NICE 2004 Anxiety: management of anxiety (panic disorder, with or without agoraphobia, and generalised anxiety disorder) in adults in primary, secondary and community care. Available online at: http://guidance.nice.org.uk/CG22/niceguidance/pdf/English

NICE 2004 Improving supportive and palliative care for Adults with cancer, London

NICE 2005 Post-traumatic stress disorder (PTSD) – the management of PTSD in adults and children in primary and secondary care. National Institute for Clinical Excellence, London

NICE 2007 Depression (amended) – management of depression in primary and secondary care: National Institute for Health and Clinical Excellence, London

Nuffield Council on Bioethics 1993 Genetic screening. Ethical issues. Nuffield Council on Bioethics, London

Office for National Statistics 2000a Trends in fertility and contraception in the last quarter of the 20th century. HMSO, London

Office for National Statistics 2000b Annual abstract of statistics 2000. HMSO, London

Office for National Statistics 2002 Living in Britain: general household survey. ONS, London

Office for National Statistics 2004 Caesarean deliveries in NHS hospitals: social trends 34. HMSO, London

Office for National Statistics 2007 Social trends 37. Office of National Statistics, London

O'Flaherty M, Ford E, Allender S et al. 2007 Coronary heart disease trends in England and Wales from 1984 to 2004: concealed levelling of mortality rates among young adults. Heart doi: 10.1136/hrt.2007.118323

O'Keefe M, Sawyer M, Robertson D 2001 Medical student interviewing skills and mother-reported satisfaction and recall. Medical Education 35: 637–644

Oliver A, Healey A, Le Grand J 2002 Addressing health inequalities. Lancet 360: 565–567

Orbell S, Hodgkins S, Sheeran P 1997 Implementation intentions and the theory of planned behaviour. Personality and Social Psychology Bulletin 23: 953–962

Orford J 2000 Excessive appetites: a psychological view of addiction, 2nd edn. Wiley, Chichester

Osman L 1998 Health habits and illness behaviour: social factors in patient self-management. Respiratory Medicine 92: 150–155

Osman LM, Russell IT, Friend JA et al. 1993 Predicting patient attitudes to asthma medication. Thorax 48: 827–830

Panskepp J 1998 Affective neuroscience: the foundations of human and animal emotions. Oxford University Press, Oxford

Parkes CM 1975 Bereavement. Studies of grief in adult life. Penguin Books, Harmondsworth

Parkes CM 1996 Bereavement. Studies of grief in adult life, 3rd edn. Tavistock Publications, London

Patterson J, Barlow J, Mockford C et al. 2002 Improving mental health through parenting programmes: block randomised controlled trial. Archives of Diseases in Childhood 87: 472–477

Peterson C, Vaillant GE, Seligman MEP 1988 Pessimistic explanatory style is a risk factor for physical illness: a thirty-five-year longitudinal study. Journal of Personality and Social Psychology 55: 23–27

Petrie KJ, Weinmen J, Sharpe N et al. 1996 Role of patients' view of their illness in predicting return to work and functioning after myocardial infarction: longitudinal study. British Medical Journal 312: 1191–1194

Petticrew M, Bell R, Hunter D 2002 Influence of psychological coping on survival and recurrence in people with cancer: systematic review. British Medical Journal 325: 1066–1069

Petty RE, Cacioppo JT 1986 The elaboration likelihood model of persuasion. In: Berowitz L (ed.) Advances in experimental social psychology. Academic Press, New York, pp. 123–205

Philo G 1999 Media and mental illness. In: Philo G (ed.) Message received. Longman, London

Pieterse ME, Seydel ER, De Vries H et al. 2001 Effectiveness of a minimal contact smoking cessation program for Dutch general practitioners: a randomised controlled trial. Preventive Medicine 32: 182–190

Phillips DP, Ruth TE, Wagner LM 1993 Psychology and survival. Lancet 342: 1142–1145

Pilnick A 2002 Genetics and society: an introduction. Open University Press, Buckingham

Platt S 1985 Measuring burden of psychiatric illness on the family. An evaluation of some rating scales. Psychological Medicine 15: 383–393

Platt S, Martin CJ, Hunt SM et al. 1989 Damp housing, mould growth and symptomatic health state. British Medical Journal 298: 1673–1678

Platt JJ, Husband SD, Taube D 1991 Major psychotherapeutic modalities for heroin addiction – a brief overview. International Journal of the Addictions 25: 1453–1477

Platt S, Pavis S, Akram G 1999 Changing labour market conditions and health: a systematic literature review (1993–98). Dublin. European Foundation for the Improvement of Living and Working Conditions. Available online at: www.eurofound.ie/publications/files/EF9915EN.pdf

Platt S, Boyle P, Crombie I et al. 2007 The Epidemiology of Suicide in Scotland 1989–2004: an examination of temporal trends and risk factors at national and local levels. Available online at: http://www.scotland.gov.uk/Publications/2007/03/01145422/0

Polivy J, Herman CP 2002 Causes of eating disorders. Annual Review of Psychology 53: 187–213

Pollock K, Grime J 2002 Patients' perceptions of entitlement to time in general practice consultations for depression: qualitative study. British Medical Journal 325: 687

Powell J 2006 Health needs assessment: a systematic approach. Available online at: http://www.library.nhs.uk/HealthManagement/ViewResource.aspx?resID=29549&tabID=290&summaries=true&resultsPerPage=10&sort=TITLE&catID=4033

Prior L 1995 Chance and modernity: accidents as a public health problem. In: Bunton R, Nettleton S, Burrows R (eds) The sociology of health promotion. Routledge, London

Puri B, Laking PJ, Treasaden IH 1996 Textbook of psychiatry. Churchill Livingstone, Edinburgh

Radcliff C, Lester H 2003 Perceived stress during undergraduate medical training: a qualitative study. Medical Education 37: 32–38

Radley A 1994 Making sense of illness: the social psychology of health and disease. Sage, London

Raistrick D, Hodgson R, Ritson B 1999 Tackling alcohol together. The evidence base for a UK alcohol policy. Free Association Books, London

Ramchandani P, Stein A, Evans J et al. 2005 Paternal depression in the postnatal period and child development: a prospective population study. Lancet 365: 2201–2205

Registrar General's Mortality Statistics 1994 HMSO, London

Registrar General 2007 Scotland's population 2006: The Registrar General's annual review of demographic trends, 152nd edn. Available online at: http://www.gro-scotland.gov.uk/files1/stats/annual-report2006/annual-report-2006.pdf

Repper J, Perkins R 2006 Social inclusion and recovery: a model for mental health services. Baillière Tindall, London

Richards M 1993 The new genetics: some issues for social scientists. Sociology of Health and Illness 15: 567–586

Richards HM, Reid ME, Watt GCM 2002 Socioeconomic variations in response to chest pain: qualitative study. British Medical Journal 324: 1308–1312

Roberts H, Smith S, Bryce C 1993 Prevention is better ... Sociology of Health and Illness 15: 447–463

Rodgers A, Corbett T, Bramley D et al. 2005 Do u smoke after txt? Results of a randomised trial of smoking cessation using mobile phone text messaging. Tobacco Control 14: 255-261

Romano JM, Turner JA, Jensen MP et al. 1995 Chronic pain patient spouse behavioral interactions predict patient disability. Pain 63: 353–360

Rose D, Fleischmann P, Wykes T et al. 2003 Patients' perspectives on electroconvulsive therapy: systematic review. British Medical Journal 326: 1363

Ross MT 2007 Safety of complementary and alternative medicine. In: Cumming AD, Simpson K, Brown D (eds) Complementary and alternative medicine: an illustrated colour text. Elsevier Churchill Livingstone, Edinburgh

Ross S, Cleland J, Macleod MJ 2006 Stress, debt and undergraduate medical student performance. Medical Education 40: 584–589

Rost K, Nutting P, Smith JL et al. 2002 Managing depression as a chronic disease: a randomised trial of ongoing treatment in primary care. British Medical Journal 325: 934

Roth A, Fonagy P 2004 What works for whom? A critical review of psychotherapy research. Guildford Publication, London

Rovelli M, Palmeri D, Vossler E et al. 1989 Compliance in organ transplant recipients. Transplantation Proceedings 21: 833–844

Royal College of Physicians and Royal College of Psychiatrists 1995 The psychological care of medical patients. Royal College of Physicians and Royal College of Psychiatrists, London

Royal College of Psychiatrists 2004 Carers and confidentiality in mental health. Issues involved in information sharing. Available online at: www.rcpsych.ac.uk/PDF/carersandconfidentiality.pdf

RSA 2007 Drugs – facing facts: the report of the RSA Commission on Illegal Drugs, Communities and Public Policy. Royal Society for the encouragement of Arts, Manufactures and Commerce, London

Rudd P, Price MG, Graham LE et al. 1986 Consequences of worksite hypertension screening: differential changes in psychosocial function. American Journal of Medicine 80: 853–861

Ruiter RAC, Abraham C, Kok G 2001 Scary warnings and rational precautions: a review of the psychology of fear appeals. Psychology and Health 16: 613–630

Ruiz JG, Mintzer MJ, Leipzig RM 2006 The impact of E learning in medical education. Academic Medicine 81: 207–212

Rushforth H 1999 Communication with hospitalised children: review and application of research pertaining to children's understanding of health and illness. Journal of Child Psychology and Psychiatry 40: 683–691

Ruston A, Clayton J, Calnan M 1998 Patients' actions during their cardiac event: qualitative study exploring differences and modifiable factors. British Medical Journal 316: 1060–1065

Sabat SR, Harré R 1992 The construction and deconstruction of self in Alzheimer's disease. Ageing and Society 12: 443–461

Sacks O 1986 The man who mistook his wife for a hat. Picador, London

Saile H, Burgemeir R, Schmidt LR 1988 A meta-analysis of studies on psychological preparation of children facing medical procedures. Psychology and Health 2: 107–132

Salkovskis PM 1989 Somatic problems. In: Hawton K, Salkovskis PM, Kirk J et al. (eds) Cognitive behaviour therapy for psychiatric problems: a practical guide. Oxford University Press, New York, pp. 235–276

Sargent RP, Shepard RM, Glantz SA 2004 Reduced incidence of admissions for myocardial infarction associated with public smoking ban: before and after study. British Medical Journal 328: 977–980

Saunders C, Sykes N 1993 The management of terminal malignant disease, 3rd edn. Edward Arnold, London

Sawdon AM, Cooper M, Seabrook R 2007 The relationship between self-discrepancies, eating disorder and depressive symptoms in women. European Eating Disorders Review 15: 207–212

Sawyer S, Drew S, Yeo M et al. 2007 Adolescents with a chronic condition: challenges living, challenges treating. Lancet 369: 1481–1489

Scambler G, Hopkins A 1986 Being epileptic: coming to terms with stigma. Sociology of Health and Illness 8: 26–43

Schachter S 1964 The interaction of cognitive and physiological determinants of emotional states. In: Berkowitz L (ed.) Advances in experimental social psychology, vol. 1. Academic Press, New York

Schaie KW 1996 Intellectual development in adulthood. In: Birren JE, Schaie KW (eds) Handbook of the psychology of aging. Academic Press, London

Scherer K 1984 On the nature and function of emotion: a component process approach. In: Scherer KR, Ekman PE (eds) Approaches to emotion. Erlbaum, Hillsdale NJ, pp. 293–317

Schnall PL, Landsbergis PA, Baker D 1994 Job strain and cardiovascular disease. Annual Review of Public Health 15: 381–411

Schwartz GE 1980 Testing the biopsychosocial model: the ultimate challenge facing behavioural medicine? Journal of Consulting and Clinical Psychology 50: 1040–1053

Schwimmer JB, Burwinkle TM, Varni JW 2003 Health-related quality of life of severely obese children and adolescents. Journal of the American Medical Association 289: 1813–1819

Scottish Executive 2000 Same as you. The Scottish Executive, Edinburgh

Scottish Executive 2005a The Scottish health survey 2003. Available online at: http://www.scotland.gov.uk/Publications/2005/12/02160336/03367

Scottish Executive 2005b Scotland's people: annual report: results from the 2003/2004 Scottish household survey. Available online at www.scotland.gov.uk/Resource/Doc/57346/0016412.pdf

Seligman MEP 1995 The effectiveness of psychotherapy: the Consumer Reports study. American Psychologist 50: 965–974

Senior P, Bhopal RS 1994 Ethnicity as a variable in epidemiological research. British Medical Journal 309: 327–330

Serpell L, Hirani V, Willoughby K et al. 2006 Personality or pathology? Obsessive-compulsive symptoms in children and adolescents with anorexia nervosa. European Eating Disorders Review 14: 404–413

Seyle H 1956 The stress of life. McGraw-Hill, New York, NY

Shalev AY 2001 Post-traumatic stress disorder. Disorder takes away human dignity and character. British Medical Journal 322: 1301, 1303–1304

Shalev AY, Schreiber S, Galai T et al. 1993 Post-traumatic stress disorder following medical events. British Journal of Clinical Psychology 32: 247–253

Shapira K, McClelland HA, Griffiths NR et al. 1970 Study of the effects of tablet colour in the treatment of anxiety states. British Medical Journal 2: 446–449

Sharpe L, Sensky T, Timberlake N et al. 2003 Long-term efficacy of a cognitive behavioural treatment from a randomised controlled trial for patients recently diagnosed with rheumatoid arthritis. Rheumatology 42: 435–441

Shaw M, Davey Smith G, Dorling D 2005 Health inequalities and New Labour: how the promises compare with real progress. British Medical Journal 330: 1016–1021

Sheeran P 2002 Intention–behavior relations: a conceptual and empirical review. European Review of Social Psychology 12: 1–36

Siderfin C 2005 Remote and rural general practice in Scotland. British Medical Journal Career Focus 331: 135–136

Sikorski J, Renfrew M, Pindoria S et al. 2003 Support for breastfeeding mothers; a systematic review. Paediatric and Perinatal Epidemiology 17: 407–417

Simpson SH, Eurich DT, Majumdar SR et al. 2006 A meta-analysis of the association between adherence to drug therapy and mortality. British Medical Journal 333: 15–18

Sinclair DA, Murray L 1998 Effects of postnatal depression on children's adjustment in school. British Journal of Psychiatry 172: 58–63

Slack MK, Brooks AJ 1995 Medication management issues for adolescents with asthma. American Journal of Health-system Pharmacy 52: 1417–1421

Snoek F, Skinner TC (eds) 2000 Psychology in diabetes care. Wiley, Chichester

Social Policy Research Unit 2004 Hearts and minds. The health effects of caring. Available online at: www.carersuk.org/ Policyandpractice/PolicyResources/Research/ HeartsMinds.pdf

Sorce JF, Emde RN, Campos J et al. 1985 Maternal emotional signaling: its effect on the visual cliff behavior of 1-year-olds. Developmental Psychology 21: 195–200

Spiegel D, Bloom JR, Kraemer HC et al. 1989 Effect of psychosocial treatment on survival of patients with metastatic breast cancer. Lancet 334: 888–891

Stanton AL, Danoff-Burg S, Cameron CL et al. 1994 Coping through emotional approach: problems of conceptualization and confounding. Journal of Social and Personality Psychology 66: 350–362

Steinberg L 2007 Risk taking in adolescence: new perspectives from brain and behavioral science. Current Directions in Psychological Science 16: 55–59

Stewart M 2001 Towards a global definition of patient centred care. British Medical Journal 322: 444–445

Stewart MA, McWhinney IR, Buck CW 1979 The doctor–patient relationship and its effect upon outcome. Journal of the Royal College of General Practitioners 29: 77–82

Stewart-Williams S 2004 The placebo puzzle: Putting together the pieces. Health Psychology 23: 198–206

Stjernsward J, Clark D 2004 Palliative medicine – a global perspective. In: Doyle D, Hanks G, Cherny N et al. (eds) Palliative medicine in the Oxford textbook of palliative medicine, 3rd edn. Oxford University Press, Oxford, pp. 1199–1224

Stock J, Cervone D 1990 Proximal goal setting and self-regulatory processes. Cognitive Therapy and Research 14: 483–498

Stone SV, McCrae RR 2007 Personality and health. In: Ayers S, Baum A, McManus C et al. (eds) Cambridge handbook of psychology, health and medicine, 2nd edn. Cambridge University Press, Cambridge, p. 155

Stone J, Aronson E, Crain AL et al. 1994 Inducing hypocrisy as a means of encouraging young adults to use condoms. Personality and Social Psychology Bulletin 20: 116–128

Stroebe M, Schut H 1999 The dual process model of coping with bereavement; rationale and description. Death Studies 23: 197–224

Stroebe W, Stroebe MS 1987 Bereavement and health: the psychological and physical consequences of partner loss. Cambridge University Press, Cambridge

Stuart-Hamilton I 1994 The psychology of ageing. Jessica Kingsley, London

Summerfield D 2001 The invention of post-traumatic stress disorder and the social usefulness of a psychiatric category. British Medical Journal 322: 95–98

Surbone A 2006 Telling the truth to patients with cancer: what truth? Lancet Oncology 7: 944–950

Talge NM, Neal C, Glover V 2007 Antenatal maternal stress and long-term effects on child neurodevelopment: how and why? Journal of Child Psychology and Psychiatry 48: 245–261

Taylor S 1986 Health psychology. Random House, New York

Taylor KM 1988 Telling bad news: physicians and the disclosure of undesirable information. Sociology of Health and Illness 10: 120–132

Tew M 1990 Safer childbirth? A critical history of maternity care. Chapman & Hall, London

Thomas K, Noble P 2007 Improving the delivery of palliative care in general practice: an evaluation of the first phase of the gold standards framework. Palliative Medicine 21: 49–53

Thorpe G 1993 Enabling more dying people to remain at home. British Medical Journal 307: 915–918

Thurstone LL 1938 Primary mental abilities. University of Chicago Press, Chicago

Tincoff R, Jusczyk PW 1999 Some beginnings of word comprehension in 6-month-olds. Psychological Science 10: 172–175

Tones K, Tilford S 1994 Health education: effectiveness, efficiency and equity. Chapman & Hall, London

Townsend P, Davidson N, Whitehead M (eds) 1992 Inequalities in health: the Black report and the health divide. Penguin, Harmondsworth

Tuckett D, Boulton M, Olsen C et al. 1985 Meetings between experts: an approach to sharing ideas in medical consultations. Tavistock, London

Tudor Hart J 1971 The inverse care law. Lancet 27: 405–412

Tuomilehto J, Lindstrom J, Eriksson JG et al. 2001 Prevention of type 2 diabetes mellitus by changes in lifestyle among subjects with impaired glucose tolerance. New England Journal of Medicine 344: 1343–1350

Turner B 1995 Medical power and social knowledge, 2nd edn. Sage, London

Twigg J, Atkin K 1991 Evaluating support to informal carers. Social Policy Research Unit, York

Twycross R 1994 Pain relief in advanced cancer. Churchill Livingstone, Edinburgh

Twycross R 1999 Introducing palliative care, 3rd edn. Radcliffe Medical Press, Oxon

Twycross R, Wilcock A 2001 Symptom management in advanced cancer, 3rd edn. Radcliffe Medical Press, Oxfordshire

UKATT research team 2005 Cost effectiveness of treatment for alcohol problems: findings of the randomised UK alcohol treatment trial (UKATT). British Medical Journal 331: 544

UK Prospective Diabetes Study Group 1998 Intensive blood-glucose control with sulphonylureas or insulin compared with conventional treatment and risk of complications in patients with type 2 diabetes (UKPDS 33). Lancet 352: 837–853

Ulstad V 2001 Coronary heart disease. In: Rosenfeld JA (ed.) Handbook of women's health: an evidence-based approach. Cambridge University Press, Cambridge, Chapter 29

Ünal B, Critchley JA, Fidan D et al. 2005 Life-years gained from modern cardiological treatments and population risk factor changes in England and Wales, 1981–2000. American Journal of Public Health 95: 103–108

Valliant GE 2003 A 60-year follow up of alcoholic men. Addiction 98: 1043–1051

Van den Bergh BRH, Mulder EJH, Mennes M et al. 2005 Antenatal maternal anxiety and stress and neurobehavioural development of the fetus and child: links and possible mechanisms: a review. Neuroscience and Biobehavioral Reviews 29: 237–258

van der Klink JL, Blonk RWB, Schene AH et al. 2001 The benefits of interventions for work-related stress. American Journal of Public Health 91: 270–276

Van Der Weyden M 2007 Challenges and change in medical training: the Australian curriculum framework for junior doctors. Medical Journal of Australia 186: 332–333

Vartiainen E, Paavola M, McAlister A et al. 1998 Fifteen-year follow-up of smoking prevention effects in the North Karelia Youth Project. American Journal of Public Health 88: 81–85

Vickers A 2000 Recent advances in complementary medicine. British Medical Journal 321: 683–686

Vincent C, Furnham A 1997 Complementary medicine: a research perspective. Wiley, Chichester

Waddell G 1998 The back pain revolution. Churchill Livingstone, Edinburgh

Wadsworth MEJ, Montgomery SM, Bartley MJ 1999 The persisting effect of unemployment on health and social well-being in men in early working life. Social Science and Medicine 48: 1491–1499

Walter T 1999 On bereavement: the culture of grief. Open University Press, Buckingham

Warr PB 1978 Work, unemployment and mental health. Oxford University Press, Oxford

Watson D, Pennebaker JW 1989 Health complaints, stress and distress: exploring the central role of negative affectivity. Psychological Review 96: 234–254

Watson JB, Raynor R 1920 Conditioned emotional responses. Journal of Experimental Psychology 3: 1–14

Watson M, Lucas C, Hoy A 2006 Adult palliative care guidance, 2nd edn. Mount Vernon and Sussex Cancer Networks and Northern Ireland Palliative Medicine Group, South West London, Surrey, West Sussex and Hampshire

Weich S, Lewis G 1998 Poverty, unemployment and common mental disorders: population based cohort study. British Medical Journal 317: 115–119

Weinstein N 1982 Unrealistic optimism about susceptibility to health problems. Journal of Behavioral Medicine 5: 441–460

Weinstein N 1984 Why it won't happen to me: perceptions of risk factors and susceptibility. Health Psychology 3: 431–457

Weinstein N 1987 Unrealistic optimism about susceptibility to health problems: conclusions from a community wide sample. Journal of Behavioural Medicine 10: 481–500

Weinstein ND, Lyon JE 1999 Mindset, optimistic bias about personal risk and health-protective behaviour. British Journal of Health Psychology 4: 289–300

Wellings K, Wadsworth J, Johnson AM et al. 1995 Provision of sex education and early sexual experience: the relation examined. British Medical Journal 311: 417–420

West P, MacIntyre S, Annandale E et al 1990 Social class and health in youth findings for the West of Scotland. Twenty-07 Study Social Science in Medicine 30: 665–673

Westergaard J, Noble I, Walker A 1989 After redundancy: the experience of economic insecurity. Polity Press, Cambridge

Westerterp KR 2006 Perception, passive overfeeding and energy metabolism. Physiology and Behavior 89: 62–65

Whalley LJ, Deary IJ 2001 Longitudinal cohort study of childhood IQ and survival up to age 76. British Medical Journal 322: 1–5

WHOQOL Group 1998 The World Health Organization quality of life assessment (WHOQOL): development and general psychometric properties. Social Science and Medicine 46: 1569–1585

Wight D, Henderson M, Raab G et al. 2000 Extent of regretted sexual intercourse among young teenagers in Scotland: a cross-sectional survey. British Medical Journal 320: 1243–1244

Wilkinson RG 1998 Unhealthy societies: the afflictions of inequality. Routledge, London

Williams RL 1973 Black intelligence test of cultural homogeneity. Newsweek, December 19th, p. 109

Williams R 1983 Concepts of health: an analysis of lay logic. Sociology 17: 185–204

Williams G 1984 The genesis of chronic illness: narrative reconstruction. Sociology of Health and Illness 6: 175–200

Williams JM, Binnie LM 2002 Children's concepts of illness: an intervention to improve knowledge. British Journal of Health Psychology 7: 129–147

Williams KE, Chambless DL, Ahrens A 1997 Are emotions frightening? An extension of the fear of fear construct. Behavioral Research and Therapy 35: 229–248

Williams C, Kitzinger J, Henderson L 2003 Envisaging the embryo in stem cell research: rhetorical strategies and media reporting of the ethical debates. Sociology of Health and Illness 25: 793–814

Williamson VK, Winn CR, Pugh ALG 1992 Public views on an extended role for community pharmacy. International Journal of Pharmacy Practice 1: 223–229

Willis E 2002 Public health and the 'new' genetics: balancing individual and collective outcomes. Critical Public Health 12: 119–138

Winterton Report 1992 Maternity services second report, vol. 1. Health Committee. HMSO, London

Woelk H 2000 Comparison of St John's wort and imipramine for treating depression: randomised controlled trial. British Medical Journal 321: 536–539

Wood W, Kallgren CA, Priesler RM 1985 Access to attitude-relevant information in memory as a determinant of persuasion: the role of message attributes. Journal of Experimental Social Psychology 21: 73–85

Woodroffe C, Glickman M, Barker M et al. 1993 Children, teenagers and health: the key data. Open University Press, Buckingham

Worden JW 1991 Grief counselling and grief therapy. A handbook for the mental health practitioner. Routledge, London

World Health Organization 1946 Constitution. World Health Organization, Geneva

World Health Organization 1948 Preamble to the Constitution of the World Health Organization as adopted by the International Health Conference, New York, 19–22 June, 1946; signed on 22 July 1946 by the representatives of 61 States (Official Records of the World Health Organization 2, 100) and entered into force on 7 April 1948.

World Health Organization Division of Mental Health 1993 WHO-QOL study protocol: the development of the World Health Organization quality of life assessment instrument (MNG/PSF/93). World Health Organization, Geneva

World Health Organization 2002a Infant and young child nutrition; global strategy for infant and young child feeding. World Health Organization, Geneva

World Health Organization 2002b Towards a common language for functioning, disability and health: ICF. WHO, Geneva, Switzerland

World Health Organization 2002c National cancer control programmes: policies and guidelines. WHO, Geneva

World Health Organization 2005 International classification of diseases, 10th revision, 2nd edn. WHO, Geneva

World Health Organization 2007 The top 10 causes of death. Fact sheet no. 310. Available online at: http://www.who.int/mediacentre/factsheets/fs310/en/index.html

World Health Organization 2008 Available online at: http://www.who.int/whosis/database/core/core_select.cfm

World Medical Association international code of medical ethics. Available online at: http://www.wma.net/e/policy/c8.htm

Yardley SJ, Davis CJ, Sheldon F 2001 Receiving a diagnosis of lung cancer: patients' interpretations, perceptions and perspectives. Palliative Medicine 15: 379–386

Yellowlees PM, Ruffin RE 1989 Psychological defences and coping styles in patients following a life-threatening attack of asthma. Chest 95: 1298–1303

Yeomans MR 2007 The role of palatability in control of food intake: implications for understanding and treating obesity. In: Cooper SJ, Kirkham TC (eds) Appetite and body weight: integrative systems and the development of anti-obesity drugs. Elsevier, pp. 247–269

Zajonc RB 1998 Emotions. In: Gilbert D, Fiske ST, Lindzey G (eds) Handbook of social psychology, 4th edn. McGraw-Hill, New York

Zellner DA, Garriga-Trillo A, Centeno S et al. 2004 Chocolate craving and the menstrual cycle. Appetite 42: 119–121

Zigler E, Valentine J 1979 Project Head Start: a legacy of the war on poverty. Free Press, New York

Index